METHODS IN MOLECULAR BIOLOGY

Series Editor
John M. Walker
School of Life and Medical Sciences
University of Hertfordshire
Hatfield, Hertfordshire, AL10 9AB, UK

For further volumes:
http://www.springer.com/series/7651

Acute Myeloid Leukemia

Methods and Protocols

Edited by

Paolo Fortina

Thomas Jefferson University, Sidney Kimmel Cancer Center, Philadelphia, PA, USA

Eric Londin

Department of Pathology, Anatomy and Cell Biology, Sidney Kimmel Medical College
Thomas Jefferson University, Philadelphia, PA, USA

Jason Y. Park

Department of Pathology, UT Southwestern Medical Center
and Children's Medical Center, Dallas, TX, USA

Larry J. Kricka

Department of Pathology, and Laboratory Medicine,
University of Pennsylvania Medical Center, Philadelphia, PA, USA

Humana Press

Editors
Paolo Fortina
Thomas Jefferson University, Sidney Kimmel Cancer Center
Philadelphia, PA, USA

Jason Y. Park
Department of Pathology
UT Southwestern Medical Center and Children's Medical Center
Dallas, TX, USA

Eric Londin
Department of Pathology, Anatomy and Cell Biology
Sidney Kimmel Medical College Thomas Jefferson University
Philadelphia, PA, USA

Larry J. Kricka
Department of Pathology and Laboratory Medicine
University of Pennsylvania Medical Center
Philadelphia, PA, USA

ISSN 1064-3745 ISSN 1940-6029 (electronic)
Methods in Molecular Biology
ISBN 978-1-4939-7140-4 ISBN 978-1-4939-7142-8 (eBook)
DOI 10.1007/978-1-4939-7142-8

Library of Congress Control Number: 2017945299

Cover illustration: Cover image courtesy of Drs. Hung S. Luu and Jason Y. Park.

Printed on acid-free paper

This Humana Press imprint is published by Springer Nature
The registered company is Springer Science+Business Media LLC
The registered company address is: 233 Spring Street, New York, NY 10013, U.S.A.

Preface

Acute myeloid leukemia (AML) is the most common type of leukemia. The Cancer Genome Atlas Research Network has demonstrated the increasing genomic complexity of AML. In addition, the network has facilitated our understanding of the molecular events leading to this deadly form of malignancy for which the prognosis has not improved over past decades. AML is a highly heterogeneous disease, and cytogenetic and molecular analysis of the various chromosome aberrations including deletions, duplications, aneuploidy, balanced reciprocal translocations, and fusion of transcription factor genes and tyrosine kinases has led to a better understanding and identification of subgroups of AML with different prognoses. Furthermore, molecular classification based on mRNA expression profiling has facilitated the identification of novel subclasses and defined high-, poor-risk AML based on specific molecular signatures. However, despite increased understanding of AML genetics, the outcome for AML patients whose number is likely to rise as the population ages has not changed significantly. Until it does, further investigation of the genomic complexity of the disease and advances in drug development are needed. In this review, leading AML clinicians and research investigators provide an up-to-date understanding of the molecular biology of the disease addressing advances in diagnosis, classification, prognostication, and therapeutic strategies that may have significant promise and impact on overall patient survival.

Philadelphia, PA, USA — Paolo Fortina
Philadelphia, PA, USA — Eric Londin
Dallas, TX, USA — Jason Y. Park
Philadelphia, PA, USA — Larry J. Kricka

Contents

Contributors

MARCO ALESSANDRINI • *Faculty of Health Sciences, Department of Immunology, and Institute for Cellular and Molecular Medicine, SAMRC Extramural Unit for Stem Cell Research and Therapy, University of Pretoria, Pretoria, South Africa*

MICHAEL ANDREEFF • *Department of Leukemia, The University of Texas MD Anderson Cancer Center, Houston, TX, USA*

ADAM BAGG • *Division of Hematopathology, Department of Pathology and Laboratory Medicine, Hospital of the University of Pennsylvania, Philadelphia, PA, USA*

RICHARD BORIACK • *Department of Pathology and Laboratory Medicine, Children's Health, Children's Medical Center, Dallas, TX, USA*

MARTIN CARROLL • *Division of Hematology & Oncology, Abramson Cancer Center, Perelman School of Medicine at the University of Pennsylvania, Philadelphia, PA, USA; Philadelphia Veterans Administration Medical Center, Philadelphia, PA, USA*

WEINA CHEN • *Department of Pathology, University of Texas Southwestern Medical Center, Dallas, TX, USA*

MICHAEL W. CRUISE • *Pathology Department, Cleveland Clinic Main Campus, Cleveland, OH, USA*

SONJA FUNK • *University of Pittsburgh School of Medicine, University of Pittsburgh Cancer Institute, Pittsburgh, PA, USA*

SAAR GILL • *Center for Cellular Immunotherapies, University of Pennsylvania, Philadelphia, PA, USA; Division of Hematology/Oncology, University of Pennsylvania, Philadelphia, PA, USA; Abramson Cancer Center, University of Pennsylvania, Philadelphia, PA, USA*

MARGARET A. GOODELL • *Department of Pediatrics, Baylor College of Medicine and Texas Children's Hospital, Houston, TX, USA; Dan L. Duncan Cancer Center, Department of Molecular and Human Genetics, Stem Cells and Regenerative Medicine Center and Center for Cell and Gene Therapy, Baylor College of Medicine, Houston, TX, USA*

YUHAN GUO • *Division of Haematology, Department of Medicine, Li Ka Shing Faculty of Medicine, The University of Hong Kong, Pokfulam, Hong Kong, China*

ANNA G. GUZMAN • *Department of Pediatrics, Baylor College of Medicine and Texas Children's Hospital, Houston, TX, USA; Dan L. Duncan Cancer Center, Department of Molecular and Human Genetics, Stem Cells and Regenerative Medicine Center and Center for Cell and Gene Therapy, Baylor College of Medicine, Houston, TX, USA*

BAI-LIANG HE • *Division of Haematology, Department of Medicine, Li Ka Shing Faculty of Medicine, The University of Hong Kong, Pokfulam, Hong Kong, China*

MARYBETH HELFRICH • *Department of Pathology and Laboratory Medicine, The Children's Hospital of Philadelphia, Philadelphia, PA, USA*

TAE HYUN HWANG • *Department of Quantitative Health Sciences, Cleveland Clinic, Cleveland, OHIO, USA; Department of Clinical Sciences, University of Texas Southwestern Medical Center, Dallas, TX, USA; Harold C. Simmons Cancer Center, University of Texas Southwestern Medical Center, Dallas, TX, USA*

CHANG-SOOK HONG • *University of Pittsburgh School of Medicine, University of Pittsburgh Cancer Institute, Pittsburgh, PA, USA*
MIRA JEONG • *Department of Pediatrics, Baylor College of Medicine and Texas Children's Hospital, Houston, TX, USA; Dan L. Duncan Cancer Center, Department of Molecular and Human Genetics, Stem Cells and Regenerative Medicine Center, Center for Cell and Gene Therapy, Baylor College of Medicine, Houston, TX, USA*
PATRICIA M. JONES • *Department of Pathology, University of Texas Southwestern Medical Center, Dallas, TX, USA; Department of Pathology and Laboratory Medicine, Children's Health, Children's Medical Center, Dallas, TX, USA*
CARL H. JUNE • *Center for Cellular Immunotherapies, University of Pennsylvania, Philadelphia, PA, USA; Abramson Cancer Center, University of Pennsylvania, Philadelphia, PA, USA*
SHARON S. KAPPALA • *Faculty of Health Sciences, Department of Immunology, and Institute for Cellular and Molecular Medicine, SAMRC Extramural Unit for Stem Cell Research and Therapy, University of Pretoria, Pretoria, South Africa*
TODD W. KELLEY • *Department of Pathology, University of Utah, Salt Lake City, UT, USA*
SAAD S. KENDERIAN • *Center for Cellular Immunotherapies, University of Pennsylvania, Philadelphia, PA, USA; Division of Hematology, Department of Medicine, Mayo Clinic, Rochester, MN, USA*
REBECCA L. KING • *Division of Hematopathology, Department of Laboratory Medicine and Pathology, Mayo Clinic, Rochester, MN, USA*
ERIC KONNICK • *Genetics and Solid Tumor Laboratory, Department of Laboratory Medicine, University of Washington, Seattle, WA, USA*
MARINA KONOPLEVA • *Department of Leukemia, The University of Texas MD Anderson Cancer Center, Houston, TX, USA*
SEAN R. LANDMAN • *Department of Computer Science and Engineering, University of Minnesota, Minneapolis, MN, USA*
ANSKAR Y.H. LEUNG • *Division of Haematology, Department of Medicine, Li Ka Shing Faculty of Medicine, The University of Hong Kong, Pokfulam, Hong Kong, China*
CHRISTINA M. LOCKWOOD • *Genetics and Solid Tumor Laboratory, Department of Laboratory Medicine, University of Washington, Seattle, WA, USA*
MARLISE R. LUSKIN • *Department of Medical Oncology, Dana-Farber Cancer Institute, Boston, Massachusetts*
HUNG S. LUU • *Department of Pathology, University of Texas Southwestern Medical Center, Dallas, TX, USA; Department of Pathology, Children's Medical Center at Dallas, Univeristy of Texas Southwestern Medical Center, Dallas, TX, USA*
ALVIN C.H. MA • *Division of Haematology, Department of Medicine, Li Ka Shing Faculty of Medicine, The University of Hong Kong, Pokfulam, Hong Kong, China*
STEPHEN R. MASTER • *Department of Pathology & Laboratory Medicine, Weill Cornell Medical College, New York, NY, USA*
MICHELE E. PAESSLER • *Department of Pathology and Laboratory Medicine, Perelman School of Medicine at the University of Pennsylvania, Philadelphia, PA, USA; Department of Pathology and Laboratory Medicine, The Children's Hospital of Philadelphia, Philadelphia, PA, USA*
NAOMI PARK • *DNA Pipelines Research and Development, Wellcome Trust Sanger Institute, Cambridge, UK*

MICHAEL S. PEPPER • *Faculty of Health Sciences, Department of Immunology, and Institute for Cellular and Molecular Medicine, SAMRC Extramural Unit for Stem Cell Research and Therapy, University of Pretoria, Pretoria, South Africa*

DINESH RAKHEJA • *Department of Pathology, University of Texas Southwestern Medical Center, Dallas, TX, USA; Department of Pathology and Laboratory Medicine, Children's Health, Children's Medical Center, Dallas, TX, USA; Department of Pediatrics, University of Texas Southwestern Medical Center, Dallas, TX, USA*

JONATHAN SCHUMACHER • *Department of Pathology, ARUP Laboratories, Salt Lake City, UT, USA*

XIANGGUO SHI • *Division of Haematology, Department of Medicine, Li Ka Shing Faculty of Medicine, The University of Hong Kong, Pokfulam, Hong Kong, China*

TIM C.P. SOMERVAILLE • *Leukemia Biology Laboratory, Cancer Research UK Manchester Institute, The University of Manchester, Manchester, UK*

EDUARD A. STRUYS • *Metabolic Unit, Clinical Chemistry, VU University Medical Center, Amsterdam, The Netherlands*

PHILIPPE SZANKASI • *Department of Pathology, ARUP Laboratories, Salt Lake City, UT, USA*

GEORGE VASSILIOU • *Haematological Cancer Genetics, Wellcome Trust Sanger Institute, Cambridge, UK*

GERALD B.W. WERTHEIM • *Department of Pathology and Laboratory Medicine, Perelman School of Medicine at the University of Pennsylvania, Philadelphia, PA, USA; Department of Pathology and Laboratory Medicine, The Children's Hospital of Philadelphia, Philadelphia, PA, USA*

THERESA L. WHITESIDE • *University of Pittsburgh School of Medicine, University of Pittsburgh Cancer Institute, Pittsburgh, PA, USA*

DANIEL H. WISEMAN • *Leukemia Biology Laboratory, Cancer Research UK Manchester Institute, The University of Manchester, Manchester, UK*

DAVID WU • *UW Hematopathology, UW Molecular Genetic Pathology, Hematopathology Laboratory, Department of Laboratory Medicine, University of Washington, Seattle, WA, USA*

ZHIHONG ZENG • *Department of Leukemia, The University of Texas MD Anderson Cancer Center, Houston, TX, USA*

Chapter 1

Molecular Malfeasance Mediating Myeloid Malignancies: The Genetics of Acute Myeloid Leukemia

Rebecca L. King and Adam Bagg

Abstract

A remarkable number of different, but recurrent, structural cytogenetic abnormalities have been observed in AML, and the 2016 WHO AML classification system incorporates numerous distinct entities associated with translocations or inversions, as well as others associated with single gene mutations into a category entitled "AML with recurrent genetic abnormalities." The AML classification is heavily reliant on cytogenetic and molecular information based on conventional genetic techniques (including karyotype, fluorescence in situ hybridization, reverse transcriptase polymerase chain reaction, single gene sequencing), but large-scale next generation sequencing is now identifying novel mutations. With targeted next generation sequencing panels now clinically available at many centers, detection of mutations, as well as alterations in epigenetic modifiers, is becoming part of the routine diagnostic evaluation of AML and will likely impact future classification schemes.

Key words Acute myeloid leukemia, 2016 WHO AML classification, Acute promyelocytic leukemia, NGS, Karyotype, FISH, RT-PCR, Epigenetics

1 Introduction

Acute myeloid leukemia (AML) is a complex and heterogeneous disease that was first subclassified in 1976 according to the French-American-British (FAB) scheme which was primarily a morphology-based system [1]. Since then, cytogenetic and molecular techniques have resulted in the discovery of numerous recurrent genetic abnormalities in AML. These recurrent genetic abnormalities have not only advanced our ability to subclassify this disease, but have in many cases provided prognostic markers and even therapeutic targets. The World Health Organization (WHO) now recognizes an AML classification which is heavily reliant on cytogenetic and molecular information [2]. While the majority of the genetic aberrations discussed in the current WHO classification rely primarily on conventional cytogenetic techniques such as karyotype or fluorescence in situ hybridization (FISH) and reverse transcriptase

Paolo Fortina et al. (eds.), *Acute Myeloid Leukemia: Methods and Protocols*, Methods in Molecular Biology, vol. 1633, DOI 10.1007/978-1-4939-7142-8_1,

polymerase chain reaction (RT-PCR)-based or conventional sequencing techniques, the literature is abound with novel mutations identified in large-scale next generation sequencing (NGS) studies. With targeted NGS panels now clinically available at many centers, detection of mutations, as well as alterations in epigenetic modifiers, is becoming part of the routine diagnostic evaluation of AML and will likely influence future classification schemes.

2 WHO Classification of AML: Recurrent Translocations and Genetic Rearrangements

A remarkable number (>300) of different, but recurrent, structural cytogenetic abnormalities have been observed in AML, some of which are highlighted in Table 1. The current (2016) WHO AML classification system incorporates numerous distinct entities associated with translocations or inversions, as well as several others associated with single gene mutations into a category entitled "AML with recurrent genetic abnormalities" [2, 3].

2.1 Acute Promyelocytic Leukemia with PML-RARA

A discussion of the relevance of genetics in AML must begin with acute promyelocytic leukemia (APL) which by far demonstrates the most compelling genotype–phenotype correlation and represents a success story for genetically targeted cancer therapy. APL is an acute leukemia of neoplastic promyelocytes that accounts for 5–10% of AML cases [2]. There are two morphologic variants, the classic hypergranular form in which the neoplastic cells have abundant pink granules and numerous Auer rods, and the microgranular variant in which the cells have bi-lobed nuclei and a paucity of granules. Both variants are associated with the *PML-RARA* t(15;17)(q24;q21) translocation in 99% of cases, with the remaining 1% demonstrating variant translocations involving the disruption of the retinoic acid receptor alpha (*RARA)* gene at 17q21. The *PML-RARA* fusion, which is not always accompanied by a grossly karyotypically evident t(15;17) translocation, is considered "disease defining," meaning that it is diagnostic of AML regardless of blast percentage [4]. In the t(15;17), the *RARA* gene is fused to the promyelocytic leukemia (*PML*) gene which encodes a protein normally localized to nuclear bodies or PODs (*P*ML *O*ncogenic *D*omains) within the nucleus. The resultant fusion protein represses transcription of genes involved in normal myeloid differentiation by freeing the cell from normal transcriptional regulatory control by physiologic levels of retinoic acid [5]. One of the remarkable success stories of modern oncology was the discovery that this blockage could be overcome by supraphysiologic levels of retinoic acid in the form of all-trans retinoic acid (ATRA) therapy [5]. Treatment with this agent has resulted in cure rates that exceed 90% in some series [6]. *FLT3*-internal tandem

Table 1
Examples of recurrent chromosomal abnormalities in acute myeloid leukemia with frequencies and prognostic relevance

Genetic lesion	Chromosomal abnormality	Frequency[a] (%)	Prognostic significance
Abnormality[b]			
Complex karyotype	Variable; ≥3 abnormalities	~10–15	Unfavorable
Monosomal karyotype	≥2 autosomal monosomies or 1 autosomal monosomy with any other structural abnormality	~5–10	Unfavorable
RUNX1-RUNX1T1	t(8;21)(q22;q22)	~5–10	Favorable
PML-RARA	t(15;17)(q24;q21)	~5–10	Favorable
MYH11-CBFB	inv(16)(p13q22)	~5–10	Favorable
KMT2A-V	t(11;v)(q23;v)	~5	Unfavorable
MLLT3-KMT2A	t(9;11)(p22;q23)	~2	Intermediate
DEK-NUP214	t(6;9)(p23;q34)	~1–2	Unfavorable
GATA2-MECOM	inv(3)(q21q26)	~1–2	Unfavorable
RBM15-MKL1	t(1;22)(p13;q13)	<1	Unfavorable
ZBTB16-RARA	t(11;17)(q23;q21)	<1	Unfavorable
NPM1-RARA	t(5;17)(q35;q21)	<1	Favorable
NUMA-RARA	t(11;17)(q13;q21)	<1	Favorable
STAT5-RARA	t(17;17)(q11;q21)	<1	Unfavorable
BCR-ABL1	t(9;22)(q34q11.2)	<1	Unfavorable
NUP98-V	t(11;V)(p15;v)	<1	Unfavorable
KAT6A-V	t(8;V)(p11;v)	<1	Unfavorable

[a]Reported frequencies have been averaged from a number of multicenter studies, and usually reflect those reported in adults <60 years
[b]*V* or *v*—variable fusion partners/chromosomal breakpoints

duplication mutations have been described in 20–40% of patients with APL; while typically associated with poor prognosis, their prognostic impact here is controversial [7].

RARA can be translocated to various gene partners other than *PML* [8] (Table 1). WHO no longer considers these variants as "definitional" of APL. From a clinical perspective, the t(11;17)(q23;q21) *ZBTB16-RARA* and t(17;17)(q11;q21) *STAT5-RARA* translocations are critical to note as they may show resistance to ATRA therapy [8–12]. In the former, the *ZBTB16* gene itself acts as a transcriptional repressor that cannot be abrogated by

ATRA. Other variants including *NPM1-RARA* t(5;17)(q35;q21) and *NUMA-RARA* t(11;17)(q13;q21) are typically ATRA responsive [8, 9, 12]. In the current diagnostic era, conventional karyotype and FISH are critical in detection of these variants, as they will be missed by RT-PCR assays targeted for the *PML-RARA* translocation.

Although the t(15;17) is easily detectable by karyotype, FISH and RT-PCR-based methods are often used for rapid diagnosis and the latter can be employed in a quantitative fashion for minimal residual disease (MRD) detection. With regard to diagnosis of the common t(15;17) translocation, the breakpoints in *RARA* are well conserved in intron 2, while there are three breakpoints in the *PML* gene in intron 3 (bcr-3), intron 6 (bcr-1), and exon 6 (bcr-2). These give rise to the short, long, and variable fusion transcripts, respectively. Since the breakpoints in exon 6 are relatively uncommon (5%), a single downstream *RARA* primer and two upstream *PML* primers can be used to detect greater than 90% of *PML-RARA* fusion transcripts [13].

2.2 Core Binding Factor AML: RUNX1-RUNX1T1 t(8;21)(q22;q22) and MYH11-CBFB inv(16)(p13q22)

AMLs involving the *RUNX1-RUNX1T1* t(8;21)(q22;q22) and *MYH11-CBFB* inv(16)(p13q22)/t(16;16)(p13;q22) abnormalities are collectively referred to as core binding factor (CBF) leukemias due to their involvement of the *CBFA2* subunit (*RUNX1*) and *CBFB* subunit, respectively. The CBF subunits form a transcriptional protein that is critical for normal hematopoiesis. As such, both of these translocations result in disruption of the transcriptional complex resulting in a fusion protein that acts in a dominant-negative fashion to repress transcription of important hematopoietic targets including *MPO*, *GMCSF*, *IL3*, and the *TRB* [14]. Like the t(15;17), these two rearrangements are diagnostic of AML regardless of blast percentage [4]. The presence of either of these translocations in adult AML imparts a favorable prognosis [15] (Table 1).

The t(8;21) is common in AML accounting for approximately 5–10% of cases [15]. These leukemias often, but not always, show a characteristic morphologic phenotype including myeloid blasts with peri-nuclear hofs and large, salmon colored granules, as well as long tapered Auer rods [2].

Detection of the t(8;21) can be easily performed using karyotype, FISH, and RT-PCR. The breakpoints cluster within a single intron of both genes, so that similar *RUNX1/RUNXT1* chimeric transcripts are usually generated in every case. Thus, a simple RT-PCR assay, using a *RUNX1* primer and an *RUNX1T1* primer, is sufficient to detect this translocation at a molecular level.

AML with inv(16)/t(16;16) accounts for 5–10% of all AML [15]. The inv(16)(p13q22) or t(16;16)(p13;q22) results in a fusion protein involving a myosin heavy chain gene (MYH11) and the beta subunit of the CBF protein complex. This rearrangement sequesters the CBFB protein in the cytoplasm impeding its ability to function normally as part of the transcription factor complex. The most common morphologic association with this type of AML is that of the former FAB M4-eo in which the blasts have a myelomonocytic phenotype and there are associated abnormal eosinophils with basophilic granules [2].

Because the inv(16) can be subtle on karyotypic analysis, RT-PCR and/or FISH testing is integral to detecting this rearrangement. Interestingly, gain of chromosome 22 is the most common secondary karyotypic abnormality in patients with inv(16), but is uncommon in other situations, and thus should alert one to the presence of an inv(16) [16]. From a molecular perspective, the breakpoints in the two genes on chromosome 16 are heterogeneous, with at least 10 different fusion transcripts generated. While 99% of breakpoints in *CBFB* occur in intron 5 of that gene, the breakpoint heterogeneity is quite marked in the *MYH11* gene, with seven different exons (7 through 13) variably included in the fusion transcripts [17]. Fortunately, the most common form—designated type A—accounts for approximately 90% of cases with this genetic fusion, while two other transcripts (types D and E) account for an additional 5% [18].

Both the t(8;21) and inv(16) impart a favorable prognosis in AML [15]. Interestingly, cases of inv(16) AML with the +22 may have an even more favorable prognosis. However, point mutations in the *KIT* and *FLT3* genes (discussed below) impart a worse prognosis in patients with t(8;21) or inv(16) [19, 20], albeit not to the degree that they will shift these CBF AMLs into a inferior prognostic category.

2.3 AML with Translocations Involving MLL (KMT2A) at 11q23

The *MLL* (*KMT2A*) gene located on chromosome 11q23 is involved in over 100 different translocations with various gene partners in AML as well as acute lymphoblastic leukemia (ALL), and myelodysplastic syndromes (MDS) [21, 22]. Of the numerous translocation partners, the most common in AML are *MLLT3* (*AF9*) on 9q21 in the t(9;11) translocation, and one of three genes (*MLLT1/ENL, ELL* or *EEN/SH3GL1*) on 19p13 in the different t(11;19) translocations [23]. In the WHO 2016 classification, the t(9;11) (p22;q23) *MLLT3-KMT2A* translocation is recognized as a distinct, genetically defined subtype of AML and accounts for 2% of adult AML but up to 10% of AML in children, especially infants [2]. Most cases demonstrate monoblastic differentiation. There is also a high rate of *KMT2A* translocations in patients who develop leukemia secondary to topoisomerase-II inhibitors (therapy-related AML) [24]. In general, *KMT2A* translocations in AML predict for poor outcomes, with the t(9;11) representing an exception with a more intermediate prognosis [15]. More recently, groups have shown that the t(6;11)(q27;q23) (*KMT2A-MLLT4/AF6*) is associated particularly with dismal prognosis [25], while the t(1;11) (9q21;q23) portends an especially good outcome, with a greater than 90% event-free survival [23].

The *KMT2A* gene codes for a histone-lysine methyltransferase protein that acts to modulate gene expression via chromatin remodeling. With its myriad translocation partners, *KMT2A* generates fusion proteins that bind histones and upregulate leukemic gene expression via DOT1L-induced methylation of the histone H3K79 [26]. Adding to the complexity of this process is the role of other transcriptional regulators, including PU.1, which acts in a fusion-gene-independent fashion to promote leukemogenesis in these leukemias [27, 28]. The breakpoints in *KMT2A* tend to cluster in a relatively small (8.3-kb) area spanning exons 5–11, referred to as a breakpoint cluster region (BCR) [21]. Interestingly, *KMT2A* translocations in de novo leukemias tend to cluster in the 5′ region of the BCR, while those in therapy-related and infant AMLs occur more often in the 3′ region [29].

Because of the many translocation partners, screening for *KMT2A* rearrangements is most effectively done by FISH using a *KMT2A* break-apart probe strategy followed by dual-fusion probes to identify the partner gene. Molecular methods can also be used to target the most common translocations.

2.4 AML with DEK-NUP 214 t(6;9)(p23;q34)

The t(6;9)(p23;q34) translocation is present in a low percentage (1–2%) of AML, and is often associated with multilineage dysplasia and basophilia [2]. Overall survival in this subgroup is poor [15, 30].

The translocation results in an oncofusion protein DEK-NUP214 that globally increases translational activity secondary to phosphorylation of the translational initiation protein EIF4E [31, 32]. Detection of this translocation can be effectively performed by karyotype, FISH, and RT-PCR, with the breakpoints clustering within a single intron in both genes, allowing for straightforward detection by RT-PCR.

2.5 AML with GATA2-MECOM inv(3)(q21q26.2) or t(3;3)(q21;q26.2)

AML with inv(3) and the related t(3;3) account for approximately 1–2% of AML cases. This genetic abnormality may arise in MDS, as well as de novo AML. Both often display megakaryocytic dysplasia, especially forms with mono- or binucleation [2]. This subtype of AML is associated with poor prognosis [15, 33].

The translocation results in the juxtaposition of a *GATA2* enhancer to the *MECOM* gene, a complex zinc finger protein that acts as a transcriptional regulator. This event results in upregulation of *MECOM* by the enhancer, thereby promoting leukemogenesis [34]. Karyotype can detect the rearrangement, although it may be missed if metaphases are of poor quality. Due to variable breakpoints, FISH is more effective in detecting the translocation than RT-PCR and acts as a useful adjunct to conventional karyotype [35].

2.6 AML with RBM15-MKL1 t(1;22)(p13;q13)

Occurring primarily in infants and children, AML with the t(1;22)(p13;q13) is rare (<1% of AML cases) [36, 37]. These leukemias typically have megakaryoblastic differentiation [36]. Although challenging to study due to their rarity, patients have an intermediate prognosis with intensive chemotherapy [38].

The t(1;22) results in an in-frame fusion of *RBM15* (1p13) and *MKL1* (22q13) that contains almost the entire coding region of both genes. *RBM15-MKL1* may modulate Notch signaling through interactions with RBPJ [39]. Detection of the translocation can be accomplished via karyotype, FISH, or RT-PCR.

2.7 AML with t(9;22)(q34;q11.2) BCR-ABL1

While AML can arise from pre-existing chronic myeloid leukemia (CML), there is increasing evidence that de novo *BCR-ABL1*-associated AML exists and represents a unique biologic category. The WHO 2016 recognizes this as a provisional entity. These patients seem to have a poor prognosis and must be recognized for appropriate inclusion of tyrosine kinase inhibitors in the therapeutic regimen [40, 41].

Detection of the t(9;22) can be performed using standard karyotype and FISH, as well as a RT-PCR, with the *BCR* breakpoint most commonly occurring after e13/e14, generating the p210 protein that is characteristic of CML, but seen less frequently in acute lymphoblastic leukemia (ALL) [40, 42]. Recent studies using array Comparative Genomic Hybridization (aCGH) suggest that loss of *IKZF1* and *CDKN2A*, common abnormalities in *BCR-ABL1*-positive ALL, is also found in this group of AMLs [41]. In addition, unique deletions of antigen receptor genes (IGH and TCR) may distinguish de novo *BCR-ABL1*-positive AML from transformed CML [41].

2.8 Other Cytogenetic Changes in AML

In addition to translocations, numerous other cytogenetic abnormalities can occur in AML (Table 1). While not all of these are recognized currently as distinct WHO entities, their presence is important to note for prognostic purposes and/or therapeutic purposes.

AML with ≥3 cytogenetic abnormalities is considered to have a complex karyotype (AML-CK) and is associated with poor prognosis. These cases most often fall into one of two WHO subgroups: AML with myelodysplasia-related changes (AML-MRC) and therapy-related AML (t-AML), the latter under the umbrella term of therapy-related myeloid neoplasms [2].

AML with a monosomal karyotype (AML-MK), defined as the presence of at least two autosomal monosomies or a single monosomy plus an additional structural abnormality, confers an extremely poor prognosis [23, 43, 44].There is considerable overlap with cases of AML-CK. AML-MK cases account for 5–10% of AML, and are enriched in patients older than 60 years [44].

Finally, a number of myelodysplasia-associated genetic abnormalities can be seen in AML, and confer an inferior prognosis.

Table 2
Cytogenetic abnormalities sufficient to diagnose AML with myelodysplasia-related changes when blasts are ≥20% in blood or bone marrow

Complex karyotype[a]
Unbalanced abnormalities
−7/del(7q)
−5/del(5q)
i(17q)/t(17p)
−13/del(13q)
del(11q)
del(12p)/t(12p)
idic(X)(q13)
Balanced abnormalities
t(11;16)(q23;p13.3)
t(3;21)(q26.2;q22.1)
t(1;3)(p36.3;q21.1)
t(2;11)(p21;q23)
t(5;12)(q33;p12)
t(5;7)(q33;q11.2)
t(5;17)(q33;p13)
t(5;10)(q33;q21)
t(3;5)(q25;q34)

[a]≥3 Abnormalities

Examples include whole or partial deletions of chromosomes 5, 7, and 17 (15). Additional abnormalities sufficient to merit classification as AML-MRC are listed in Table 2.

3 Somatic Mutations in AML

In addition to the chromosomal abnormalities discussed above, a number of somatic mutations have been identified in AML, and the rate of discovery is increasing with the introduction of NGS technology. These include *FLT3* abnormalities, *KMT2A* partial tandem duplications, and *NPM1, DNMT3A, CEBPA, RUNX1, KIT, ASXL1, TET2, IDH1/IDH2, WT1,* and *RAS* mutations. Evaluation for mutations in a number of these genes such as *FLT3,*

NPM1, and *CEPBA* is now standard of care in the workup of AML, due to their prognostic and indeed diagnostic significance. Mutations in these genes overlap with several of the genetically defined categories listed above (although they are enriched in the 45% of AMLs that are cytogenetically normal), but in the case of *NPM1* and *CEPBA*, also have earned their own WHO diagnostic categories. *RUNX1* mutated cases have additionally been recognized as a provisional diagnostic entity in the WHO 2016. In addition to these, a number of the genes listed above have already been shown to have prognostic, and in some cases potentially therapeutic, relevance [Table 3].

Nearly all AMLs have mutations in one of nine categories of genes grouped by their biologic function, including transcription factor fusions (18% of cases); the gene encoding nucleophosmin/*NPM1* (27%); tumor-suppressor genes (16%); DNA-methylation–related genes (44%); signaling genes (59%); chromatin modifying genes (30%); myeloid transcription factor genes (22%); cohesin-complex genes (13%); and spliceosome-complex genes (14%) [45–48]. Patterns of cooperation and mutual exclusivity suggested strong biologic relationships among several of the genes and categories. For example, *FLT3*, *NPM1*, and *DNMT3A* tend to occur together, while transcription factor fusions and mutations of *NPM1*, *RUNX1*, *TP53*, and *CEBPA* are mutually exclusive [46]. In addition, many of the genes discussed below, as well as those listed in Table 3, show enrichment in specific morphologic or genetically defined AML subgroups such as *KIT* mutations in CBF AMLs.

3.1 NPM1 Mutations

Nucleophosmin (*NPM1*) is the most commonly mutated gene in cytogenetically normal (CN) AML. The WHO 2016 recognizes AML with mutated *NPM1* as a distinct entity [3]. The protein functions as a nuclear phosphoprotein that actively shuttles between the nucleus and cytoplasm and interacts as a chaperone with a number of tumor suppressors (CDKN2A/p14ARF and P53) [49]. The most common *NPM1* mutation (80% of cases) results in a 4 base pair duplication in the coding region of exon 12 (50). Mutations in *NPM1* alter tryptophan residues required for proper nucleolar localization and create a nuclear export signal at the C-terminus of the protein [50]. Consequently, the mutant nucleophosmin protein is sequestered in the cytoplasm, and through dimerization, causes the sequestration of the wild-type protein as well. Because of its role as a chaperone protein, this leads to the mislocalization of p14ARF and ultimately to the inhibition of p53 activity [49].

Approximately 40% of *NPM1* mutated AMLs also harbor *FLT3* internal tandem duplication (*FLT3*-ITD) mutations (see below), a feature which seems to significantly affect the prognostic relevance of *NPM1* [51]. Those with *NPM1* mutations and without

Table 3
Examples of recurrent mutations in AML

Gene target	Approximate frequency in AML[a] (%)	Prognostic significance	Putative consequence/ altered biologic mechanism	Associations (morphologic, genetic, or demographic)
NPM1	25–30	Favorable	Cytoplasmic mislocalization; dysregulated P53	Cup-like nuclear invaginations CD34-*FLT3-ITD*
DNMT3A	20	Unfavorable	Epigenetic	[b]
FLT3-ITD	15	Unfavorable	↑Signal transduction	Cup-like nuclear invaginations
WT1	10–15	Unclear/unfavorable	↓Transcription	–
RAS	10–15	None	↑Signal transduction	CBF AML
TET2	10–15	Unfavorable	DNA methylation	–
CEBPA	10	Favorable (when bialleic)	↓Transcription	Coexpression of T-cell antigens
IDH1	10	Unclear	Oncometabolite/DNA methylation	Monosomy 8 Cup-like nuclear invaginations
IDH2	10	Unclear	Oncometabolite/DNA methylation	Cup-like nuclear invaginations
ASXL1	10	Unfavorable	Chromatin modification	AML-MRC
TP53	5–10	Unfavorable	DNA damage repair	Complex karyotype
Cohesins (*STAG1/2, SMC1A, SMC3, RAD21*)	5–10	Unclear/unfavorable	Chromatid separation	Down syndrome
RUNX1	5–10	Unfavorable	↓Transcription	Minimal differentiation
ND4	5	Favorable	Electron transport	–
PHF6	5	Unfavorable	Epigenetic	Males
U2AF1	5	Unfavorable	Spliceosome	AML-MRC
FLT3-TKD	5	None/unclear	↑Signal transduction	–
KIT	5	Unfavorable	↑Signal transduction	CBF AML
KMT2A-PTD	5	Unfavorable	Chromatin modification	Trisomy 11
CBL	1	Unclear	↑Signal transduction	CBF AML

AML acute myeloid leukemia, *CBF* Core binding factor, *PTD* partial tandem duplication, *MRC* myelodysplasia-related changes

[a]Mutation frequency of some mutations may be up to twofold higher in CN AML

[b]High dose daunorubicin improves outcomes for patients with *DNMT3A* mutations

FLT3-ITD mutations have an overall favorable prognosis, similar to the *CBF* AMLs [51]. In fact, the presence of an *NPM1* mutation seems to supersede the negative prognostic value of multilineage dysplasia in the absence of cytogenetic abnormalities [52]. In contrast, *NPM1* mutations in the presence of the *FLT3*-ITD have a poor prognosis. Evaluation of newly diagnosed AML for *NPM1* mutations has become standard of care at most centers.

3.2 FLT3 Mutations

FLT3 is a receptor tyrosine kinase whose activation via ligand binding and homodimerization results in phosphorylation of downstream effectors in the STAT5 and MAPK signaling pathways [53]. Through these pathways, FLT3 acts to affect growth induction and apoptosis inhibition. Mutations in the *FLT3* gene occur in one of two ways: internal tandem duplication (ITD) of the juxtamembranous (JM) domain and a missense mutation in the tyrosine kinase activation domain (TKD), typically at amino acid D835 [53, 54]. Functionally both lead to constitutive activation of the tyrosine kinase and thus a pro-growth and anti-apoptotic signal for the cell. The ITD is more common, occurring in 25–30% of AMLs (again enriched in CN AML), with the TKD point mutation occurring in 5% [54]. Interestingly only the ITD mutation seems to have prognostic relevance [54].

The *FLT3*-ITD mutation is associated with poor overall survival in AML, and this influence is usually independent of a number of previously discussed recurrent cytogenetic abnormalities [54]. It is important to determine the allelic ratio of mutant:wild-type DNA, as this affects its prognostic impact. As noted above, the *FLT3*-ITD often co-occurs with the *NPM1* mutation, with the badness of the former trumping the goodness of the latter.

Because of its prognostic relevance, testing for *FLT3* mutations in all new AMLs is critical and a number of PCR-based assays are available. Targeted therapies against *FLT3* have been developed and may prove a useful adjunct to more conventional chemotherapy [55].

3.3 CEPBA Mutations

CEPBA (CCAT enhancer binding protein alpha) encodes a leucine zipper transcription factor that homodimerizes to regulate granulocytic differentiation. Mutations result in increased cellular proliferation and inhibition of differentiation, thus promoting myeloid leukemogenesis. Mutations typically occur as either N-terminal frame shift that acts in a dominant-negative fashion or as C-terminal in-frame deletions/insertions that affect DNA binding [56]. Only when mutations are biallelic and different does their presence predict for a favorable prognosis [57].

CEPBA mutations occur in 15–18% of CN AML, and approximately 10% of AML cases, overall. However, up to 45% of these, in some series, are monoallelic [57]. In the 2016 WHO classification, AML with biallelic mutation of *CEPBA* is recognized as a distinct entity [3]. Also important to note is that the presence of biallelic *CEPBA* mutations now supersedes the presence of multilineage dysplasia in cases of AML without concurrent MDS-associated cytogenetic abnormalities [3, 58].

3.4 RUNX1 Mutations

The *RUNX1* gene, located at 21q22, has been previously discussed with regard to its involvement in t(8;21)-associated AML. Distinct from these cases, inactivating point mutations can be found in the *RUNX1* gene in 5–10% of AMLs [59]. In contrast to the favorable prognosis imparted by the t(8;21), *RUNX1* point mutations predict for worse overall survival and therapy resistance [59]. AML with *RUNX1* mutations is now recognized as a provisional entity in the WHO 2016 [3]. However, these cases should only be classified as such in the absence of MDS-related cytogenetic abnormalities or other recurrent translocations shown in Tables 1 and 2 [3].

3.5 KIT Mutations

KIT mutations are especially common in core binding factor AMLs (t(8;21) and inv.(16)), occurring in approximately 20% of these cases. *KIT* mutations typically occur in exons 8 or 17 resulting in constitutive activation of the tyrosine kinase [20]. The presence of a *KIT* mutation in these cases is associated with a poor prognosis [20].

3.6 MLL (KMT2A) Mutations

KMT2A is another gene implicated not only in structural rearrangements but also in cryptic abnormalities. Mutations in *KMT2A* are usually partial tandem duplication (PTD) and occur in approximately 10% of CN AMLs, but they are especially enriched in the setting of trisomy 11 where they occur in 90% of cases. The *KMT2A* PTD is readily detected by RT-PCR and is associated with an unfavorable outcome [60].

4 Germline Predisposition

Although most AMLs are sporadic diseases, a subset may be familial [61]. The 2016 WHO classification includes acknowledgement of AML and other myeloid neoplasms in which there is a germ line mutation or predisposition syndrome (Table 4). The underlying predisposing genetic lesion should be included in the diagnosis of these rare cases.

Table 4
Genetic predisposition to AML

Gene	Syndrome	Other hematologic malignancies	Other hematologic manifestations	Nonhematologic manifestations
CEBPA	Familial AML with mutated *CEBPA*	–	–	–
DDX1	Familial AML with mutated *DDX41*	MDS, CMML	–	–
RUNX1	Familial platelet disorder with propensity to myeloid malignancies	MDS, T-ALL	Thrombocytopenia, bleeding propensity	Eczema
ANKRD26	Thrombocytopenia 2	MDS	Thrombocytopenia, bleeding propensity	–
ETV6	Thrombocytopenia 5	MDS, CMML, B-ALL, PCM	Thrombocytopenia	Possible Risk for solid tumors
GATA2	Familial MDS/AML with mutated *GATA2*	MDS, CMML	MonoMAC syndrome	Lymphedema, hearing loss, extragenital warts
Numerous[a]	Fanconi anemia	MDS	Aplastic anemia	Developmental delay, renal and skeletal abnormalities, SCC of head, neck, anogenital region
Numerous[b]	Telomere syndromes (dyskeratosis congenita)	MDS	Macrocytosis, aplastic anemia	Pulmonary and hepatic fibrosis, SCC of head, neck, anogenital region
Unknown	Down syndrome	B-ALL, MDS	Cytopenias, transient abnormal myelopoiesis	Numerous

[a]Genes that are implicated in the development of Fanconi anemia include *FANCA, FANCB, FANCC, BRCA2, FANCD2, FANCE, FANCF, FANCG, FANCI, BRIP1, FANCL, FANCM, PALB2, RAD51C*, and *SLX4*

[b]Genes that are implicated in the development of telomere syndromes include *TERC, TERT; CTC1, DKC1, NHP2, NOP10, RTEL1, TINF2, WRAP53, ACD*, and *PARN*

5 Beyond the Genome: Epigenetic Changes in AML

The most common epigenetic mechanisms include histone modification and DNA CpG methylation. While a number of gene mutations in AML impact these functions, global changes in DNA methylation have also been described in AML and may provide the basis for subclassification in the future [47, 62, 63].

One specific gene, *DNMT3A,* is a DNA methyltransferase that is mutated in ~20% of AMLs resulting in increased cellular proliferation. Mutations in this gene have been shown to impact methylation patterns in AML [64, 65]. While most studies have shown *DNMT3A* mutation to be a poor prognostic marker, others have refuted this association [64, 65]. Interestingly, however, *DNMT3A* mutations (in particular the most frequent one, R882) may persist in remission without adversely affecting prognosis [66].

DNA hydroxymethylation is one mechanism by which CpG methylation can be reversed. Several genes involved in this process, such as *TET2*, *IDH1*, and *IDH2,* are commonly mutated in AML.

Genes affecting histone proteins, common targets of epigenetic changes, are frequently mutated in AML. The *MLL/KMT2A* gene encodes an epigenetic modifier of histone proteins and is involved in both mutations and translocations in AML. Another protein, ASXL1, is also involved in methylation of histone proteins, and *ASXL1* is mutated in ~10% of AMLs. These mutations are associated with AML-MRC and generally show a poor prognosis [48]. Finally, *EZH2* codes for a catalytic enzyme involved in methylation of histone tails. *EZH2* mutations have been described in AML, albeit rarely [67].

6 Conclusion

In this era of NGS and other molecular technologies, our rate of discovery of new genetic aberrations in AML has skyrocketed, and complemented our already extensive knowledge about the cytogenetic landscape in this disease. This newfound wealth of information has not only impacted classification schemes but also provided new insights into disease pathogenesis and options for targeted therapy.

References

1. Bennett JM, Catovsky D, Daniel MT et al (1976) Proposals for the classification of the acute leukaemias. French-American-British (FAB) co-operative group. Br J Haematol 33(4):451–458
2. Swerdlow S, Campo E, Harris NL et al (2008) WHO classification of tumours of haematopoietic and lymphoid tissues, vol 2, 4th edn. IARC Press, Lyon
3. Arber DA, Orazi A, Hasserjian R et al (2016) The 2016 revision to the World Health Organization classification of myeloid neoplasms and acute leukemia. Blood 127(20): 2391–2405
4. Foucar K, Anastasi J (2015) Acute myeloid leukemia with recurrent cytogenetic abnormalities. Am J Clin Pathol 144(1):6–18

5. Degos L (1992) All-trans-retinoic acid treatment and retinoic acid receptor alpha gene rearrangement in acute promyelocytic leukemia: a model for differentiation therapy. Int J Cell Cloning 10(2):63–69
6. Abla O, Ribeiro RC (2014) How I treat children and adolescents with acute promyelocytic leukaemia. Br J Haematol 164(1):24–38
7. Molica M, Breccia M (2015) FLT3-ITD in acute promyelocytic leukemia: clinical distinct profile but still controversial prognosis. Leuk Res 39(4):397–399
8. Adams J, Nassiri M (2015) Acute Promyelocytic leukemia: a review and discussion of variant translocations. Arch Pathol Lab Med 139(10): 1308–1313
9. Brunel V, Lafage-Pochitaloff M, Alcalay M, Pelicci PG, Birg F (1996) Variant and masked translocations in acute promyelocytic leukemia. Leuk Lymphoma 22(3–4):221–228
10. Jansen JH, Lowenberg B (2001) Acute promyelocytic leukemia with a PLZF-RARalpha fusion protein. Semin Hematol 38(1):37–41
11. Guidez F, Parks S, Wong H et al (2007) RARalpha-PLZF overcomes PLZF-mediated repression of CRABPI, contributing to retinoid resistance in t(11;17) acute promyelocytic leukemia. Proc Natl Acad Sci U S A 104(47):18694–18699
12. Redner RL (2002) Variations on a theme: the alternate translocations in APL. Leukemia 16(10):1927–1932
13. Rossi V, Levati L, Biondi A (2006) Diagnosis and monitoring of PML-RARA-positive acute promyelocytic leukemia by qualitative RT-PCR. Methods Mol Med 125:115–126
14. Sinha C, Cunningham LC, Liu PP (2015) Core binding factor acute myeloid leukemia: new prognostic categories and therapeutic opportunities. Semin Hematol 52(3): 215–222
15. Grimwade D, Hills RK, Moorman AV et al (2010) Refinement of cytogenetic classification in acute myeloid leukemia: determination of prognostic significance of rare recurring chromosomal abnormalities among 5876 younger adult patients treated in the United Kingdom Medical Research Council trials. Blood 116:354–365
16. Wong KF, Kwong YL (1999) Trisomy 22 in acute myeloid leukemia: a marker for myeloid leukemia with monocytic features and cytogenetically cryptic inversion 16. Cancer Genet Cytogenet 109(2):131–133
17. Costello R, Sainty D, Lecine P et al (1997) Detection of CBFbeta/MYH11 fusion transcripts in acute myeloid leukemia: heterogeneity of cytological and molecular characteristics. Leukemia 11(5):644–650
18. Claxton D, Xie QS, Patel S, Deisseroth AB, Kornblau S (1996) The gene product of CBFB-MYH11. Leukemia 10(9):1479–1485
19. Paschka P, Du J, Schlenk RF et al (2013) Secondary genetic lesions in acute myeloid leukemia with inv(16) or t(16;16): a study of the German-Austrian AML study group (AMLSG). Blood 121(1):170–177
20. Paschka P, Marcucci G, Ruppert AS et al (2006) Adverse prognostic significance of KIT mutations in adult acute myeloid leukemia with inv(16) and t(8;21): a cancer and leukemia group B study. J Clin Oncol 24(24): 3904–3911
21. Schoch C, Schnittger S, Klaus M et al (2003) AML with 11q23//MLL abnormalities as defined by the WHO classification: incidence, partner chromosomes, FAB subtype, age distribution, and prognostic impact in an unselected series of 1897 cytogenetically analyzed AML cases. Blood 102:2395–2402
22. Meyer C, Hofmann J, Burmeister T et al (2013) The MLL recombinome of acute leukemias in 2013. Leukemia 27(11): 2165–2176
23. Balgobind BV, Raimondi SC, Harbott J et al (2009) Novel prognostic subgroups in childhood 11q23/MLL-rearranged acute myeloid leukemia: results of an international retrospective study. Blood 114(12):2489–2496
24. Fianchi L, Pagano L, Piciocchi A et al (2015) Characteristics and outcome of therapy-related myeloid neoplasms: report from the Italian network on secondary leukemias. Am J Hematol 90(5):E80–E85
25. Krivtsov AV, Armstrong SA (2007) MLL translocations, histone modifications and leukaemia stem-cell development. Nat Rev Cancer 7(11):823–833
26. Chen CW, Koche RP, Sinha AU et al (2015) DOT1L inhibits SIRT1-mediated epigenetic silencing to maintain leukemic gene expression in MLL-rearranged leukemia. Nat Med 21(4):335–343
27. Zhou J, Wu J, Li B et al (2014) PU.1 is essential for MLL leukemia partially via crosstalk with the MEIS/HOX pathway. Leukemia 28(7):1436–1448
28. Aikawa Y, Yamagata K, Katsumoto T et al (2015) Essential role of PU.1 in maintenance of mixed lineage leukemia-associated leukemic stem cells. Cancer Sci 106(3):227–236
29. Emerenciano M, Meyer C, Mansur MB, Marschalek R, Pombo-de-Oliveira MS (2013) The distribution of MLL breakpoints corre-

lates with outcome in infant acute leukaemia. Br J Haematol 161(2):224–236
30. Tarlock K, Alonzo TA, Moraleda PP et al (2014) Acute myeloid leukaemia (AML) with t(6;9)(p23;q34) is associated with poor outcome in childhood AML regardless of FLT3-ITD status: a report from the Children's oncology group. Br J Haematol 166(2): 254–259
31. Ageberg M, Drott K, Olofsson T, Gullberg U, Lindmark A (2008) Identification of a novel and myeloid specific role of the leukemia-associated fusion protein DEK-NUP214 leading to increased protein synthesis. Genes Chromosomes Cancer 47(4):276–287
32. von Lindern M, Breems D, van Baal S, Adriaansen H, Grosveld G (1992) Characterization of the translocation breakpoint sequences of two DEK-CAN fusion genes present in t(6;9) acute myeloid leukemia and a SET-CAN fusion gene found in a case of acute undifferentiated leukemia. Genes Chromosomes Cancer 5(3):227–234
33. Lugthart S, Groschel S, Beverloo HB et al (2010) Clinical, molecular, and prognostic significance of WHO type inv(3)(q21q26.2)/t(3;3)(q21;q26.2) and various other 3q abnormalities in acute myeloid leukemia. J Clin Oncol 28(24):3890–3898
34. Yamazaki H, Suzuki M, Otsuki A et al (2014) A remote GATA2 hematopoietic enhancer drives leukemogenesis in inv(3)(q21;q26) by activating EVI1 expression. Cancer Cell 25(4):415–427
35. Shearer BM, Sukov WR, Flynn HC, Knudson RA, Ketterling RP (2010) Development of a dual-color, double fusion FISH assay to detect RPN1/EVI1 gene fusion associated with inv(3), t(3;3), and ins(3;3) in patients with myelodysplasia and acute myeloid leukemia. Am J Hematol 85(8):569–574
36. Lion T, Haas OA (1993) Acute megakaryocytic leukemia with the t(1;22)(p13;q13). Leuk Lymphoma 11(1–2):15–20
37. Carroll A, Civin C, Schneider N et al (1991) The t(1;22) (p13;q13) is nonrandom and restricted to infants with acute megakaryoblastic leukemia: a pediatric oncology group study. Blood 78(3):748–752
38. Inaba H, Zhou Y, Abla O et al (2015) Heterogeneous cytogenetic subgroups and outcomes in childhood acute megakaryoblastic leukemia: a retrospective international study. Blood 126(13):1575–1584
39. Mercher T, Raffel GD, Moore SA et al (2009) The OTT-MAL fusion oncogene activates RBPJ-mediated transcription and induces acute megakaryoblastic leukemia in a knockin mouse model. J Clin Invest 119(4):852–864
40. Soupir CP, Vergilio JA, Dal Cin P et al (2007) Philadelphia chromosome-positive acute myeloid leukemia: a rare aggressive leukemia with clinicopathologic features distinct from chronic myeloid leukemia in myeloid blast crisis. Am J Clin Pathol 127(4):642–650
41. Nacheva EP, Grace CD, Brazma D et al (2013) Does BCR/ABL1 positive acute myeloid leukaemia exist? Br J Haematol 161(4):541–550
42. Konoplev S, Yin CC, Kornblau SM et al (2013) Molecular characterization of de novo Philadelphia chromosome-positive acute myeloid leukemia. Leuk Lymphoma 54(1): 138–144
43. Moon JH, Lee YJ, Seo SK et al (2015) Outcomes of allogeneic hematopoietic cell transplantation in acute myeloid leukemia patients with monosomal karyotypes. Acta Haematol 133(4):327–335
44. Weinberg OK, Ohgami RS, Ma L et al (2014) Acute myeloid leukemia with monosomal karyotype: morphologic, immunophenotypic, and molecular findings. Am J Clin Pathol 142(2):190–195
45. Murati A, Brecqueville M, Devillier R et al (2012) Myeloid malignancies: mutations, models and management. BMC Cancer 12:304
46. Meyer SC, Levine RL (2014) Translational implications of somatic genomics in acute myeloid leukaemia. Lancet Oncol 15(9): e382–ee94
47. Genomic and epigenomic landscapes of adult de novo acute myeloid leukemia (2013) N Engl J Med 368(22):2059–2074
48. Ohgami RS, Ma L, Merker JD et al (2015) Next-generation sequencing of acute myeloid leukemia identifies the significance of TP53, U2AF1, ASXL1, and TET2 mutations. Mod Pathol 28(5):706–714
49. Colombo E, Marine JC, Danovi D, Falini B, Pelicci PG (2002) Nucleophosmin regulates the stability and transcriptional activity of p53. Nat Cell Biol 4(7):529–533
50. Boissel N, Renneville A, Biggio V et al (2005) Prevalence, clinical profile, and prognosis of NPM mutations in AML with normal karyotype. Blood 106(10):3618–3620
51. Thiede C, Koch S, Creutzig E et al (2006) Prevalence and prognostic impact of NPM1 mutations in 1485 adult patients with acute myeloid leukemia (AML). Blood 107(10): 4011–4020
52. Diaz-Beya M, Rozman M, Pratcorona M et al (2010) The prognostic value of multilineage dysplasia in de novo acute myeloid leukemia

patients with intermediate-risk cytogenetics is dependent on NPM1 mutational status. Blood 116(26):6147–6148

53. Stirewalt DL, Radich JP (2003) The role of FLT3 in haematopoietic malignancies. Nat Rev Cancer 3(9):650–665
54. Thiede C, Steudel C, Mohr B et al (2002) Analysis of FLT3-activating mutations in 979 patients with acute myelogenous leukemia: association with FAB subtypes and identification of subgroups with poor prognosis. Blood 99(12):4326–4335
55. Grunwald MR, Levis MJ (2015) FLT3 tyrosine kinase inhibition as a paradigm for targeted drug development in acute myeloid leukemia. Semin Hematol 52(3):193–199
56. Pabst T, Mueller BU, Zhang P et al (2001) Dominant-negative mutations of CEBPA, encoding CCAAT/enhancer binding protein-alpha (C/EBPalpha), in acute myeloid leukemia. Nat Genet 27(3):263–270
57. Green CL, Koo KK, Hills RK et al (2010) Prognostic significance of CEBPA mutations in a large cohort of younger adult patients with acute myeloid leukemia: impact of double CEBPA mutations and the interaction with FLT3 and NPM1 mutations. J Clin Oncol 28(16):2739–2747
58. Bacher U, Schnittger S, Macijewski K et al (2012) Multilineage dysplasia does not influence prognosis in CEBPA-mutated AML, supporting the WHO proposal to classify these patients as a unique entity. Blood 119(20): 4719–4722
59. Gaidzik VI, Bullinger L, Schlenk RF et al (2011) RUNX1 mutations in acute myeloid leukemia: results from a comprehensive genetic and clinical analysis from the AML study group. J Clin Oncol 29(10):1364–1372
60. Dohner K, Tobis K, Ulrich R et al (2002) Prognostic significance of partial tandem duplications of the MLL gene in adult patients 16 to 60 years old with acute myeloid leukemia and normal cytogenetics: a study of the acute myeloid leukemia study group Ulm. J Clin Oncol 20(15):3254–3261
61. DiNardo CD, Bannon SA, Routbort M et al (2016) Evaluation of patients and families with concern for predispositions to hematologic malignancies within the hereditary hematologic malignancy clinic (HHMC). Clin Lymphoma Myeloma Leuk 16(7): 417–428
62. Wertheim GB, Smith C, Luskin M et al (2015) Validation of DNA methylation to predict outcome in acute myeloid leukemia by use of xMELP. Clin Chem 61(1):249–258
63. Figueroa ME, Lugthart S, Li Y et al (2010) DNA methylation signatures identify biologically distinct subtypes in acute myeloid leukemia. Cancer Cell 17(1):13–27
64. Ley TJ, Ding L, Walter MJ et al (2010) DNMT3A mutations in acute myeloid leukemia. N Engl J Med 363:2424–2433
65. Yan XJ, Xu J, Gu ZH et al (2011) Exome sequencing identifies somatic mutations of DNA methyltransferase gene DNMT3A in acute monocytic leukemia. Nat Genet 43(4):309–315
66. Bhatnagar B, Eisfeld AK, Nicolet D et al (2016) Persistence of DNMT3A R882 mutations during remission does not adversely affect outcomes of patients with acute myeloid leukaemia. Br J Haematol 175(2):226–236
67. Lindsley RC, Mar BG, Mazzola E et al (2015) Acute myeloid leukemia ontogeny is defined by distinct somatic mutations. Blood 125(9):1367–1376

Chapter 2

Cytochemical Staining

Michele E. Paessler, Marybeth Helfrich, and Gerald B.W. Wertheim

Abstract

Historically, the diagnosis and classification of acute leukemia involved morphologic review of blasts in the peripheral blood and bone marrow smears and cytochemical staining. Cytochemical stains, which are enzymatic colorimetric reactions that occur in the cells of interest, were necessary to assign and confirm myeloid and lymphoid lineage. In the current WHO 2008 Classification of leukemia, immunophenotyping and cytogenetic analysis have largely replaced cytochemical staining in the characterization of acute leukemias. Nonetheless, cytochemical testing remains a useful adjunct assay for the proper classification of acute leukemia in a number of diagnostic settings. This chapter reviews the principles of the most common cytochemical stains, their procedures and guides to interpretation, and results in acute myeloid leukemia.

Key words Acute myeloid leukemia, Bone marrow, Cytochemical stains

1 Introduction

Acute leukemia is characterized by a proliferation of immature hematopoietic elements (i.e., blasts) that undergo a maturation arrest and do not develop into fully differentiated cells (i.e., neutrophils, monocytes, lymphocytes) [1]. The diagnosis of acute leukemia relies on distinguishing blasts with myeloid differentiation from those with lymphoid differentiation. The current WHO classification system broadly segregates acute leukemia into acute myeloid (AML), B-lymphoblastic (B-ALL), and T-lymphoblastic (T-ALL) leukemia, with subclasses therein [2]. Accurate phenotypic characterization of acute leukemia as myeloid or lymphoid is essential for proper treatment; therapy for AML and ALL is markedly distinct [3, 4]. Current classification of leukemia relies heavily on the immunophenotypic profile of leukemic cells [2]. Thus, antibody-based detection of specific B-cell, T-cell, and myeloid markers is essential at diagnosis; the methods for detection include flow cytometry of fresh cells or immunohistochemistry of formalin fixed paraffin embedded (FFPE) tissue. Additionally, in-depth genetic analysis using massively parallel DNA sequencing

Paolo Fortina et al. (eds.), *Acute Myeloid Leukemia: Methods and Protocols*, Methods in Molecular Biology, vol. 1633,
DOI 10.1007/978-1-4939-7142-8_2, © Springer Science+Business Media LLC 2017

techniques is being developed for the classification based on recurrent mutations [5]. However, the earliest techniques for lineage assignment (and the techniques on which much of the classification of acute leukemia is based) involve cytochemical stains for cellular components that characterize different hematopoietic lineages [6]. These include stains for the myeloid markers myeloperoxidase (MPO), Sudan Black B (SBB), and chloroacetate esterase (CAE); the monocytic and megakaryocytic marker of nonspecific esterase (NSE); acid phosphatase (AP), which shows a typical pattern in T cells; and periodic acid Schiff stain (PAS), which identifies B lymphoblasts and atypical erythroid precursors.

Cytochemical stains are based on chemical colorimetric reactions that occur within the cells of interest. These reactions rely on either substrates within the cells (such as PAS and Sudan Black B staining) or enzymatic activity that the cells possess (such as myeloperoxidase or chloroacetate esterase activity) [6]. The stains used in leukemia classification deposit a colored product at the site of the reaction that can be fixed (chemically cross-linked) in place and then examined by light microscopy. The presence, intensity, and pattern of staining—taken in context with morphologic, immunophenotypic, and clinical assessments—can indicate the lineage of the leukemic cells.

Most diagnostic laboratories do not routinely perform cytochemical stains on peripheral blood smears or bone marrow aspirates from patients with acute leukemia. Instead, immunophenotypic results from either flow cytometry or immunohistochemistry are usually sufficient for accurate classification of myeloid, B-lymphoid of T-lymphoid acute leukemia. However, cytochemistry has not been entirely replaced by immunophenotypic assays. Cytochemistry has the advantage over flow cytometry in that it provides simultaneous examination of cellular differentiation and morphology. Thus, these cytochemical stains may be useful when fresh aspirate material is not available for flow cytometry or when flow cytometry yields inconclusive results. Additionally, they may be used in assessing immature cells that cannot be readily distinguished from their more mature forms by routine flow cytometry (such as promonocytes vs. mature monocytes). Although immunohistochemical staining of marrow biopsy cores may allow pathologists to circumvent the need for cytochemical stains on these occasions, there are certain instances in which this staining may be unreliable or not possible. These include immunohistochemical stains for myeloperoxidase [7], which have been shown to yield false positive results, or bone marrow studies of infants with leukemia for whom biopsies are frequently not obtained. Thus, although not frequently performed, cytochemical testing continues to remain a useful adjunct assay for the proper classification of acute leukemia [8].

2 Materials

Unless otherwise described, all reagents are stored at room temperature (20–26 °C).

2.1 Equipment

1. Staining rack.
2. Mini-Coplin jar (10 mL) or Coplin jar (60 mL).
3. Water bath set to 37 °C and shielded from light.
4. Incubator/oven.
5. #1 Whatman filter paper.

2.2 Reagents for Multiple Stains

1. Formaldehyde, 37%.
2. Ethanol. Dilute with ddH_2O to make 70% ethanol.
3. Acetone.
4. Sodium nitrite. Make 100 mM and 4% w/v solutions with ddH_2O.
5. Potassium phosphate, monobasic, KH_2PO_4.
6. Sodium phosphate, dibasic, Na_2HPO_4.
7. Buffered formalin/acetone fixative: 20 mg Na_2HPO_4; 100 mg KH_2PO_4; 30 mL ddH_2O; 45 mL Acetone; 25 mL 37% Formaldehyde. Na_2HPO_4 and KH_2PO_4 are added to ddH_2O and mix until dissolved prior to adding acetone and formaldehyde. Store at 4 °C.
8. Cytoseal 60 mounting medium (Thermo Scientific #8310-4).

2.3 Reagents for Specific Stains

2.3.1 MPO

1. Hydrogen peroxide 3%.
2. Trizmal buffer pH 6.3 (Sigma-Aldrich #903C). Discard if turbidity develops.
3. Trizmal working buffer. Mix 50 mL of Trizmal buffer pH 6.3 with 450 mL of ddH_2O.
4. Peroxidase Indicator Reagent (Sigma-Aldrich #3901), prealiquoted in vials. Store at 4 °C.
5. Acid Hematoxylin solution (Sigma-Aldrich #2652).

2.3.2 Sudan Black B

Sudan Black B staining system (Sigma-Aldrich #308B). Contains Sudan Black B staining reagent and Gill's #3 hematoxylin solution. Sudan Black B stain may be returned to stock bottle and reused. When control is no longer positive, discard stock bottle. Protect hematoxylin from light.

2.3.3 CAE/NSE

1. Hydrochloric acid, HCl, 37%.
2. Pararosaniline base.
3. Methyl Green.

4. Sodium fluoride, NaF.
5. 2-Methoxyethanol, ethylene glycol monomethyl ether.
6. *N,N*-Dimethylformamide.
7. Alpha-Naphthyl acetate.
8. Naphthol AS-D Chloroacetate.
9. Fast Blue BB Base (Sigma-Aldrich #F3378). Store at −20 °C.
10. 1/15 M Na_2HPO_4 stock buffer. Dissolve 9.5 g Na_2HPO_4 in 900 mL ddH_2O. Add ddH_2O to 1 L.
11. 1/15 M KH_2PO_4 stock buffer. Dissolve 9.1 g KH_2PO_4 in 900 mL ddH_2O. Add ddH_2O to 1 L.
12. 1/15 M Phosphate working buffer, pH 7.4. Mix 80.4 mL of 1/15 M Na_2HPO_4 stock buffer with 19.6 mL of 1/15 M KH_2PO_4 stock buffer.
13. 1/15 M Phosphate working buffer, pH 6.3. Mix 22.4 mL of 1/15 M Na_2HPO_4 stock buffer with 77.6 mL of 1/15 M KH_2PO_4 stock buffer.
14. Sodium Nitrite solution: dissolve 4 g of sodium nitrite in distilled water. Bring to final volume of 100 mL. No expiration date. Good until cloudy.
15. 4% Pararosaniline solution: Dissolve 1 g pararosaniline in 5 mL of concentrated HCl with gentle warming. Slowly add 20 mL distilled water with constant stirring. Allow to cool. Filter when cool. No expiration date.
16. 1% Methyl Green Solution (Methyl Violet Free): Add 1 g methyl green to 100 mL distilled water. Mix well and filter before initial use. No expiration date. May be returned to container and reused until the time required to obtain an adequate stain exceeds 15 min.

2.3.4 Acid Phosphatase

1. Citrate solution (Sigma-Aldrich #915).
2. Citrate/acetone/formaldehyde fixative. To 25 mL Citrate Solution, add 65 mL acetone and 8 mL of 36% formaldehyde. Place in glass bottle and cap tightly. Store at 4 °C. Warm to room temperature prior to use.
3. 2.5 M Acetate solution, pH 5.2 (Sigma-Aldrich #3863). Store at 4 °C. Discard if turbidity develops.
4. Naphthol AS-BI Phosphoric acid solution (Sigma-Aldrich #1802). Store at −20 °C. Warm to 37 °C and mix well prior to use. Discard if reagent turns yellow.
5. Fast garnet GBC base solution (Sigma-Aldrich #3872). Store at 4 °C.
6. Methylene Blue solution (Sigma-Aldrich #1808). Store tightly capped.

7. Methylene Blue counterstain: Add 1 mL methylene blue solution to 9 mL of ddH_2O. Mix well. Prepare fresh.
8. Aqua-mount mounting medium (VWR #41799–008).

2.3.5 PAS

1. Formalin/Alcohol fixative. Mix 10 mL of 36% formaldehyde with 90 mL of 100% ethanol. Store in a tightly sealed glass bottle.
2. Periodic acid (Sigma-Aldrich #375810). Dissolve 1 g periodic acid in 100 mL of ddH_2O.
3. Schiff's reagent (Sigma-Aldrich #3952016). Store in refrigerator (2–4 °C) in tightly sealed container protected from light. Discard if solution turns pink. Warm to room temperature (20–26 °C) before use.
4. Mayer's Hematoxylin stain (Sigma-Aldrich #MHS16). Filter before use with Whatman #1 filter paper. Store protected from light.

3 Procedure

3.1 General Procedure for All Stains

Coverslips or slide smears prepared from peripheral blood, bone marrow aspirate, or body fluid that is either non-anticoagulated or anticoagulated with heparin or EDTA. For body fluids, cytocentrifuge preparations may be used. If the specimen is not anticoagulated, slides or coverslips must be made immediately after the specimen is collected from the patient. Preparations from anticoagulated specimens should be made within 2 h of specimen collection. Smears should be air dried, stored at room temperature, and protected from light and humidity until staining is performed. If properly stored, these smears are stable for at least 2 months [9].

For quality control, freshly prepared coverslip smears of nonleukemic bone marrow or peripheral blood should be stained as positive controls each time a patient sample is evaluated. If the control cells are not positive, reagents should be replaced (*see* **Note 1**). The control results should be reported to document they were performed.

The evaluation of the patient samples requires identification of the blast cells present. These are the only cells that are reported as positive or negative. A description of the staining pattern should be given, as should the percentage of the positive blasts. Positive normal cells are not reported.

3.2 Procedures for Specific Stains

3.2.1 MPO Principle

Myeloperoxidase is present in neutrophils, monocytes, and their precursors but not in lymphoid cells [10]. The MPO stain is highly specific and a positive stain is sufficient for reporting myeloid differentiation (i.e., AML Acute myeloid leukemia (AML) or acute leukemia Leukemia of ambiguous lineage) [2]. Classical methods for determining the presence of myeloperoxidase involved the use of benzidine or diaminobenzidine, which are highly carcinogenic. In 1977, Hanker et al. described the use of p-phenylenediamine and catechol to detect the presence of peroxidase [11].

3.2.2 Procedure

1. Prewarm 50 mL of Trizmal Dilute Buffer in 37 °C water bath.
2. Place smears in Coplin jar and fill with formalin/alcohol fixative. Incubate at room temperature for 30 s. Appropriately discard fixative and wash smears three times with ddH_2O.
3. Prepare Peroxidase Indicator Reagent solution by adding 1 vial of Peroxidase Indicator Reagent and 0.2 mL of 3% hydrogen peroxide to the prewarmed Trizmal Dilute Buffer. Mix thoroughly.
4. Add Peroxidase Indicator Reagent solution to Coplin jar with fixed smears. Protect from light (*see* **Note 2**) and incubate for 30 min at 37 °C. After incubation, properly discard the reagent and wash smears three times with ddH_2O.
5. Add Acid Hematoxylin solution to Coplin jar with fixed smears. Incubate for 15 min at room temperature. After incubation, properly discard the stain and wash smears three times with ddH_2O.
6. Air-dry and mount with Cytoseal 60.

3.2.3 Expected Results (Tables 1 and 2)

Although myeloperoxidase is generally considered a marker for cells of myeloid lineage, monocytic cells may also display weak positivity [10, 12]. Neutrophils and their precursors should show brown-black cytoplasmic granulation that should be darker than background staining of the red blood cells. Monocytes may be weakly positive while lymphocytes and red cell precursors are negative.

Table 1
Stain and counterstain colors

Stain	Positive	Counterstain
Sudan Black	Black	Purple
Myeloperoxidase	Dark brown	Purple
PAS	Red	Purple
Acid phosphatase	Red	Green
CAE	Blue	Green
α-Napthyl acetate	Red brown	Green
ANA-Megka	Red brown	Green
α-Napthyl butyrate	Red brown	Green

Table 2
Expected results

	Sudan Black	Myeloperoxidase	PAS	Acid Phos	CAE	α-Napthyl Acetate	α-Napthyl acetate w NaF	ANA-Megka	ANA-Megka w NaF	α-Napthyl butyrate
Normal cell lines										
Promyelocyte	+/++	+/++	+/+	+/++	+/++	−/+	−/+	−	−	−
Neutrophil	++	++	+++	+	+/++	−/+	−/+	−	−	−
Monocyte	−/+	−/+	+	++	−	+++	−	+/++	−	+/++
Lymphocyte	−	−	−	−/++	−	−/+	−/+	−/+	−/+	−/+
Erythroblast	−	−	−	+	−	−/+	−/+	−	−/+	−
AML without maturation	+	+	+ Fine granular	+	−/+	−/+	Not inhibited	−	−	−
AML with maturation	++	++	+ Fine granular	+	+	−/+	Not inhibited	−	−	−
Acute myelomonocytic	+	+	+	+	−/+	+	Inhibited	+	Inhibited	+
Acute monoblastic/ monocytic leukemia	−/+	−	+	+	−	++	Inhibited	++	Inhibited	++
Acute erythroid leukemia	−	−	+	focal	−	−/+	−/+	−/+	−/+	−
Acute megakaryoblastic leukemia	−−	−	+	+	−−	−/+	Inhibited	+ Punctate	Not inhibited	−

Peroxidase activity may be decreased or absent in the mature neutrophils of patients with myelodysplastic syndromes or acute myeloid leukemia (*see* **Note 3**) [13]. MPO staining may also be used to diagnose hereditary myeloperoxidase deficiency in which all neutrophils and monocytes are deficient but eosinophils are unaffected [14]. In cases of homozygous deficiency, neutrophil peroxidase is undetectable, whereas heterozygous cases show decreased staining relative to normal controls.

3.3 Sudan Black B

3.3.1 Principle

Sudan Black B stains several lipids including phospholipids and neutral fats that are contained in the granules of the neutrophil series [15]. Since cells that are committed to lymphoid maturation do not contain these granules, lymphoblasts typically are negative, whereas cells undergoing myeloid maturation will be positive. Sudan Black B is, therefore, a useful adjunct for myeloperoxidase and CAE stains.

3.3.2 Procedure

1. Place smears into slots in the Coplin jar. Fill Coplin jar with buffered formalin/acetone fixative solution and incubate for 1 min at room temperature. Appropriately discard fixative and wash smears three times with ddH_2O.
2. Fill Coplin jar with Sudan Black B Staining Reagent and stain for 15 min at room temperature. Appropriately discard staining reagent and wash smears three times with ddH_2O.
3. Fill Coplin jar with 70% ethanol. Incubate for 2 min at room temperature. Appropriately discard and wash smears three times with ddH_2O.
4. Counterstain by filling the Coplin jar with Gill #3 Hematoxylin solution. Incubate for 15 min at room temperature. Return stain to bottle when done. Wash smears three times with ddH_2O.
5. Air-dry and mount with Cytoseal 60.

3.3.3 Expected Results (Tables 1 and 2)

Maturing myeloid precursors will show black or dark blue intracellular staining at the site of primary and secondary granule formation. Although Sudan Black B is generally considered to be a myeloid marker, monocytic appearing cells may display weak positivity [16]. This usually occurs in myelomonocytic leukemia. Normal lymphocytes do not stain with Sudan Black B, yet several reports have documented rare instances of B lymphoblastic leukemia that stain for Sudan Black B [17]. Hence, Sudan Black B staining should be interpreted in the context of other phenotypic results.

3.4 NSE/CAE Principle

Cytochemical reactions for esterases distinguish between the cells of the monocyte series and the neutrophil series. The leukocyte esterases hydrolyze an ester derived from naphthalene to release a naphthol compound, which then combines with the diazonium salt present in the reaction mixture to form a colored precipitate at the site of enzyme activity [10]. The reaction for nonspecific esterases using alpha-naphthyl acetate as the substrate is strongly positive in monocytes and monocyte precursors and demonstrates a punctate positivity pattern in megakaryocytes and megakaryocyte precursors [10]. A sodium fluoride (NaF) inhibition step may be incorporated into the nonspecific esterase stain procedure to allow distinction between monocytic and megakaryocytic lineages, since NaF completely inhibits the monocytic enzyme while the megakaryocyte enzyme is only partially inhibited [10, 18]. The reaction using naphthol AS-D chloroacetate as substrate is positive in neutrophils and neutrophil precursors and negative in monocytes and monocyte precursors.

3.4.1 Procedure

1. Place smears in slots of two Coplin jars, one marked NSE and the other marked NaF.
2. Fill both jars with *cold* buffered Formalin/Acetone Fixative and incubate for 30 s. Appropriately discard fixative and wash smears three times with ddH_2O.
3. Air-dry for 15 min.
4. Prepare hexazotized pararosaniline by mixing 100 μL of 4% Sodium Nitrite solution with 100 μL 4% pararosaniline solution (*see* **Note 4**). Let stand at room temperature for at least 1 min before adding to the incubation mixture.
5. Prepare incubation mixtures for nonspecific esterase. Label two conical tubes as NSE and NSE/NaF. Add the reagents in Table 3 in the order listed, mixing well after each addition. Assure that solids have dissolved prior to proceeding to the next addition (*see* **Note 5**).
6. Filter solutions through #1 filter paper into new conical tubes (*see* **Note 6**).

Table 3
Nonspecific esterase staining (NSE)

	NSE	NSE/NAF
α-Naphthyl acetate	10 mg	10 mg
Ethyleneglycolmonomethyl ether	0.5 mL	0.5 mL
1/15 M phosphate buffer pH 6.3	9.5 mL	9.5 mL
Hexazotized pararosaniline	0.05 mL	0.05 mL
Sodium fluoride	None	15 mg

Table 4
Chloroacetate esterase staining (CAE)

Naphthol AS-D chloroacetate	1 mg
N,N-dimethylformamide	0.5 mL
1/15 M phosphate buffer pH 7.4	9.5 mL
Fast Blue BB	5 mg

7. Add solutions to the appropriate Coplin jars with smears and incubate at 37 °C for 50 min. Appropriately discard staining solution and wash smears three times with ddH_2O.
8. Prepare the CAE incubation mixture by adding the reagents in Table 4 in the order listed, mixing well after each addition. As with the NSE mixture, be sure that all solids are dissolved prior to the next addition (*see* **Note 7**).
9. Add the CAE incubation mixture to Coplin jars containing smears stained for NSE. Incubate for 10 min at room temperature. Appropriately discard staining solution and wash smears three times with ddH_2O.
10. Prepare dilute counterstain by adding 1 mL of 1% Methyl Green to 9 mL of ddH_2O. Fill Coplin jars containing the NSE and CAE stained smears with dilute methyl green. Incubate at room temperature for 5 min. Properly discard the stain and wash smears three times with ddH_2O.
11. Air-dry and mount with Cytoseal 60.

3.4.2 Expected Results (Tables 1 and 2)

These two esterase stains are used primarily to distinguish AML of granulocytic, monocytic, and megakaryocytic lineages [19, 20]. CAE is present in the granules myeloid cells and is insensitive to NaF inhibition. The pattern of CAE staining should parallel those of Sudan Black and Peroxidase, both in normal and leukemic myeloid cells. Normal myeloblasts are negative for CAE, but myeloblasts in some cases of AML are positive. CAE is negative in eosinophils, lymphocytes, plasma cells, erythroblasts, megakaryocytes, and mature monocytes.

NSE stain is strongest in monocytes, macrophages, megakaryocytes, and platelets. Weak activity is present in granulocytes and T lymphocytes (*see* **Note 8**). Activity in monocytes and macrophages is completely inhibited by sodium fluoride, while stain is retained, though diminished in intensity, in granulocytes and megakaryocytes.

3.5 Acid Phosphatase

3.5.1 Principle

Acid phosphatase in hematopoietic cells can hydrolyze a variety of hydroxynaphtholic anilides, releasing insoluble naphthols, which couple efficiently at acid pH with diazonium salts [19, 21]. The resultant product forms a colored precipitate at the enzyme location.

3.5.2 Procedure

1. Prewarm a bottle of ddH_2O at 37 °C.
2. Place smears into a Coplin jar. Fill Coplin jar with Citrate/Acetone/Formaldehyde Fixative. Incubate at room temperature for 30 s. Properly discard the fixative and wash smears three times with ddH_2O.
3. Prepare the incubation mixture by mixing 0.2 mL of sodium nitrite solution to 0.2 mL of fast garnet GBC base solution. Mix gently and let stand for at least 2 min.
4. Add the incubation mixture above to 7.6 mL of prewarmed ddH_2O.
5. Add 1 mL acetate solution.
6. Add 1 mL Naphthol AS-BI Phosphoric acid solution and mix well (*see* **Note 9**).
7. Fill the Coplin jar containing the samples, with fresh mixture from **step 8**. Cap tightly and place in the 37 °C incubator for 1 h. Properly discard the staining solution and wash smears three times with ddH_2O.
8. Make methylene blue counterstain by adding 1 mL methylene blue solution to 9 mL ddH_2O and mix well.
9. Add the dilute methylene blue counterstain to the Coplin jar and incubate for 2 min at room temperature. Properly discard the staining solution and wash smears three times with ddH_2O.
10. Air-dry and mount with Aqua-mount (*see* **Note 10**).

3.5.3 Expected Results (Tables 1 and 2)

Acid phosphatase activity is indicated by red granular precipitate and is diffusely positive in the cytoplasm of most cells of the hematopoietic system. Moderate staining is seen in plasma cells, megakaryocytes, and monocytes. Weak reactions are present normally in the myeloid series. Histiocytes and osteoclasts should be strongly granular positive. Very little acid phosphatase activity is present in erythroid precursors. In T-cell leukemia acid phosphatase is characteristically strong and localized in the Golgi area, so focal (dot-like) staining of the blasts suggests T-cell lineage [22]. Megakaryoblasts may also show focal staining [20, 23]. Correlation with other phenotyping assays is necessary for definitive lineage assignment.

3.6 PAS Principle

Periodic acid oxidizes cellular glycols and related compounds to their cognate aldehydes. These aldehydes can then react with the Schiff's reagent (leukofuchsin) releasing fuchsin [24]. These reactions result in bright pink staining of the cellular component that originally contained the oxidizable compounds. In blood and bone marrow cells, glycogen is the compound primarily responsible for PAS staining.

3.6.1 Procedure

1. Place smears into slots in the Coplin jar.
2. Fill the Coplin jar with formalin/alcohol fixative and incubate for 5 min at room temperature. Properly discard the fixative and wash smears three times with ddH_2O.
3. Fill the Coplin jar with the periodic acid solution and incubate for 15 min at room temperature. Properly discard the acid solution and wash smears three times with ddH_2O.
4. Fill the Coplin jar with Schiff's reagent and incubate for 15 min at room temperature. Properly discard the Schiff's reagent and wash smears three times with ddH_2O.
5. Fill the Coplin jar with Mayer's Hematoxylin and incubate for 15 min at room temperature. Properly discard the stain and wash smears three times with ddH_2O.
6. Air-dry and mount with Cytoseal 60.

3.6.2 Expected Results (See Table 1)

Mature neutrophils, megakaryocytes, and platelets normally stain intensely pink or red. Monocyte cytoplasm stains faintly pink and may contain fine or course granules. Myeloblasts and normal erythroid cells do not stain. Cytoplasmic staining increases with the increasing maturity of the myeloid cells.

In AML, staining is variable and largely depends on the differentiation state of the blasts. Acute promyelocytic leukemia will show more intense staining of the leukemic cells than AML with minimal differentiation. Intense staining is also seen in acute megakaryoblastic leukemia. In contrast to normal erythroid precursors, which do not stain with PAS, large areas of PAS positivity can be seen in the erythroid cells of MDS and acute erythroleukemia [6]. Large granular staining can be seen in the cytoplasm of B lymphoblasts (i.e., block positivity) [25].

4 Notes

1. For the PAS stain, Schiff's reagent is labile and is the most likely reagent to cause negative results in the control reaction. Replacing this reagent only and testing control smears is likely to correct falsely negative PAS staining.
2. This reaction is extremely light sensitive. Care must be taken to ensure that the smears to be stained are protected from any prolonged exposure to light, which may render them falsely negative.
3. Whereas a positive MPO stain is sufficient for determination of myeloid differentiation, a negative myeloperoxidase stain should never be considered pathognomonic of acute nonmyelocytic leukemia (i.e., lymphoblastic leukemia).

4. The solution should be golden brown with rim of small bubbles at the top.
5. On addition of the phosphate buffer the solution will turn milky white; if it turns purple, properly discard and start anew.
6. The solutions will be clear and pale gold after filtering.
7. On addition of the phosphate buffer the solution may turn faintly milky white. The addition of the Fast Blue BB will make the mixture yellow after mixing and blue on standing after time.
8. NSE staining is highly sensitive to reaction conditions. Undesired reactivity may occur if the reaction conditions are not followed carefully. Increasing the incubation period and altering the pH or temperature may give false positive results. Stains should be interpreted in the context of other phenotypic results.
9. Solution should be amber. Formation of precipitate indicates reagent deterioration.
10. Cytoseal 60 cannot be used with acid phosphatase stain.

References

1. Jaffe ES, Vardiman JW, Campo E et al (2011) Hematopathology. Saunders/Elsevier, Philadelphia, PA
2. Swerdlow SH, Harris NL, Jaffe ES et al (2008) WHO classification of tumours of haematopoietic and lymphoid tissue. IARC, Lyon
3. O'Donnell MR, Abboud CN, Altman J et al (2012) Acute myeloid leukemia. J Natl Compr Cancer Netw 10(8):984–1021
4. Alvarnas JC, Brown PA, Aoun P et al (2012) Acute lymphoblastic leukemia. J Natl Compr Cancer Netw 10(7):858–914
5. Ley TJ, Ding L, Raphael BJ et al (2013) Genomic and epigenomic landscapes of adult de novo acute myeloid leukemia. N Engl J Med 368(22):2059–2074. doi:10.1056/NEJMoa1301689
6. Altman AJ (1985) Cytologic diagnosis of the acute nonlymphoid leukemias. I. Morphologic, cytochemical, and ultrastructural features. Am J Pediatr Hematol Oncol 7(1):21–44
7. Arber DA, Snyder DS, Fine M et al (2001) Myeloperoxidase immunoreactivity in adult acute lymphoblastic leukemia. Am J Clin Pathol 116(1):25–33. doi:10.1309/hdue-dn2e-b72e-jk99
8. Mhawech P, Buffone GJ, Khan SP et al (2001) Cytochemical staining and flow cytometry methods applied to the diagnosis of acute leukemia in the pediatric population: an assessment of relative usefulness. J Pediatr Hematol Oncol 23(2):89–92
9. Yam LT, Li CY, Crosby WH (1971) Cytochemical identification of monocytes and granulocytes. Am J Clin Pathol 55(3):283–290
10. Li CY, Lam KW, Yam LT (1973) Esterases in human leukocytes. J Histochem Cytochem 21(1):1–12
11. Hanker JS, Yates PE, Metz CB et al (1977) A new specific, sensitive and non-carcinogenic reagent for the demonstration of horseradish peroxidase. Histochem J 9(6):789–792
12. Resnitzky P, Shaft D, Yaari A et al (1994) Distinct intracellular lysozyme content in normal granulocytes and monocytes: a quantitative immunoperoxidase and ultrastructural immunogold study. J Histochem Cytochem 42(11):1471–1477
13. Seo IS, Li CY, Yam LT (1993) Myelodysplastic syndrome: diagnostic implications of cytochemical and immunocytochemical studies. Mayo Clin Proc 68(1):47–53
14. Lanza F, Latorraca A, Musto P et al (1991) Cytochemically unreactive neutrophils from subjects with myeloperoxidase (mpo) deficiency show a complex pattern of immunoreactivity with anti-mpo monoclonal antibodies: a flow cytometric and immunocytochemical study. Ann Hematol 63(2):94–100

15. Horobin RW (1981) Structure-staining relationships in histochemistry and biological staining. Part 3: some comments on the intentional and artifactual staining of lipids. Acta Histochem Suppl 24:237–246
16. Grande M (1977) Monocytic differentiation of cluster cells in agar culture of normal human bone marrow. A cytochemical investigation. Biomedicine 26(5):326–330
17. Behm FG (1990) Morphologic and cytochemical characteristics of childhood lymphoblastic leukemia. Hematol Oncol Clin North Am 4(4):715–741
18. Kass L (1979) Cytochemistry of esterases. CRC Crit Rev Clin Lab Sci 10(2):205–223
19. Elghetany MT, MacCallum JM, Davey FR (1990) The use of cytochemical procedures in the diagnosis and management of acute and chronic myeloid leukemia. Clin Lab Med 10(4):707–720
20. Pombo De Oliveira MS, Gregory C, Matutes E et al (1987) Cytochemical profile of megakaryoblastic leukaemia: a study with cytochemical methods, monoclonal antibodies, and ultrastructural cytochemistry. J Clin Pathol 40(6):663–669
21. Rodak BF, Fritsma GA, Keohane E (2011) Hematology: clinical principles and applications, 4th edn. Saunders, Philadelphia, PA
22. Catovsky D, Costello C (1979) Cytochemistry of normal and leukaemic lymphocytes: a review. Basic Appl Histochem 23(4):255–270
23. Srivastava BI, Rossowski W, Minowada J (1983) Cytochemical comparison of immunologically characterized human leukaemia/lymphoma cell lines representing different levels of maturation. Br J Cancer 47(6):771–779
24. Turgeon M (2004) Clinical hematology: theory and procedures, 4th edn. Lippincott Williams & Wilkins, Philadelphia, PA USA
25. Hayhoe FG, Quagliono D, Flemans RJ (1960) Consecutive use of Romanowsky and periodic-acid-Schiff techniques in the study of blood and bone-marrow cells. Br J Haematol 6:23–25

Chapter 3

Immunohistochemistry in Acute Myeloid Leukemia

Michael W. Cruise

Abstract

The World Health Organization's Classification of Tumours of Haematopoietic and Lymphoid Tissues (Swerdlow et al. (eds) WHO Classification of tumours of haematopoietic and lymphoid tissues, 4th edn. WHO Press, Lyon, 2008) created a classification scheme incorporating genetic, molecular, morphologic, and immunophenotypic characteristics. The diagnosis of acute myeloid leukemia requires equal to or greater than 20% blasts (except in some cases with specific cytogenetic abnormalities or in erythroleukemia). The diagnostic work up typically includes morphologic, cytochemical, and immunophenotypic features. This generally includes evaluation of the peripheral blood, bone marrow aspirate, and bone marrow trephine biopsy. As stated in the WHO Classification of Tumours of Haematopoietic and Lymphoid Tissues, "the contribution of an adequate bone marrow biopsy cannot be over stated" (Swerdlow et al. (eds) WHO Classification of tumours of haematopoietic and lymphoid tissues, 4th edn. WHO Press, Lyon, 2008). The evaluation of the bone marrow biopsy provided the necessary material for immunohistochemical studies used for both diagnosis and prognosis.

The following text will focus on the utilization of immunohistochemical studies in the classification of acute myeloid leukemia. Other methodologies will be discussed elsewhere in this volume.

Key words AML, Immunohistochemistry, Protocol, Classification, Bone marrow biopsy

1 Introduction

The acute leukemia/lymphomas are characterized broadly as acute myeloid leukemia, lymphoblastic leukemia/lymphoma, and acute leukemia of ambiguous lineage. Acute myeloid leukemia (AML) can be further subclassified into AML with recurrent genetic abnormalities, AML with myelodysplasia, and AML not otherwise specified. The last category, AML not otherwise specified, can be further subdivided by morphologic and immunophenotypic profile.

Generally the first task is determining if there are sufficient number/percentage of blasts. The diagnosis of acute myeloid leukemia requires equal to or greater than 20% blasts (or blasts equivalents). The gold standard for blast evaluation is determining the percentage of blasts in a 500-cell differential count of the bone marrow aspirate or 200-cell differential of the peripheral blood.

Paolo Fortina et al. (eds.), *Acute Myeloid Leukemia: Methods and Protocols*, Methods in Molecular Biology, vol. 1633, DOI 10.1007/978-1-4939-7142-8_3,

However, there are conditions in which bone marrow biopsy and immunohistochemical stains are required, especially when a bone marrow aspirate cannot be obtained or is hemodiluted. For the identification of blasts, the most helpful immaturity markers are CD34, CKIT/CD117, and Tdt. Generally these markers are strongest in undifferentiated cells with expression decreasing with maturation. In cases where the aspirate is poor or there is a dry tap, immunohistochemical staining of the bone marrow core biopsy can in fact yield an increased blast count resulting in the diagnosis of AML. Generally CD117 has a similar expression pattern as CD34 but in various specimens and diagnosis, one tends to be more sensitive [2, 3]. Tdt is generally useful in acute lymphoblastic leukemia/lymphoma (ALL), while CD117 is generally limited to AML (only rarely seen in T-ALL). CD34 can be seen in both AML and ALL but generally more limited expression, as it is only present in approximately 50% of AML cases [4]. As such, it is usually beneficial to stain for multiple markers.

In addition to assessing blasts counts, immunohistochemical staining is useful in the classification of the lineage of the blasts (Table 1) and further subclassification of the process. The WHO classifies cytoplasmic CD3 as the lineage marker for T cells. However, other T-cell associated antigens can be expressed on AML. Specifically CD7 can be expressed on approximately 10–20% of AML and CD2 is often expressed in acute promyelocytic leukemia [5]. The WHO classifies myeloid lineage markers as myeloperoxidase or evidence of monocytic differentiation with at least two of the following: nonspecific esterase, CD11c, CD14, CD64, or

Table 1
Requirements for assigning lineage to a blast

Myeloid lineage
– Myeloperoxidase, or
– Monocytic differentiation (at least 2 of the following: nonspecific esterase, CD11c, CD14, CD64, lysozyme)
T lineage
– Cytoplasmic CD3 (monoclonal antibodies to CD3 epsilon chain; IHC with polyclonal anti-CD3 antibody may react with CD3 zeta chain, which is not T cell–specific); or
– Surface CD3 (rare in mixed phenotype acute leukemia)
B lineage (multiple antigens required)
– Strong CD19 with at least 1 of the following strongly expressed: CD79a, cytoplasmic CD22, CD10; or
– Weak CD19 with at least 2 of the following strongly expressed: CD79a, cytoplasmic CD22, CD10

Adapted from 2008 Tumours of Haematopoietic and Lymphoid Tissues [1]

lysozyme. However, generally only CD14 and lysozyme are readily utilized by immunohistochemistry. B cell lineage is a little less specific requiring the testing of multiple antigens (CD19, CD22, CD79a, and CD10).

Further classification of the lesions requires determining the differentiation of the neoplastic cells and immunohistochemical stains remain a power tool for this purpose (Table 2). The typical markers of myeloid differentiation are myeloperoxidase, CD33, and CD13; however CD117, CD15, and CD56 can also suggest myeloid differentiation (especially in the absence of lymphoid markers). Monocytic differentiation can be highlighted by CD14, CD68 (clones PG-M1 and KP1), lysozyme, and CD163. Additionally CD4 (on CD3 negative cells) can be used as a monocytic marker. Erythroid differentiation can be demonstrated by expression of Glycophorin A (CD235a) or by hemoglobin A, and megakaryocytic differentiation can be highlighted by expression of CD42b, CD41, CD61, and von Willebrand factor (factor VIII-related Ag).

While cytogenetic and molecular findings can be entity defining, many have unique immunophenotypic findings. The typical immunophenotypic findings are outlined in Table 3 and some key findings are briefly highlighted below. Specifically here we will focus on acute myeloid leukemia not otherwise specified (AML NOS). AML with minimal differentiation is the most immature of the AML NOS subtypes and typically expresses only early antigens such as CD34 and CD117. There are no morphology or cytochemical features to differentiate AML with minimal differentiation from acute lymphoblastic leukemia, thus requiring immunophenotyping for a diagnosis. Additionally, this subtype can demonstrate TdT expression in up to 20–50% of cases [6]. The AML with minimal differentiation is often positive for CD33. While it is negative for myeloperoxidase by cytochemistry, a subset of the blasts may be positive for myeloperoxidase by immunohistochemistry. Even though the blasts can be positive for TdT they are negative for cCD3, CD79a, PAX5, and CD22.

Table 2
Markers of differentiation

Precursor	CD34, CD117, TdT, CD10, CD3, CD19
Myeloid	Myeloperoxidase, CD13, CD33, HLA-DR, CD117
Erythroid	Glycophorin A, hemoglobin A
Megakaryocytic	CD41, CD42b, CD61, von Willebrand factor (factor VIII-related Ag)
Monocytic	CD14, CD68, CD163

Table 3
WHO classification of AML and their typical immunoprofile

AML with recurrent genetic abnormalities	Typical immunohistochemical phenotype
AML with t(8;21); RUNX1-RUNX1T1	CD34+, HLA-DR+, MPO+, CD13+, CD33 wk., CD15+, PAX5+, Tdt+/−
AML with inv.(16) or t(16;16); CBFB-MYH11	Often multiple blast population CD34, CD117, often CD2+, either (CD13+, CD33+, CD15+, MPO+) or (CD14+, CD4+, CD68+)
APL with t(15;17); PML-RARA	CD34 wk., HLA-DR wk. to −, CD33+, CD13+/−, CD117 −/+
AML with t(9;11); MLLT3-MLL	CD34 wk. to −, CD117 wk. to -, CD33+ CD4+, HLA-DR+
AML with t(6;9); DEK-NUP214	CD34+, CD117+, MPO+, CD13+, CD33+, CD38+, HLA-DR+, Tdt+/−
AML with inv.(3) or t(3;3); RPN1-EVI1	CD34+, CD13+, CD33+, HLA-DR+, CD7+, CD41+/−, CD61+/−
AML with t(1;22)(p13;q13); RBM15-MKL1	CD34−, CD13+, CD33+, HLA-DR−, CD41+, CD61+, CD42+/−
Acute myeloid leukemia, not otherwise specified	
AML with minimal differentiation	CD34+, CD38+, HLA-DR+, CD13+, CD117+, CD33+/−, TdT+/−, CD7 −/+
AML without maturation	CD34+/−, CD117+ HLA-DR+/−, CD13+, CD33+ CD15−, CD14−, CD7+/−
AML with maturation	CD34sub, CD117 sub, positive for one or more of the following: CD13, CD33, CD15; CD14-, CD7+/−
Acute myelomonocytic leukemia	Mixed blast population, subpopulation CD34+ and/or CD117+, HLA-DR+, variable for CD13, CD33, CD15; subpopulation positive for CD14, CD4, CD68, CD163, and lysozyme.
Acute monoblastic/monocytic leukemia	MPO wk. to −, lysozyme+, CD117+/−, CD34+/−, CD33+, CD13+, CD15, CD163+, CD68+
Erythroleukemia, erythroid/myeloid	Two blast population: (1) MPO −, glycophorin+, hemoglobin+, (2) morphology and phenotype of AML with minimal differentiation.
Pure erythroid leukemia	CD117+, HLA-DR−, CD34−, glycophorin A+/−, hemoglobin A+/−
Acute megakaryoblastic leukemia	CD34−, CD45−, tdt−, MPO −, CD41+, CD61+, CD42 −/+
Acute basophilic leukemia	CD13+/−, CD33+/−, CD123+, CD34+, HLA-DR+, CD117−, CD25−, mast cell tryptase-
Acute panmyelosis with myelofibrosis	CD34+, CD13+/−, CD33+/−, CD117+/−, MPO+, lysozyme+, CD61+/−, CD42b+/−, glycophorin A+/−, hemoglobin A

sub subpopulation is positive, *wk.* weak to negative expression, *MPO* myeloperoxidase, + positive, − negative, +/− often positive but can be negative, −/+ often negative but can be positive

The next category of acute myeloid leukemia without maturation includes markers of myeloid differentiation including myeloperoxidase and often will express CD13, CD33, along with immaturity markers CD34 and CD117. As the name implies they are negative for markers of maturation including CD15, CD14, CD68, and CD163. They can however have aberrant expression of CD7 and a small percentage have been reported to express CD2, CD4, or CD56. Acute myeloid leukemia with maturation (FAB M2) expresses myeloid differentiation markers including myeloperoxidase, CD13, and/or CD33. Since there is maturation generally only a part of the blasts will express CD34 or CD117. Generally these blasts are also positive for CD15 without expression of monocytic markers CD14, CD68, CD163, or CD4. Additionally while CD7 can be expressed they are usually negative for CD2 and CD56. It should be noted that definitive differentiation between AML with and without maturation can be challenging by tissue immunohistochemistry and generally is used to correlate with the flow cytometry results.

The next two categories under AML NOS include those with at least some monocytic differentiation. The acute myelomonocytic leukemia has two to three blast populations, one demonstrating monocytic differentiation, another with neutrophilic differentiation and often a population of immature blasts. The immature blast population expresses CD34 and/or CD117 with occasional CD7 expression. The monocytic population expresses monocytic differentiation with one or more of the following: CD14, CD4, CD68, CD163, and lysozyme (muramidase). The myeloid or neutrophilic blasts will have expression of myeloperoxidase as well as CD13, CD33, or CD15. The next category, acute monoblastic and monocytic leukemia, is an AML in which greater than 80% of the blasts are of the monocytic lineage with only a minor neutrophilic component. As this is a more mature AML, the blasts are less likely to be CD34 positive but generally retain CD117 expression. There is generally variable expression of myeloid markers, myeloperoxidase, CD13, CD33, and CD15. The blasts also express markers of monocytic differentiation including CD4, CD14, CD68, CD163, and/or lysozyme.

Acute erythroid leukemia can exist either as an erythroid and myeloid process (greater than or equal to 50% erythroid precursors and greater than or equal 20% myeloblast in the non-erythroid component) or as a pure erythroid leukemia (greater than or equal to 80% of the bone marrow cells). The erythroid and myeloid process demonstrates a population of erythroblasts that express markers of erythroid differentiation including hemoglobin-A and glycophorin-A and only have focal CD34 expression and are generally negative for myeloperoxidase. Additionally, the myeloid blasts are generally immature with expression similar to AML with minimal differentiation.

Acute megakaryoblastic leukemia is a leukemia with greater than 20% blasts in which 50% or more of the blasts demonstrates megakaryocyte lineage. This type of leukemia can have extensive bone marrow fibrosis and as such there can be limited material collected by aspirate. As such immunohistochemistry on the bone marrow biopsy may be the only method to determine the immunophenotype and percentage of blasts. The blasts are variable positive for CD117 and CD34 and can be positive for CD13 and CD33. The blasts are generally negative for TdT and myeloperoxidase. The megakaryoblasts typical express CD41 and/or CD61. The mature megakaryoblasts can also express factor VIII and/or CD42. CD31 can be helpful and was once thought to be lineage specific for megakaryocytes; however, CD31 can be seen on other AML and vascular lesions.

In cases of acute panmyelosis with myelofibrosis there is often a dense bone marrow fibrosis and the aspirates are generally dry (low cellularity) and insufficient for evaluation by aspirate smear or by flow cytometry. Often immunohistochemical staining of the bone marrow biopsy is the only way to determine the presence of and the immunophenotypic profile of the blasts and confirm the diagnosis. The blast population generally expresses precursor markers CD34 and/or CD117 along with myeloid markers CD13 and CD33, and however is usually negative for myeloperoxidase. Specifically, immunohistochemistry is generally the only method to determine that blasts exceed the 20% threshold needed for the diagnosis. This is a panmyelosis with multilineage proliferation, generally of the megakaryocytic (CD61, CD41, Factor VIII) and the erythroid (hemoglobin A, Glycophorin) lineages.

While we will not discuss in depth the immunophenotype of the AML with recurrent genetic abnormalities, they are listed in Table 3. However, we will discuss aberrant expression of PAX5 in AML. Specifically, PAX5 is typically a B-cell maker; however the expression of PAX5 in AML is correlated with the t(8;21) translocation [7].

There are areas of caution when utilizing certain antibodies by immunohistochemistry. One example would be CD15: while this antibody can be used to determine blast differentiation, the high expression in the normal granulocytes can make interpretations of the stain in tissue section very challenging. Another problematic antibody is HLA-DR. This antibody is extremely usefully by flow cytometry; however the antibody has had variable success in immunohistochemical evaluation of tissue sections. As newer clones become available this marker may become more useful. Additionally, other myeloid markers CD13 and CD33 tend to be less sensitive by immunohistochemistry as compared to flow cytometry [8]. Two additional markers that are not typically used by flow cytometry for the evaluation of AML but can be utilized by immunohistochemistry are CD99 and CD43. Up to 95% of acute myeloid leukemia are positive for CD43, which can be extremely helpful, especially in extramedullary lesions (myeloid sarcoma) [9]. Additionally, AML/myeloid sarcoma can be CD99 positive and as such the possibility of AML should be considered in cases of small round blue cell tumors with CD99 expression [6].

In summary, for the work up of a possible acute myeloid leukemia the important first step is evaluation of the aspirate and bone marrow biopsy. The morphologic differential of the blast populations will dictate the panel performed. Several staining algorithms for working up possible AML cases have been published [8, 10]. Generally most panels include blast markers CD34, CD117, and TdT. If the blasts are immature then markers for B cell, T cell, and myeloid lineage are performed (as seen in the tables). Once the blasts have demonstrated a myeloid lineage, then differentiation markers can be exploited. Multiple markers must be utilized in order to render the correct lineage and diagnosis. Correlation with other ancillary studies must be performed. Below are detailed methodologies for both manual and automated systems.

2 Materials

2.1 Manual Antigen Retrieval

1. Sodium citrate buffer: 10 mM Sodium citrate, pH 6.0. Add 2.94 g Tri-sodium citrate (dihydrate) to 1 L of distilled water. Mix to dissolve and then adjust pH to 6.0 with 1 N HCl. Store at room temperature for 3 months.
2. ETDA buffer: 1 mM EDTA, adjusted to pH 8.0. Add 0.37 g EDTA (ethylenediaminetetraacetic acid) to 1 L of distilled water. Mix to dissolve and then adjust pH to 8.0 with NaOH. Store at room temperature for 3 months.
3. Tris-EDTA buffer: 10 mM Tris Base (tris(hydroxymethyl)aminomethane), 1 mM EDTA solution, 0.05% Tween 20, pH 9.0. To 1 L of distilled water add 1.21 g of Tris base and 0.37 g EDTA. Mix to dissolve and then adjust pH to 9.0. Finally add 0.5 mL of Tween 20 and mix well.

2.2 Manual Wash

1. 10× TBS: To 900 mL of distilled water add 24 g of Tris–HCL (tris(hydroxymethyl)aminomethane hydrochloride), 5.6 g of Tris base, and 88 g NaCl. The solution is mixed until dissolved and then pH is adjusted to 7.6 with HCl or NaOH. Finally adjust volume with distilled water to a final volume of 1 L. Store at room temperature for 3 months.
2. TBST: 1× Tris-buffered saline, 0.1% Tween 20. Add 100 mL of TBS 10× to 900 mL distilled water and mix. Then check to ensure pH is 7.6 and adjust if needed. Finally add 1 mL of Tween 20 and mix well.

2.3 Blocking Solution

1. Preferred blocking solution is 2.5% serum from the species of the secondary reagent. In the manual method below we utilize 2.5% horse serum. While part of the ImmPRESS™ detection kits are utilized in the methods below, an alternative can be 2.5% horse serum in TBS (2.5 mL of horse serum in 97.5 mL of 1× TBS) or 1% BSA in TBS blocking solution (1 g immunohistochemical grade bovine serum albumin (Vector laboratories, Burlingame, CA, USA) with 100 mL of TBS).

2.4 Antibody Diluent

2.5% serum from the species of the secondary reagent. In the manual method below we utilize 2.5% horse serum in TBS. Alterative one could utilize 1× TBS with 0.1% immunohistochemical grade bovine serum albumin.

2.5 Peroxidase Block

Make up fresh and add 30 mL of 30% hydrogen peroxide solution (Fisher Chemical, Waltham, MA, USA) to 270 mL distilled water.

2.6 Avidin/Biotin Blocking

Avidin/Biotin Blocking Kit (Vector laboratories, Burlingame, CA, USA).

2.7 Detection System

ImmPRESS™ reagent HRP Universal Antibody (Anti-Mouse IgG/Anti-Rabbit IgG, Peroxidase) Polymer Detection Kit (made in horse) (Vector laboratories).

2.8 Chromogen Reagent

ImmPACT DAB Peroxidase (HRP) Substrate (Vector laboratories).

2.9 Automated Systems

1. Reaction Buffer (10×): Tris-based buffer (pH 7.5 ± 0.2) (Ventana, Tucson, AZ, USA). Make 1× reaction buffer by mixing the 2 L bottle with 18 L of distilled water (1 part diluted with 9 parts). Check pH with a test strip, acceptable range is 7.3–7.7.
2. Liquid coverslip (Ventana).
3. EZ Prep (10×): aqueous-based detergent solution with preservative (Ventana). Make 1× buffer by diluting 2 L of EZ Prep Concentrate with 18 L of distilled water.
4. CC1 Predilute: tris-based buffer with a slightly basic pH (8.5) (Ventana).
5. CC2 Predilute: citrate buffer at a slightly acidic pH (6) (Ventana).
6. Protease 2; endopeptidase containing approximately 0.1 mg/mL alkaline protease enzyme activity (Ventana).
7. Antibody Diluent: (0.3% protein in 0.1 M phosphate buffered saline pH 7.3) (Ventana).

8. optiView DAB IHC Detection kit: OptiView Peroxidase Inhibitor (3.0% hydrogen peroxide solution), OptiView HQ Universal Linker (cocktail of goat anti-mouse IgG and IgM, and goat anti-rabbit with covalently attached hapten), OptiView HRP Multimer (mouse monoclonal anti-hapten-labeled HRP tertiary antibody), OptiView H_2O_2 (0.04% H_2O_2), OptiView DAB (0.2% of 3,3′-diaminobenzidine tetrahydrochloride), and OptiView Copper (copper sulfate (5 g/L) in an acetate buffer) (Ventana).
9. OptiView Amplification Kit: containing OptiView Amplifier (tyramide with a linker containing hapten), OptiView Amplification Multimer (mouse anti-HQ-HRP), and OptiView Amplification H_2O_2 (0.04% H_2O_2) (Ventana).

2.10 General Purpose Reagents

1. Xylene histology grade (Cardinal Health, Dublin, OH, USA)
2. Reagent-grade alcohol: 100%, 95%, 80%, and 70% (Cardinal Health, Dublin, OH, USA).
3. Mayer's Hematoxylin with Lillie's Modification (Dako, Carpinteria, CA, USA).
4. Bluing Solution (Dako).
5. Decalcification Solution: EDTA in weak hydrochloric acid (Thermo Fisher Scientific, Waltham, MA, USA).
6. Zinc-formalin containers (Poly Scientific R&D Corp., Bay Shore, NY, USA).
7. Cytoseal (Thermo Fisher Scientific).
8. SUPERFROST PLUS Microscope Slide (VMR, Radnor, PA, USA).

3 Methods

The general method for immunohistochemical stain consists of sample preparation including fixation and sectioning onto charged slides, followed by deparaffinization of the sections. Next the antigens must be retrieved, by unmasking and restoring the antigen's epitope and antibody binding site. Nonspecific protein interactions must be blocked (generally utilizing serum from the same species as the secondary antibody) as well as endogenous peroxidase activity must be inhibited. Subsequently the tissue sections are incubated with a primary antibody against the antigen of interest and then followed by incubation with a secondary antibody/detection system against the species of the primary antibody. Then the sections are incubated with a chromogen, typically 3,3′-diaminobenzidine (DAB), that creates insoluble precipitate that can be visualized under light microscopy.

3.1 Special Consideration for Bone Collection and Processing

Typically, a bone marrow specimen consists of aspirate with smears, touch prep slides of bone marrow core, the bone marrow core biopsy, and clot formed from the aspirate.

1. Bone marrow clot: Set aside approximately 1 cm^3 of bone marrow aspirate and allow to clot. Next place the clot in a filter bag/between filter paper and place into a biopsy cassette and then fix the specimen in 10% formalin.
2. The biopsies are processed per standard protocol, dehydrated and placed into paraffin.
3. The biopsies are sectioned at 4 μm, placed on charged slides, and baked at 60 °C for 1 h.
4. Bone marrow core biopsy: The bone marrow core biopsies are placed in Zinc-formalin. The biopsies are fixed for 2 h (or at least 30 min).
5. The biopsies are placed in biopsy cassettes and rinsed in distilled water for 5 min.
6. The biopsy is placed into decalcification solution (*see* Subheading 2) for 30 min followed by rinsing in distilled water for 30 min and placed in 10% formalin.
7. The biopsies are processed per standard protocol, dehydrated and placed into paraffin.
8. The biopsies are sectioned at 4 μm, placed on charged slides, and baked at 60 °C for 1 h.

3.2 Manual Immunohistochemical Staining

1. The formalin fixed paraffin embedded sections must be deparaffinized and rehydrated. We typically utilize TissueTek™ slide racks and reagent containers (however other similar products could be utilized). Place slides in slide holder and move through slide dishes as follows: (a) Xylene—3 changes of 5 min each, (b) 100% Alcohol—2 changes of 3 min each; (c) 95% Alcohol—2 min; (d) 70% Alcohol—2 changes for 2 min each; (e) Distilled Water—2 changes for 2 min each.
2. For antigen retrieval utilize the Decloaking™ chamber (Biocare medical, Concord, CA, USA), or similar pressure cooker system.
3. Add 500 mL of distilled water to the reaction chamber. Move the slides into aluminum slide dish and fill with 250 mL antigen retrieval solution (*see* **Note 1**). Place three slide-staining dishes (up to 72 slides) into the reaction chamber. (Always use three dishes; if no slides in dish then fill with 250 mL distilled water. This ensures consistent temperature changes and retrieval results.)
4. As a quality control measure, steam monitor strips should be utilized as well as pH strips in order to verify that the retrieval solution reached the appropriate temperature and maintain the appropriate pH.

5. Attach the Decloaking chamber lid and seal. Start the Decloaking chamber. Standard protocol increases the temperature of the reaction chamber up to 125 °C and then holds it for 30 s followed by cooling to 90 °C. At this point the lid can be opened and the containers removed from the reactive chamber and allowed to cool for an additional 20 min at room temperature.
6. Wash the slides twice with distilled water for 5 min.
7. Place slides in freshly made 3% H_2O_2 solution and incubate for 10 min at room temperature in order to block endogenous peroxidase.
8. Wash the slides twice with distilled water for 5 min each, then wash in TBST for 5 min.
9. Wipe slide around tissue section with Kimwipes™ (or similar product) and add blocking solution and incubate for 30 min at room temperature in a humidified chamber (*see* **Note 2**) to inhibit the tissue from drying out. Alternatively, the slide around the tissue can be marked with a hydrophobic pen. Optionally, if using a streptavidin biotin detection system then after protein block, a biotin block must be performed, which can be done with the Avidin/Biotin Blocking Kit (Vector laboratories) (*see* **Note 3**).
10. Drain the blocking solution and add 1–3 drops of the Avidin D solution to cover the tissue sections and incubate for 15 min. Then rinse in TBST for 5 min.
11. Drain the blocking solution and add 1–3 drops of the biotin solution to cover the tissue sections and incubate for 15 min. Then rinse in TBST for 5 min.
12. Drain slides and add primary antibody to tissue sections (*see* **Note 4**).
13. Wash slides three times with TBST (5 min each on a shaker).
14. Incubate the sections for 30 min with ImmPRESS™ reagent directed against primary antibody (secondary antibodies conjugated to horseradish peroxidse enzyme polymer) (*see* **Note 5**).
15. Wash slides three times with TBST (5 min each on a shaker).
16. Add freshly prepared ImmPACT™ DAB Peroxidase Substrate by adding 1 drop (approximately 30 μL) of ImmPACT™ DAB Chromogen concentrate to 1 mL ImmPACT™ DAB Diluent and mixing well. This substrate is added to the section and incubated until stain develops (generally 2–10 min). Optimal time must be determined experimentally.
17. Rinse sections with distilled water.
18. Stain tissue sections for 60 s with hematoxylin (Dako). Then rinse in water until excess reagent is removed.

19. Place in bluing buffer (Dako) until stain is blue (approximately 30 s).
20. Rinse in distilled water.
21. Sections are dehydrated by passing racks through two changes of 95% alcohol and three changes of 100% alcohol, followed by three changes of xylene.
22. Coverslip slides with permanent mounting media such as Cytoseal or similar reagent.

3.3 Automatic Procedure (See Note 6)

The protocol below represents steps utilizing the Ventana Benchmark™ XT (Ventana Benchmark; Ventana, Tucson, AZ, USA). The benchmark system utilizes a Liquid Cover Slip (LCS) solution during each step. The LCS consists of an inert low density, paraffinic hydrocarbon and mineral oil, that forms a layer over the aqueous solution on the slide to prevent evaporation.

1. The slides are placed on the slide carousel and the loaded tray of antibodies and reagents are placed on the instrument.
2. From the Benchmark's main screen, start the run and follow the prompts until the instrument starts to scan the bar codes for the slides and reagents. Typical program includes the following steps.
3. Removal of paraffin by combining heat, a mild detergent solution (EZ Prep) combined with vortex mixing and rinsing.
4. Antigen retrieval utilizing Ventana's proprietary regents for HIER: cell conditioning 1 (Tris containing solution, pH 8.5) or cell conditioning 2 (citrate buffer, pH 6.0) with standard antigen retrieval for 64 min at 100 °C. Alternatively Protease 2 (endopeptidase containing approximately 0.1 mg/mL alkaline protease enzyme activity) applied for 4 min at 36 °C.
5. Slides are washed with Ventana reaction buffer (Tris-based buffer, pH 7.5).
6. Block endogenous peroxidase activity with OptiView Peroxidase Inhibitor (Ventana) and incubate for 4 min, followed by rising with reactive buffer.
7. Primary antibody applied and incubated (*see* **Note 4**).
8. Slides are washed with Ventana reaction buffer (Tris-based buffer, pH 7.5).
9. The antigen is detected using the OptiView DAB IHC Detection kit.
10. Slides are incubated with OptiView HQ Universal Linker (cocktail of HQ (hapten)-labeled goat anti-mouse IgG and IgM, and goat anti-rabbit) for 8 min. Wash with reaction buffer.

11. Incubate with OptiView HRP Multimer (mouse monoclonal anti-HQ-labeled HRP tertiary antibody) for 8 min. Wash with reaction buffer.
12. Incubate OptiView Amplifier (tyramide with a linker containing HQ hapten) and OptiView Amplification H_2O_2 (0.04% H_2O_2) for 8 min. Rinse with reaction buffer.
13. Incubate OptiView Amplification Multimer (mouse anti-HQ-HRP) for 8 min. Rinse with reaction buffer.
14. OptiView H_2O_2 (0.04% hydrogen peroxide in a phosphate buffer solution) and OptiView DAB for 8 min. Rinse with reaction buffer.
15. OptiView Copper (contains copper sulfate in an acetate buffer) for 4 min, then rinse with reaction buffer.
16. Counterstain with Hematoxylin II (Ventana) for 4 min. Rinse with reaction buffer.
17. Add bluing reagent for 4 min. Rinse with reaction buffer.
18. After the run is complete, the slides are removed from the slide tray and placed in a rack in warm tap water containing a mild dish detergent with gentle agitation to remove remaining liquid coverslip.
19. Rinse slides in running tap water until all soap is removed.
20. Sections are dehydrated by passing racks through two changes of 95% alcohol and three changes of 100% alcohol, followed by three changes of xylene.
21. Coverslip slides with Cytoseal or similar reagent.

3.4 Quality Control

All staining should be done with appropriate negative and positive controls run in parallel. This allows for determination of nonspecific staining as well as ensuring that the immunoreactivity and specificity of the targeted antigen being tested. It is often advantageous to have the positive control tissue and the sample on the same slide. All reagents should be used by their expiration dates and discarded if any visual contamination is seen. Data sheets and product inserts will generally contain information on the storage, dilution, and stability of the reagents.

3.5 Validation and CLIA Standards

While outside of the scope of this paper, two publications from the College of Pathology have evaluated and made recommendation on the best practices for immunohistochemical assay validation [11, 12]. Recently the documentation requirements by the CAP and CLIA for validation of immunostains have become more stringent.

4 Notes

1. The process of fixation cross-links the proteins causing methylene bridges of the tissue and this process will often mask/hide the antigen epitopes. In order to detect the antigen this process must be partly reversed. This is accomplished by utilizing two broad categories of antigen retrieval. The first utilizes enzymatic approaches and the second utilizes heat and various pH solutions. The enzymatic approach typically utilizes Proteinase K, Trypsin, and Pepsin. However this method generally suffers from low success rate and has the potential of destroying both the antigen of interest and the tissue morphology. The heat-induced methods typical utilize one of three retrieval solutions, sodium citrate buffer pH 6, EDTA pH 8, or Tris-EDTA buffer pH 9. The slides are heated in one of these heat-induced epitope retrieval solutions generally using a pressure cooker, a microwave, or a vegetable steamer. While these can be performed offline, many of the automated systems can perform the antigen retrieval online.
2. Humidity chamber: In order to reduce evaporation and avoid drying of the tissue incubations should be carried out in a humidified chamber. After rehydration, drying at any stage will lead to nonspecific binding and high background staining. A humidity chamber can be created from a shallow, plastic box with a sealed lid and wet paper towels in the bottom. Plastic serologic pipettes can be cut to the length of the chamber and placed 4 cm apart so that the slides rest in a level position on the raised surface. The slides must be kept off the wet paper and kept level so that the reagents will not drain off.
3. Biotin block: Many systems will utilize a strept(avidin)-biotin detection system in order to amplify the signal. However, possible endogenous strept(avidin) binding sites must be blocked. This can be accomplished by incubating the tissue with strept(avidin) to bind up the endogenous biotin, followed by strept(avidin) to bind up any additional strept(avidin) binding sites.
4. Primary antibody: The selection and work up of this step is arguably the most important in the creation of clean crisp antigen staining. The dilution of the primary antibody must be experimentally determined. Generally datasheets from the primary antibodies have recommended dilutions that are generally good starting point. Although some primary antibodies are supplied in ready-to-use or prediluted formats, many are also provided in concentrated aliquots. Primary antibodies are typically incubated at room temperature for 30 min but can be incubated overnight at 4 °C. Typically when done overnight the amount of antibody used can be significantly reduced (higher antibody dilution). Table 4 lists antibodies that are often utilized in the

Table 4
List of common antibodies used for AML workup. These are recommended starting points for straining work-up. These were determined on a Ventana automated staining platform. Each individual laboratory must clinically determine the protocol conditions

Antibody	Catalog #	Clone	Vendor	Epitope retrieval	Antibody dilution	Ab incubation time (min)/ temp (°C)
CD2	MU438-UC	AB75	Biogenex	CC1	1:10	16/37
CD3	790–4341	2GV6	Ventana	CC1	Predilute	8/37
CD4	NCL-CD4-1F6	1F6	Leica	CC1	1:10	24/37
CD5	MU430-UC	4C7	Biogenex	CC1	1:10	8/RT
CD7	CM158 CK	LP15	Biocare	CC1	1:50	32/RT
CD10	NCL-CD10–270	56C6	Leica	CC1	1:5	20/37
CD15	MU302-UC	BRA4F1	Biogenex	CC1	1:40	20/37
CD20	M0755	L26	Dako	CC1	1:200	32/37
CD22	MS-1087S	FPC1	Thermo Scientific	CC2	1:10	16/37
CD31	M0823	JC/70A	Dako	CC1	1:20	16/37
CD33	NCL-L-CD33	PWS44	Leica	CC1	1:25	20/37
CD34	134 M-18	QBEnd/10	Cell Marque	–	Predilute	16/37
CD43	M0786	DF-T1	Dako	CC1	1:25	8/37
CD45	M0701	2B11, PD7/26	Dako	–	1:100	16/37
CD56	CD56-1B6	1B6	Leica	CC1	1:100	56/RT
CD57	MU314-UC	NK-1	Biogenex	CC1	1:80	12/37
CD61	CD61–308	2f2	Leica	CC1	1:100	16/37
CD68	790–2931	KP-1	Ventana	CC1	Predilute	16/37
CD68	M0876	PG-M1	Dako	CC1	1:10	16/37
CD71	NCL-CD71–309	10F11	Leica	CC2	1:40	20/RT
CD79a	M7050	JCB117	Dako	CC1	1:20	20/37
CD99	199 M-18	H036–1.1	Cell Marque	CC2	Predilute	32/42
CD117 (c-kit)	A4502	polyclonal	Dako	CC1	1:500	16/37
CD123	554,527	7G3	BD Biosciences	CC1	1:250	16/37
CD163	VP-C374	10D6	Vector	CC1	1:1600	16/37
Factor VIII	A0082	Polyclonal	Dako	–	1:200	16/37

(continued)

Table 4 (continued)

Antibody	Catalog #	Clone	Vendor	Epitope retrieval	Antibody dilution	Ab incubation time (min)/ temp (°C)
Hemoglobin-A	AR021-5R	Polyclonal	Biogenex	–	Predilute	8/RT
Muramidase	A0099	Polyclonal	Dako	Prot 2	1:100	4/37
Myeloperoxidase	289A-78	Polyclonal	Cell Marque	–	Predilute	8/RT
PAX-5	610,863	24	BD Biosciences	CC1	1:20	44/RT
TdT	E19234	Polyclonal	Spring bioscience	CC1	1:20	8/RT

work up of acute myeloid leukemia cases. As a starting point Table 4 also includes the antigen clone/manufacture, antigen retrieval conditions, and time and condition for the primary antibody incubation. These were worked up on a Ventana Benchmark platform and again the best conditions will vary from method to method and platform to platform.

A useful reference is the Nordic immunohistochemical Quality Control (NordiQC)—http://www.nordiqc.org/. This website provides information on the performances of multiple antibody clones utilized over multiple staining platforms at various institutions utilizing various antigen retrieval methods and antibody dilutions. This provides an excellent starting point; however the precise conditions must be experimentally determined for your laboratory setup.

5. There are several secondary systems that can be utilized to detect the primary antibody. While a secondary antibody directly linked to an enzyme can be used, this often does not yield a significant signal and so amplification of the signal is required. This can be in the form of a (strept)avidin-biotin complex in which the secondary antibody is biotinylated and subsequently incubated with (strept)avidin-biotin complex with reporter enzyme. Another amplification method utilizes tyramide signal amplification (TSA). In short, this utilizes tyramide linked biotin or hapten molecules. This is added after incubation with horseradish peroxidase (HRP) secondary or tertiary reagent. The HRP converts the tyramide into a reactive species that covalently deposits in the immediate area creating additional binding sites and amplification of the signal. Additionally, several systems utilize a secondary antibody linked to a polymer providing multiple attached enzymes or binding sites.

6. Automated staining: Automated-staining platforms have greatly increased the efficiency and capacity of immunohistochemical laboratories. Many can perform all components of the procedure from deparaffinization to cover slipping. There are multiple platforms available and while we discuss one of Ventana's platforms we do no specifically endorse this platform over others. A recent review [13] compares the pros and cons of several of the available automated immunohistochemical platforms and may be helpful in the evaluation of the different systems.

References

1. Swerdlow S, Campo E, Harris N et al (eds) (2008) WHO classification of tumours of haematopoietic and lymphoid tissues, 4th edn. WHO Press, Lyon
2. Rizzatti EG, Garcia AB, Portieres FL et al (2002) Expression of CD117 and CD11b in bone marrow can differentiate acute promyelocytic leukemia from recovering benign myeloid proliferation. Am J Clin Pathol 118(1):31–37
3. Dunphy CH, O'Malley DP, Perkins SL et al (2007) Analysis of immunohistochemical markers in bone marrow sections to evaluate for myelodysplastic syndromes and acute myeloid leukemias. Appl Immunohistochem Mol Morphol 15(2):154–159
4. Dunphy CH, Polski JM, Evans HL et al (2001) Evaluation of bone marrow specimens with acute myelogenous leukemia for CD34, CD15, CD117, and myeloperoxidase. Arch Pathol Lab Med 125(8):1063–1069
5. Lewis RE, Cruse JM, Sanders CM et al (2007) Aberrant expression of T-cell markers in acute myeloid leukemia. Exp Mol Pathol 83(3):462–463
6. Kang LC, Dunphy CH (2006) Immunoreactivity of MIC2 (CD99) and terminal deoxynucleotidyl transferase in bone marrow clot and core specimens of acute myeloid leukemias and myelodysplastic syndromes. Arch Pathol Lab Med 130(2):153–157
7. Valbuena JR, Medeiros LJ, Rassidakis GZ et al (2006) Expression of B cell-specific activator protein/PAX5 in acute myeloid leukemia with t(8;21)(q22;q22). Am J Clin Pathol 126(2):235–240
8. Olsen RJ, Chang CC, Herrick JL et al (2008) Acute leukemia immunohistochemistry: a systematic diagnostic approach. Arch Pathol Lab Med 132(3):462–475
9. Yang F, Tran TA, Carlson JA et al (2000) Paraffin section immunophenotype of cutaneous and extracutaneous mast cell disease: comparison to other hematopoietic neoplasms. Am J Surg Pathol 24(5):703–709
10. Dunphy CH (ed) (2015) Integrated Hematopathology: morphology and FCI with IHC, Revised edn. Hong Kong, ASCP Press
11. Hardy LB, Fitzgibbons PL, Goldsmith JD et al (2013) Immunohistochemistry validation procedures and practices: a College of American Pathologists survey of 727 laboratories. Arch Pathol Lab Med 137(1):19–25
12. Fitzgibbons PL, Bradley LA, Fatheree LA et al (2014) Principles of analytic validation of immunohistochemical assays: guideline from the College of American Pathologists Pathology and Laboratory Quality Center. Arch Pathol Lab Med 138(11):1432–1443
13. Prichard JW (2014) Overview of automated immunohistochemistry. Arch Pathol Lab Med 138(12):1578–1582

Chapter 4

Immunophenotyping by Multiparameter Flow Cytometry

Weina Chen and Hung S. Luu

Abstract

Multiparameter flow cytometry has become an indispensable tool for the diagnosis and classification of acute myeloid leukemia (AML). The basic method relies on the unique ability to detect immunophenotypic abnormalities on discrete subpopulations. The primary roles in the initial assessment of AML are to determine the immaturity of the leukemic population, define the lineage and the immunophenotypic aberrancies in blasts, and identify characteristic immunophenotypic features to predict important recurrent cytogenetic and genetic abnormalities and prognosis. The established immunophenotypic profile, a baseline "fingerprint," is used for follow-up assessment of residual disease. This chapter provides an overview of procedures for specimen processing, staining, and immunophenotyping of AML and describes our strategy for data analysis supplemented with illustrative case examples.

Key words Immunophenotyping, Flow cytometry, Acute myeloid leukemia, Cytogenetics, Residual disease

1 Introduction

Acute myeloid leukemia (AML) is a heterogeneous group of clonal hematopoietic stem cell disorders characterized by a proliferation of immature myeloid cells (i.e., myeloid blast) showing features of granulocytic, monocytic, erythroid, or megakaryocytic differentiation [1]. Flow cytometry (FC) immunophenotypic analysis is a rapid method for diagnosis and classification of AML, with results potentially available within just a few hours after the specimen is received. The principal component in the initial assessment of putative acute leukemia is to confirm the immaturity of the population of interest, define lineage (myeloid or lymphoid), and characterize immunophenotypic aberrancy distinct from normal myeloid progenitors. The established baseline immunophenotypic "fingerprint" is subsequently used for assessment of residual diseases in the follow-up samples [2–4].

AML is currently defined by the presence of ≥20% of myeloid blasts by morphologic assessment in the bone marrow (BM) or/

Paolo Fortina et al. (eds.), *Acute Myeloid Leukemia: Methods and Protocols*, Methods in Molecular Biology, vol. 1633, DOI 10.1007/978-1-4939-7142-8_4, © Springer Science+Business Media LLC 2017

and peripheral blood (PB), except in cases harboring a t(15;17), t(8;21), or inv(16), by 2008 World Health Organization (WHO) classification [1]. These cases are diagnosed as AML regardless of the blast count. FC may be helpful in blast enumeration in PB. However, blast enumeration in the BM is hampered due to multiple factors. These include inevitably variable degree of hemodilution, under-representation of nucleated red cells due to red cell lysis, loss of blasts during the specimen processing, potential imprecise blast gating strategy, and the instrument detection threshold for specimen acquisition. Therefore, morphologic evaluation in PB and BM is the gold standard for blast enumeration.

Myeloid blasts in various subtypes of AML may include myeloblasts, monoblasts, megakaryoblasts, erythroblasts, and blast equivalents including promyelocytes and promonocytes. Analytical strategies on these myeloid blasts may vary accordingly. Identification of myeloblasts is generally straightforward as the blasts typically express immature cell markers (CD34 or/and CD117), and frequently fall into the so-called "blast gate" [low CD45 and intermediate side scatter (SSC) on CD45 vs. SSC plot]. However, analysis on other types of myeloid blasts lacking these features can be challenging, in particular those blasts with monocytic differentiation (promonocytes and monoblasts) in acute monocytic leukemia or promyelocytes in acute promyelocytic leukemia. Potential pitfalls in interpretation and analytical approaches to the various myeloid blasts are presented.

Several composite immunophenotypic attributes can predict important recurrent cytogenetic abnormalities and have prognostic significance. For instance, blasts in AML with t(8;21) often express CD19, and in some cases CD56 and Tdt [5, 6]. Blast equivalents/promyelocytes in acute promyelocytic leukemia with t(15;17) frequently lack CD34 and HLA-DR but have high SSC [7, 8]. These immunophenotypic features should prompt a timely cytogenetic study for confirmation followed by targeted treatment in acute promyelocytic leukemia. These two genetically defined AMLs have a favorable prognosis.

Furthermore, FC is able to establish the baseline immunophenotypic "fingerprint" that can be used for follow-up assessment of residual disease including minimal residual disease (MRD). This is based on the assumption that the panel at diagnosis is sufficiently broad to confidently identify immunophenotypic aberrancies in order to discriminate abnormal myeloid blasts from normal myeloid progenitors in the background of the complex mixtures of cell populations, particularly in BM. While debate exits as to the blast percentage cut-off of greatest clinical significance and the optimal time for MRD assessment, multiple studies have demonstrated that MRD detected at the levels between 0.01 and 0.1% of white cells at either end of induction or consolidation is prognostically relevant and is associated with poorer outcome [9–15].

The applications of FC in diagnosing AML are constantly changing secondary to technological advancement and employment of higher color (currently up to 10-color) FC. A variety of flow cytometers and analytic software are used in different laboratories, and therefore, the composition of antibody panels and the analytical approach may differ. This chapter provides an approach for diagnosing and classifying AML using a 4-color BD FACSCalibur flow cytometer with BD CellQuest Pro acquisition software, and describes analytical strategy for data interpretation using CytoPaint Classic (Leukobyte) or BD Paint-A-Gate software.

2 Materials

Reagents are generally used as provided by the manufacturer with in-house validation prior to use.

2.1 Buffers and Cell Staining Reagents

2.1.1 PAB Stock and Working Solution Preparation

PBS/Azide/BSA (PAB) 10× Stock (1% PAB): Add 50.0 g of bovine serum albumin (BSA) to the 4500 mL of clinical laboratory reagent water (CLRW). Add 22.75 g of Sodium Azide to the mixture. Add 500 mL of 10× Dulbecco's Phosphate Buffered Saline (DPBS) to the mixture. Stir the mixture for at least 4 h. Adjust the pH of solution to 7.3 ± 0.1 using either NaOH or HCL. Filter sterilize the solution using the 100 mL filter system sets. Stock solution expiration date is 2.5 years at 2–8 °C.

PAB 1× Working solution: Add 1000 mL of 1% (10×) PAB solution to 8100 mL of water (CLRW). Add 900 mL of 10× DPBS stock solution to the mixture. Mix thoroughly. Working solution expiration date is 1 month at 2–8 °C.

Paraformaldehyde (PFA) 1% solution: Aliquot 100 mL of PFA (concentration of 10%) into a 1000 mL volumetric flask. Add 900 mL sterile PBS to a final volume of 1000 mL. Place parafilm over the flask and mix thoroughly. Transfer the 1% PFA solution into sterile 500 mL glass bottles. Expiration date is 3 month at 2–8 °C.

2.2 5% Newborn Calf Serum (NCS) Preparation

Heat inactivation of the Hyclone Newborn Calf Serum: Thaw the serum 3–4 days before use in the refrigerator (2–8 °C), and mix the contents of the bottle thoroughly. Place the bottle of serum into a water bath containing sufficient water to immerse the bottle above the serum level and set it to 56 °C. Swirl the bottle every 5 min to ensure uniform heating of the serum. Monitor the temperature of the water bath and begin timing for 30 min when the temperature reaches 56 °C. Cool the bottle of serum in an ice bath immediately after removing from the 56 °C water bath. Let it sit for 20 min and place it in the fridge until use. Add the heat inactivated NCS to RPMI by aseptically pipetting 25 mL NCS into 500 mL bottle of RPMI. Cap the bottle and mix. Expiration date is 1 month at 2–8 °C.

2.3 Buffered Ammonium Chloride (NH_4Cl) Solution

Ammonium Chloride Concentrate Solution (10×): Measure 500 mL of water (CLRW) into a 1000 mL volumetric flask. Add the following reagents into the 1000 mL flask: 80 g of NH_4Cl; 10 g of $KHCO_3$ (potassium bicarbonate); 3.7 g of EDTA (ethylenediaminetetraacetic acid). Mix the solution using a magnetic stirrer and stir bar until reagents are dissolved. Add 500 mL of water (CLRW) for a total volume of 1000 mL. Adjust the pH to 7.2–7.3 using either NaOH or HCl. Filter sterilize using 1000 mL filter sterilization unit (0.22 μm PES filter). This results in a 10× stock that can be stored at 4 °C for 6 months.

Ammonium Chloride Working Solution (1×): Dilute the Ammonium Chloride Concentrate Solution (10×) 1:10. The following is a suggested volume. Add 50 mL of NH_4Cl concentrate solution into a 500 mL bottle. Add 450 mL of water (CLRW). Prepare fresh working solution daily.

2.4 Monoclonal Antibody Panels

The antibody panels for diagnosing AML require sufficient breadth of markers, in a cost-effective manner, to cover a variety of lymphoid and myeloid antigens as well as antigens associated with cell immaturity. At initial diagnosis, such a panel will confidently identify abnormal myeloid blasts, rule out mixed phenotype acute leukemia (MPAL), and establish an immunophenotypic profile for disease follow-up.

It is imperative to titer antibodies for optimal signal-to-noise ratio under the conditions to be used. Antibodies are preferentially precocktailed to ensure consistent high-quality performance (*see* **Note 1**). Table 1 lists our proposal of the 4-color antibody combination alongside the various populations assessed in each tube. Notably, myeloid blasts are assessed in every tube. In the cases where acute erythroid or megakaryoblastic leukemia is suspected by virtue of CD36(+)/CD64(−) on myeloid blasts, a subsequent reflex panel to add the relevant lineage-associated antigens (CD41, CD61, CD71, and glycophorin A) is instituted.

3 Methods

The preanalytical phase, involving specimen collection and delivery, is perhaps the most important phase of the whole process to ensure consistently a high-quality assay. PB and BM aspirates are anticoagulated with ethylenediaminetetraacetic acid (EDTA) or sodium heparin, transported at room temperature, and processed in a timely manner (i.e., ideally within 48 h of collection). The procedure outlined below is generic and uses up-front bulk lysis followed by staining (*see* **Note 2**).

It is critical to appropriately set up instrumentation including optimization, standardization, and compensation. These topics are beyond the scope of this chapter, but are essential to the success of

Table 1
Four-color (FITC/PE/PerCP/APC) combination of monoclonal antibodies for acute myeloid leukemia

FITC/PE/PerCP/APC	Assessments
Surface markers	
CD10/CD22/CD20/CD34	Assess CD34+ progenitors including myeloid blasts and early stage hematogones; B-cell maturation (CD10 vs. CD20, and CD20 vs. CD34)
CD34/CD14/CD45/CD38	Assess CD38 and CD45 on myeloid blasts; monocytes; plasma cells (CD45 vs. CD38)
*polyλ/polyκ/CD20/CD19	Assess B-cell markers on myeloid blasts; B-lineage cells including hemetogones, mature B cells and plasma cells
CD36/CD64/CD45/CD34	Assess CD36 and CD64 on myeloid blasts; monocytes (CD36+/CD64+); erythroid and megakaryocytic cells (CD36+/CD64−)
CD16/CD56/CD45/CD11b	Assess asynchronous expression of CD11b and CD16 on myeloid blasts; CD56 expression on granuolocytes, monocytes, and blasts; granulocyte maturation (CD11b vs. CD16); NK cells; plasma cells (CD45 vs. CD56)
CD8/CD5/CD3/CD4	Assess T cell antigens on myeloid blasts; T cells; monocytes (CD4)
CD15/CD33/CD45/CD34	Evaluate asynchronous expression of CD15 on myeloid blasts; CD33 on myeloid blasts; monocytes; granulocytes
CD2/CD117/CD45/CD34	Assess CD2 and CD117 on myeloid blasts; promeylocytes and early erythyroids (CD34−/CD117+); CD2 on CD117(bright+) mast cells
CD7/CD13/HLA-DR/CD34	Assess CD13 and HLA-DR on myeloid blasts; monocytes; T/NK cells
Intracellular (ic) markers	
G1/G1/CD45/CD34	Control for MPO and icCD79a
MPO/CD79a/CD45/CD34	Assess MPO and icCD79a on myeloid blasts; MPO for mixed phenotype acute leukemia
G1/G2a/G1/CD45	Control for Tdt, icCD22 and icCD3
TdT/CD22/CD3/CD45	Assess Tdt on myeloid blasts; icCD3 and icCD22 for mixed phenotype acute leukemia

In routine screening, only polyclonal Ig Abs are used. In lymphoma work-up cases, or cases with initial polyclonal Abs revealing abnormal findings (such as lack of surface Ig expression), monoclonal Abs (in conjunction with switched fluorochromes) are used. This combined use of polyclonal and monoclonal Abs will increase the likelihood of detecting surface light chain restriction in B-cell lymphomas.

FC analysis. Readers are referred to other resources on these topics [16, 17]. For routine tests, 500,000 cells are stained with appropriate amounts of antibodies and 30,000–50,000 events are collected for analysis. For MRD tests, 1–2 million cells are stained with appropriate amounts of antibodies and up to approximately 500,000 events are collected.

3.1 PB and BM Specimen Processing for Immunophenotypic Analysis

1. Partially decant anticoagulated PB or BM specimen into a sterile 50 mL conical.
2. If the sample is BM, add an equal amount of NH_4Cl and vortex to break up the particles. If the sample is PB proceed to the next step.
3. Dilute BM or PB sample with NH_4Cl to a final 1:10 dilution.
4. Place sample on specimen rocker for 10 min at room temperature (20–25 °C).
5. Centrifuge for 8 min (290 relative centrifugal force, Brake On).
6. Decant supernatant and vortex to resuspend the pellet.
7. Add 50 mL of PAB Wash Buffer and mix.
8. Centrifuge for 8 min (290 relative centrifugal force, Brake On).
9. Decant supernatant and examine cell pellet for complete lysis. (If predominance of red cells is observed, vortex to resuspend the pellet, add 20 mL NH_4Cl, centrifuge for 8 min (290 relative centrifugal force), return to **step 6**).
10. Vortex to resuspend the cells.
11. Add 40 mL of PAB Wash Buffer and mix.
12. Centrifuge for 8 min (290 relative centrifugal force, Brake On).
13. Decant supernatant and vortex to resuspend cell pellet.
14. Add 1 mL to 50 mL of 5% NCS based on the size of the cell pellet. The target concentration is about 1×10^6 cells/mL (*see* **Note 3**).
15. Mix the sample well and check for visible particulate matter.
16. Filter with nylon mesh if necessary.
17. Perform a cell count using the Coulter A^cT diff 2 Analyzer.

    (Refrigerated cell suspensions are stable for up to 1 week.)

3.2 Surface Marker Staining of Cell Suspension

1. Place the appropriate amount of cell suspension (500,000 cells for routine test) in each 12 × 75 mm tube (1–2 million cells for MRD test).
2. Add 2–3 mL 1XPAB wash buffer.
3. Centrifuge (1.9 relative centrifugal force) for 1 min and carefully decant.

4. Add the appropriate amount of monoclonal antibodies (e.g., 40 μL) to each tube.
5. Gently vortex each tube.
6. Incubate for 20 min in the refrigerator (2–8 °C) in the dark.
7. Add 2–3 mL 1XPAB wash buffer.
8. Centrifuge (1.9 relative centrifugal force) for 1 min and carefully decant.
9. Add 250 μL of 1% PFA to each tube.
10. Gently vortex each tube.
11. Run immediately on the Flow Cytometer or cap and refrigerate (2–8 °C) and run within 1 h.

3.3 Intracellular (IC) Marker Staining

1. Pipette the appropriate amount (μL) of cell suspension in each tube.
2. Add 2–3 mL PAB wash buffer.
3. Centrifuge (1.9 relative centrifugal force) for 1 min and carefully decant.
4. Add 100 μL of CALTAG Fix & Perm Solution A, and gently vortex.
5. Incubate 15 min in the dark at room temperature (20–25 °C).
6. Add 2–3 mL PAB wash buffer.
7. Centrifuge (1.9 relative centrifugal force) for 1 min and carefully decant.
8. Add 100 μL of CALTAG Fix & Perm Solution B.
9. Add the appropriate amount of monoclonal antibodies/cocktail (e.g., 40 μL) to each tube.
10. Gently vortex each tube.
11. Incubate all markers, **except TdT**, for 20 min in the dark at room temperature (20–25 °C). TdT requires 30 min.
12. Add 2–3 mL PAB wash buffer.
13. Centrifuge (1.9 relative centrifugal force) for 1 min and carefully decant.
14. Add 250 μL of 1% PFA to each tube.
15. Gently vortex each tube.
16. Run immediately on the Flow Cytometer or cap and refrigerate (2–8 °C) and run within 1 h.

3.4 Data Analysis and Interpretation

It is essential to interpret FC results in the context of the clinical presentation, and the morphologic findings from direct smears, touch imprints, and/or cytocentrifuged prepared slides of the submitted tissue. This is not only for assessment of specimen quality in

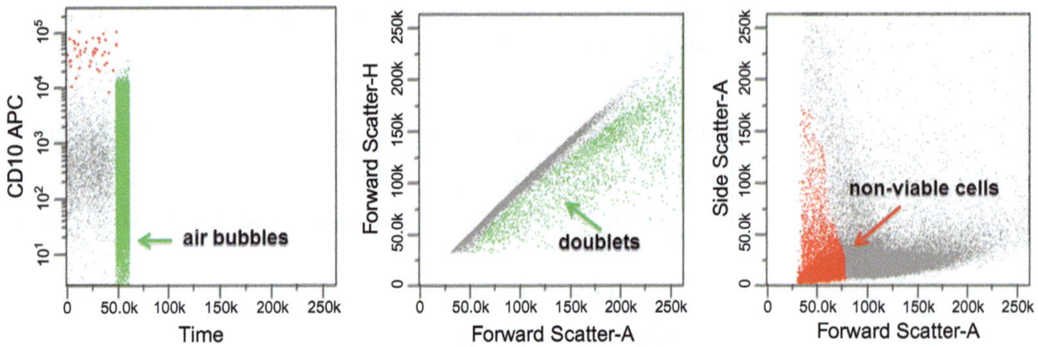

Fig. 1 Assessment of data quality and minimization of artifacts. The first step is to evaluate data over time to exclude air aspirated following exhaustion of sample. The second step is to evaluate forward scatter area over height (FSC-A and FSC-H) to exclude doublets and aggregates. The third step is to evaluate forward scatter over side scatter (FSC-A and SSC-A) to exclude very low forward scatter events that typically represent membrane damage from cellular degeneration

terms of cell viability and cellularity but also for identification of population(s) of interest. In some cases (especially certain monocytic leukemias that lack specific immunphenotypic markers of immaturity), morphology may be the most important clue that a population of cells is indeed immature.

The initial FC assessment should focus on data quality to minimize artifacts by removal of air bubble artifacts, doublets and aggregates, and nonviable cells. The first step is to evaluate data over time to exclude events corresponding to air aspirated following exhaustion of sample (Fig. 1). The second step is to evaluate forward scatter area over height (FSC-A and FSC-H) to exclude doublets and aggregates. The third step is to evaluate forward scatter area over side scatter area (FSC-A and SSC-A) to exclude very low forward scatter events that generally represent cellular debris and degenerated cells. An alternative method for removing nonviable cells is the addition of a DNA-binding dye, such as 7-amino-actinomycin D (i.e., 7-AAD). Degenerated cells demonstrate characteristic light scatter and staining patterns and are excluded from further evaluation. However, caution must be exercised to ensure that such exclusion of "nonviable cells" does not entirely exclude the population of interest, especially in cases with highly proliferative neoplasms where cell degeneration is rapid.

3.5 Analysis Strategy and Identification of Blast Population(s)

The diagnosis of AML by FC involves identifying the myeloid blast population that demonstrates immaturity, myeloid lineage differentiation, and immunophenotypic aberrancies [2–4]. The critical component is to identify the immature myeloid blasts, which may sometimes be a difficult endeavor. While CD34, an early stem cell and progenitor marker, remains a very important marker of immaturity, many AMLs are CD34(−), especially acute promyelocytic leukemia (APL), acute monocytic leukemia, or megakaryocytic leukemia.

One of the commonly employed strategies to define blasts is to gate the population in the blast gate [low CD45 and intermediate side scatter (SSC) on CD45 vs. SSC plot]. The events in this preselected region are subsequently analyzed for expression of various antigens [18, 19]. While myeloid blasts fall into this gated region in many cases, the gating strategy is potentially imprecise for multiple reasons. First, the commonly used blast gate may not be specific as it variably contains other marrow elements, including hypogranular granulocytes, atypical monocytes, hematogones, basophils, and plasmacytoid dendritic cells [20]. The presence of these contaminating populations, particularly in cases with a low blast count, may lead to a misinterpretation of the immunophenotypic profile on myeloid blasts and hamper subsequent MRD assessment. Second, the commonly used blast gate may not be sensitive in cases where blasts show much dimmer or brighter CD45 expression or have higher SSC than normal. In these scenarios, the blasts would fall outside of the "blast gate". This is often the case in acute monocytic leukemia where neoplastic immature monocytes have brighter expression of CD45. Furthermore, the immature monocytes frequently show a continuous pattern of differentiation into mature monocytes [21], creating difficulty in the separation of these two populations (Fig. 2a). Similarly, blasts that have higher SSC, such as in acute promyelocytic leukemia (APL), may also fall outside of typical blast region. Taken together, relying exclusively on traditional blast gating (low CD45 and intermediate SSC) to isolate blasts may inadvertently underestimate or overestimate the blast population(s) or lead to inaccurate characterization. Therefore, the CD45/SSC blast gate is used more effectively in combination with other myeloid lineage-specific and non-lineage-specific markers as well as CD34/CD117 to accurately isolate and define the blasts.

We advocate a multiparameter *cluster* analysis method that involves identifying multiple populations in ungated data. The populations are defined based on *cluster* formation, antigen expression, and the light scatter characteristics, all the available information in a given tube. These clusters represent distinct cell populations. Arbitrary colors are assigned to individual populations ("color" the populations). This allows simultaneous visualization of all definable populations and assessment of their immunophenotypic profile for all antigens in a given tube. In such a system, the populations of interest can be better defined, discriminated, and characterized not only from one another (Fig. 2b) but also from normal populations (*see* example Case 1 at follow-up). The latter provides reference levels of antigen expression on normal cells, which facilitates the detection of subtle shifts in the intensity of antigens in neoplastic myeloid cells. Therefore, the

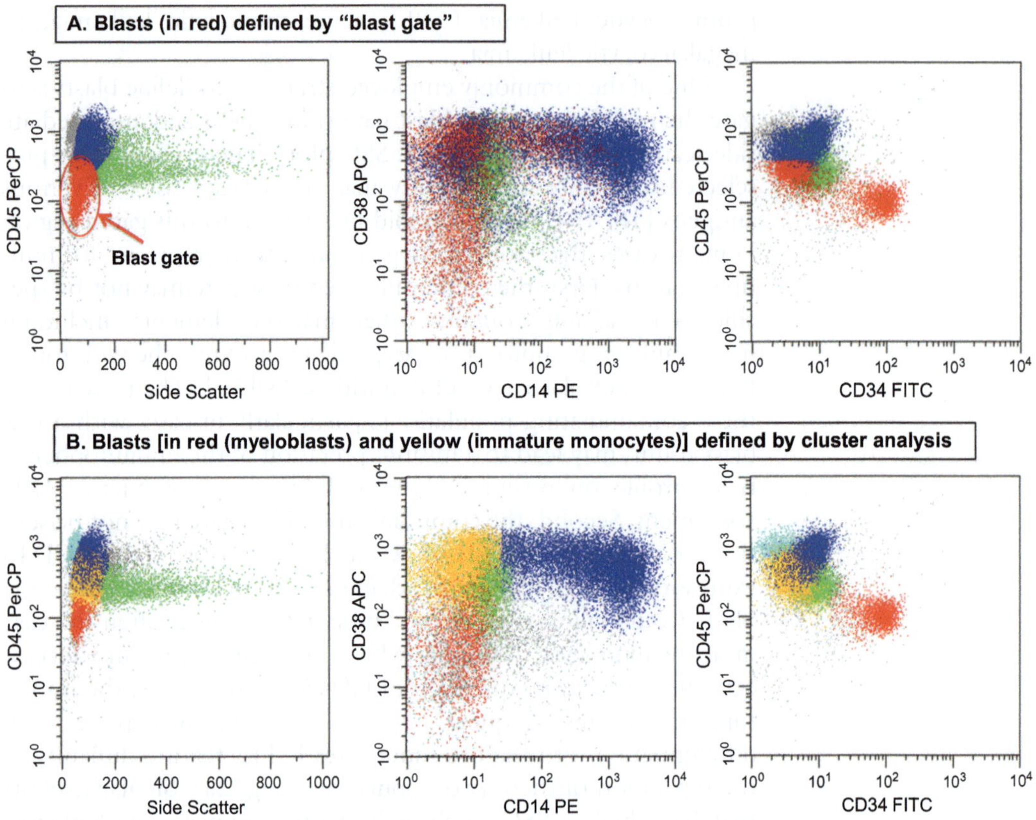

Fig. 2 Myeloid blast gating strategy: blast gate versus cluster analysis. In this example case of acute myelomonocytic leukemia in bone marrow, myeloid blasts are composed of two subsets, CD34(+) myeloblasts (in *red*) and CD34(−) monoblasts/promonocytes (in *yellow*). The immature monocytic cells have brighter CD45 and continuously differentiate into mature monocyte (in *blue*). (**a**) The separation of myeloid blast populations (in *red*, including both myeloblasts and immature monocytes) from mature monocytes (in *blue*) by CD45/SSC blast gate is indistinct. Consequently, the characterization of the immunophenotype on the immature cells is compromised. (**b**) In contrast, cluster analysis is able to define CD34(+) myeloblasts (in *red*), and distinguish CD38(strong+)/CD14(−) immature monocytes (in *yellow*) from CD38(strong+)/CD14(+) mature monocytes (in *blue*). Therefore, the characterization of the immunophenotype on the immature cells is more reliable. Granulocytes are painted in *green*, lymphocytes in light *blue*

cluster analysis approach is very useful for analyzing complex immunophenotypic patterns within complex cellular mixtures particularity in bone marrow or peripheral blood, and is especially suitable for assessment of residual disease at follow-up.

3.6 Determination of Immaturity, Myeloid Lineage, and Immunophenotypic Aberrancy

Determination of immaturity on a population of interest is intimately associated with the strategy of isolating myeloid blasts as explained in the above section. The following list is the proposed markers of immaturity or the patterns suggestive of immaturity (*see* **Note 4**):

Markersof immaturity: CD34(+) with or without CD117(+); CD117(+)/CD34(−) with high SSC (indicative of promyelocytes in acute promyelocytic leukemia), or with moderate SSC.

Patterns suggestive of immaturity: CD14(− to dim+) in monocytic cells, suggestive of immature monocytes (monoblasts/promonocytes); immature monocytes are often CD34(−) and variably CD117(−) [21]; Population falling into the blast gate (with caution, *see* above); CD36(+)/CD64(−) in nonerythroid population and falling into or close to the blast gate region (indicative of megakaryocytic or erythroid blasts).

Myeloid lineage-associated antigens include CD11b, CD13, CD14, CD15, CD33, CD36, CD41, CD61, CD64, CD65, CD71 (usually bright), CD117, glycophorin A (CD235a) (*see* **Note 5**), and myeloperoxidase (MPO). Commonly aberrant non-myeloid lineage-associated antigens include non-lineage-specific markers (CD38, CD45, CD123, and HLA-DR), and lymphoid lineage-associated markers (CD2, CD4, CD5, CD7, CD19, CD56, Tdt) (*see* **Note 6**).

Characterization of the immunophenotypic aberrancies on neoplastic myeloid blasts requires a thorough knowledge of the highly regular and reproducible patterns of antigen expression on normal myeloid progenitors, maturing myelomonocytic cells, and reactive or regenerative myelomonocytic populations, which is beyond the scope of this chapter. Briefly, normal myeloblasts express immature cell markers (CD34, CD117), pan-myeloid markers (CD13 and CD33), non-lineage-specific markers [strong CD38, moderate CD45 (similar to the level on granulocytes), and HLA-DR], and lack significant expression of later-stage mature myeloid markers or lymphoid markers. Immunophenotypic aberrancies of leukemic myeloid blasts in AML, similar to other myeloid stem cell neoplasms (in myelodysplastic syndrome and myeloproliferative neoplasm) [22, 23], typically include:

- Abnormally increased or decreased expression of antigens normally on CD34+ myeloblasts (e.g., diminished CD38 and CD45; diminished to loss of CD13 or CD33).
- Abnormally homogeneous expression of antigens that normally show coordinate variation in expression in CD34+ myeloblasts [e.g., abnormally homogeneous expression of CD38 on myeloid blasts; significant expression of MPO in myeloblasts].
- Asynchronous antigen expression (e.g., expression of later stage of myeloid markers, CD11b, CD15, or CD64, on leukemic myeloid blasts).
- Aberrant expression of non-myeloid lineage antigens [aberrant expression of T-cell antigens (e.g., CD2, CD7, or CD56) or B-cell antigen (e.g., CD19) on leukemic myeloid blasts].

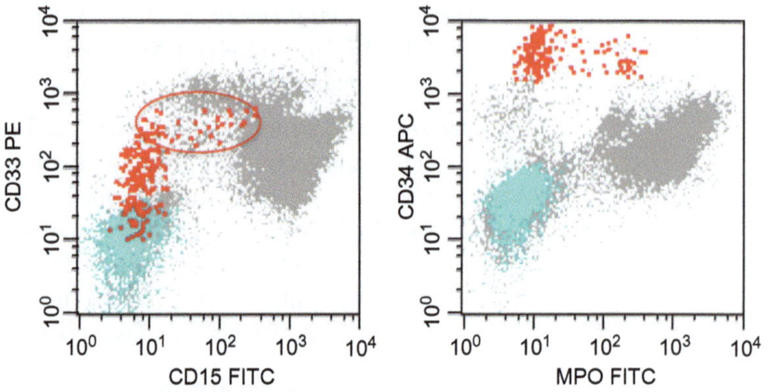

Fig. 3 The pattern of CD15 and MPO expression on normal CD34(+) myeloblasts in bone marrow. A small proportion of normal myeloblasts (in red) expressing CD15 coupled with a bright expression of CD33 (bridging into promyelocytes, in the circle), and MPO. Lymphocytes are painted in light *blue*

Notably, the majority of normal myeloblasts lack expression of CD15 but gain expression during the later stage of maturation as they differentiate into promyelocytes (the subset of CD33(bright+)/CD15(+) myeloblasts in the circle, Fig. 3). In our experience, only a small proportion of normal myeloblasts, approximately 20%, expresses MPO by FC [24]. Therefore, a significant expression of MPO on myeloid blasts is indicative of aberrancy.

Furthermore, background granulocytes and monocytes often demonstrate variable degrees of immunophenotypic abnormalities in AML. These include decreased SSC on granulocytes (suggestive of hypogranulation), altered granulocyte maturation (distorted pattern of antigen expression on the plots of CD13/CD16, CD11b/CD64, and CD11b/CD16, or lack of CD10), and expression of CD56 on granulocytes and monocytes.

3.7 Case Examples to Illustrate the Analytical Strategy

Analytical strategies on myeloid blasts and blast equivalents may vary depending on the lineage differentiation, granulocytic, monocytic, erythroid, or megakaryocytic differentiation. The following cases highlight the key points in data interpretation.

Case 1: AML with t(8;21) at Diagnosis and day 29 Follow-Up

This is a typical straightforward case of AML at diagnosis (Fig. 4a). Leukemic myeloblasts (in red) express CD34, CD117, fall into the characteristic blast gate on CD45/SSC, and express myeloid markers (CD13 and CD33), B-lymphoid marker (CD19) and CD56. Notably, the expression of CD19 with or without CD56 is characteristically associated with t(8;21). Recognizing this association of aberrant CD19 in t(8;21) AML is important to avoid misclassification as mixed phenotype acute leukemia.

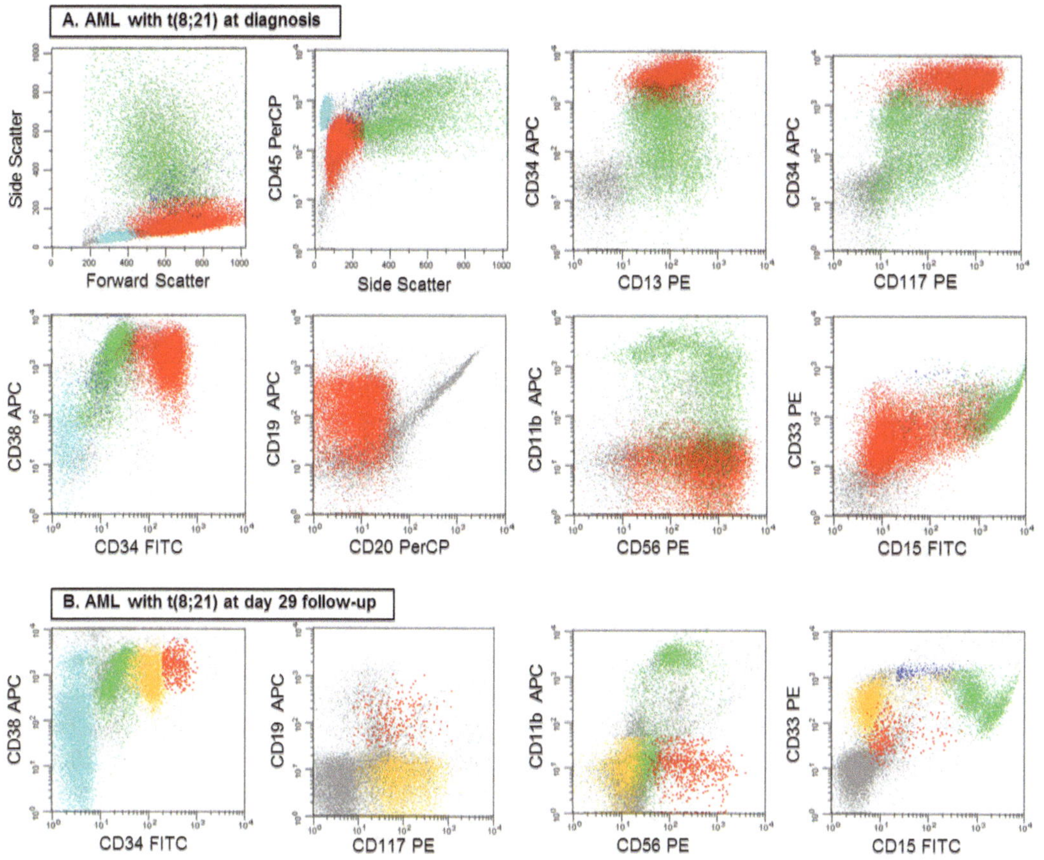

Fig. 4 AML with t(8;21) at diagnosis and day 29 follow-up. (**a**) At diagnosis, leukemic myeloblasts (in *red*) in bone marrow express CD34, CD117, CD13, CD15(partial+), CD33, CD19, CD56, and fall into the characteristic blast gate on CD45/SSC. The notable immunophenotypic aberrancies are CD19(+), CD33(dim+), CD34(bright+), CD45(dim+), and CD56(+). (**b**) At day 29 follow-up in bone marrow sample, there are two populations of CD34(+) myeloblasts, one expanded subset of normal myeloblasts (in *yellow*) and the other a much smaller subset of residual neoplastic myeloblasts (1.4% of total events) that demonstrate an aberrant immunophenotype essentially identical to that at diagnosis. Granulocytes are painted in *green*, monocytes in *dark blue*, lymphocytes in *light blue*

The aberrant immunophenotypic signature, CD19(+), CD33 (dim+), CD34 (bright+), CD45(dim+), and CD56(+) and in some cases aberrant expression of other B-lineage markers CD79a and CD22, is very helpful in assessment of MRD at day 29 (Fig. 4b). Close examination reveals two populations of CD34(+) myeloblasts, one expanded subset of normal myeloblasts (in yellow) following granulocyte-colony stimulating growth factor treatment, and the other, a much smaller subset of residual neoplastic myeloblasts (in red) that demonstrate an aberrant immunophenotype essentially identical to that at diagnosis. This case illustrates that cluster analysis is capable of dissecting complex cellular subsets and detecting subtle immunophenotypic shifts using the normal myeloblasts as an internal control population.

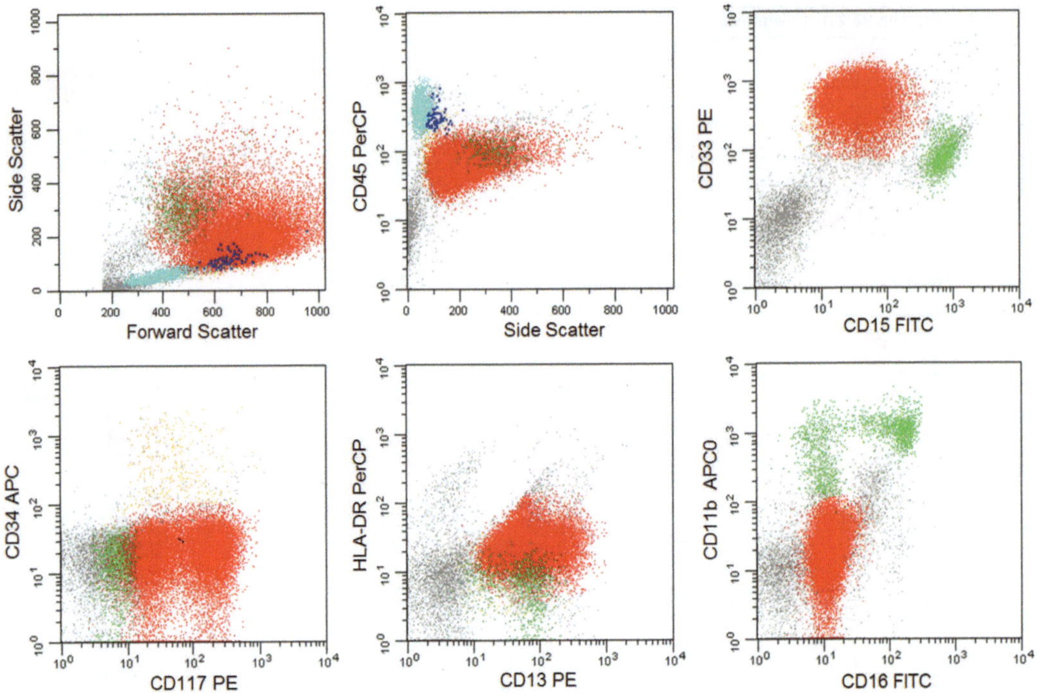

Fig. 5 Acute promyelocytic leukemia (APL) with t(15;17). An example case of APL in bone marrow demonstrates a characteristic immunophenotype in leukemic promyelocytes (in *red*): high SSC, CD15(dim+), CD33(homogeneously and bright +), CD34(−), CD117(partial +), and HLA-DR(−). Lack of CD11b(−) and CD16(−) indicates a maturation arrest. Granulocytes are painted in *green*, monocytes in *dark blue*, lymphocytes in *light blue*

It is important to be aware that the leukemic blasts may undergo immunophenotypic shifts following treatment [25, 26]. Consequently, MRD detection should examine abnormal myeloid blasts, not only showing an identical immunophenotype to that described at diagnosis but also showing immunophenotypic deviation from that of normal myeloid progenitors.

Case 2: Acute Promyelocytic Leukemia with t(15;17)

This case illustrates a characteristic immunophenotypic feature in leukemic promyelocytes in acute promyelocytic leukemia with t(15;17):highSSC,CD34(−),CD15(dim+),CD33(homogeneously and bright +), CD117(partial +), and HLA-DR(−) (Fig. 5) (*see* **Note 7**). Due to a high SSC that is likely related to cytoplasmic complexity including hypergranularity, blasts frequently fall outside of the typical blast gate. The diagnosis can be potentially challenging if CD117 expression is dim or negative. There needs to be a high level of vigilance for this entity in cases in which there is a large population of granulocytes lacking maturation. Expression of CD34 and CD2 (not in this case) is typically present in the microgranular variant. While these immunophenotypic attributes are

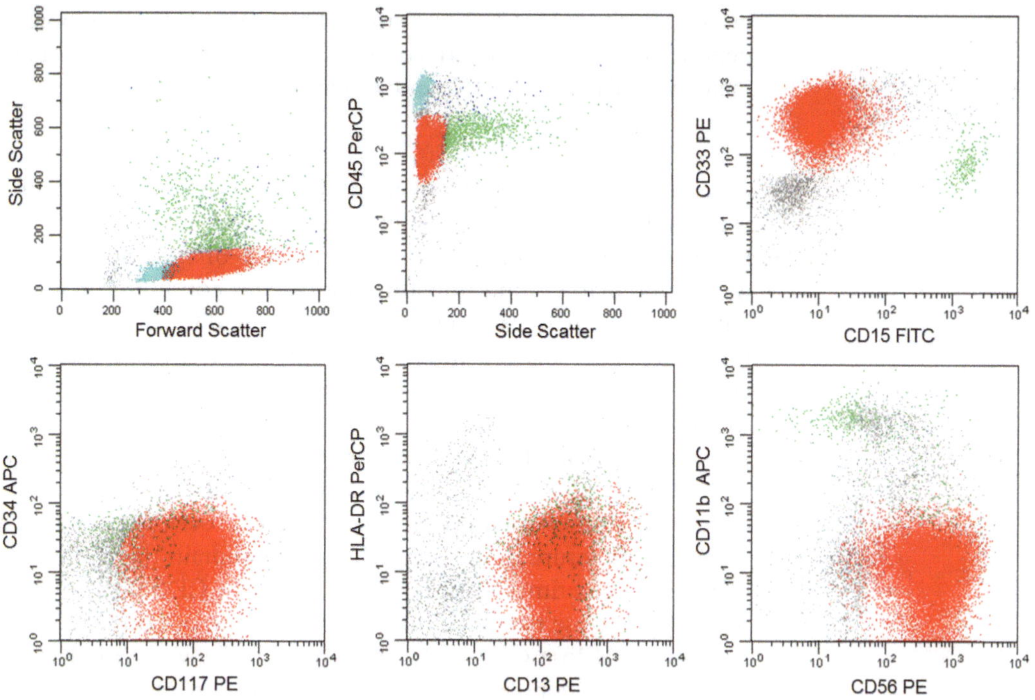

Fig. 6 AML with cup-like nuclei (lack of CD34 and HLA-DR). An example case of AML with cup-like nuclei in peripheral blood demonstrates a characteristic immunophenotype in myeloblasts (in *red*): low SSC, CD15(−), CD33(+), CD34(−), CD117(+), and HLA-DR(−). Low SSC and CD56(+) can be helpful in distinguishing this entity from acute promyelocytic leukemia. Granulocytes are painted in *green*, lymphocytes in *light blue*

highly suggestive of acute promyelocytic leukemia, a timely cytogenetic/fluorescence in situ hybridization (FISH) or molecular study confirmation is crucial in reaching a final diagnosis, such that a targeted treatment with all-trans retinoic acid (ATRA) and chemotherapy can be initiated promptly. The consequence of delay in diagnosis is potentially fatal due to disseminated intravascular coagulopathy.

Case 3: AML with cup-like Nuclei (Lack of CD34 and HLA-DR)

AML with cup-like nuclei (the so-called fishmouth nuclei) frequently has characteristic immunophenotypic features, as illustrated in this case (Fig. 6). The immunophenotype in these leukemic myeloblasts is somewhat similar to that of acute promyelocytic leukemia (e.g., lack of CD34 and HLA-DR). However, in contrast to acute promyelocytic leukemia, SSC is not increased, such that the blasts typically fall into the blast gate. In addition, these blasts tend to express CD56, which is not common in the conventional type of acute promyelocytic leukemia. One caveat is that micrograndular variants occasionally show CD56 expression. If there is any doubt regarding the differential diagnosis of acute promyelocytic leukemia versus AML with cup-like nuclei, a prompt evaluation for t(15;17) is required. This AML entity has unique genetic features, characterized by a normal karyotype and high incidence of *FLT3*, *NPM1*, and *IDH*mutations [27–29].

Case 4: Acute Myelomonocytic Leukemia

Analysis of acute myeloid leukemia with monocytic differentiation is generally much more challenging than typical AML, as discussed in the above section, due to frequent lack of *specific* immature monocytic markers and immature monocytes continuously differentiating into mature monocytes, making it difficult to separate immature from mature monocytic cells. Nevertheless, there are clues to the presence of an expanded population of immature monocytic cells, as illustrated in this example case (Fig. 7). The myeloid blasts in this case are composed of two subsets: one is CD34(+) myeloblasts (in red), and the other is immature monocytic cells (monoblasts/promonocytes, the subset of cells painted in blue). Immature monocytic cells often maintain the expression of CD15 (sometimes bright), CD33 (bright), CD36 and CD64, to the levels close to normal mature monocytes, but downregulate to completely lose CD14 [21, 30]. It is readily apparent that the monocytic cell population defined by the coexpression of CD15/CD33 and CD36/CD64 is much larger than that defined by the

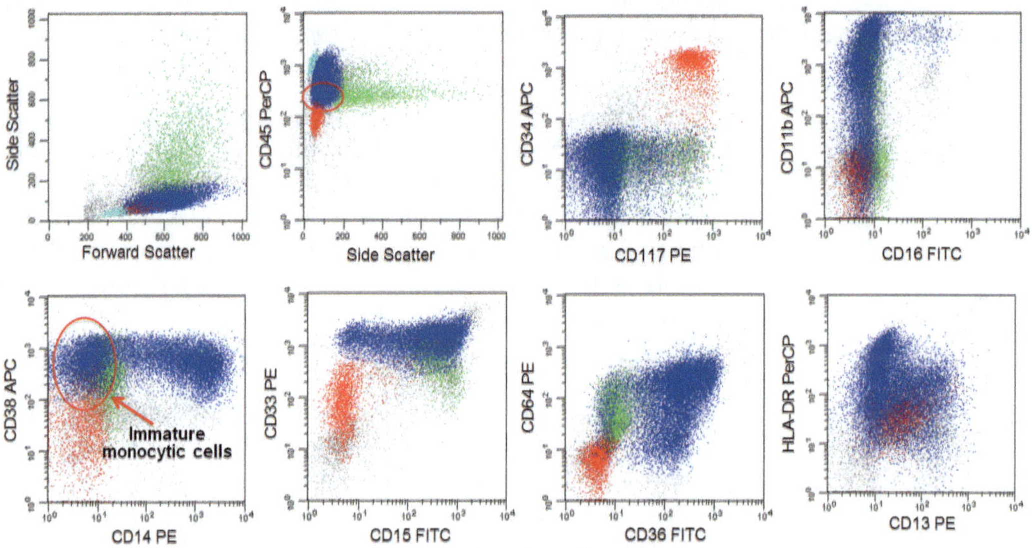

Fig. 7 Acute myelomonocytic leukemia. An example case of acute myelomonocytic leukemia in bone marrow demonstrates a characteristic immunophenotype: the myeloid blasts composed of two subsets, one CD34(+) myeloblasts (in *red*), and the other immature monocytic cells (monoblasts/promonocytes, a subset of cells painted in *blue*). Immature monocytes maintain the expression of CD15, CD33 (*bright*), CD36, and CD64, to the levels close to normal mature monocytes, but downregulate to completely lose CD14. CD15 expression is increased, and CD11b and CD13 expression are decreased in the immature monocytic cells. Granulocytes are painted in *green*, lymphocytes in *light blue*

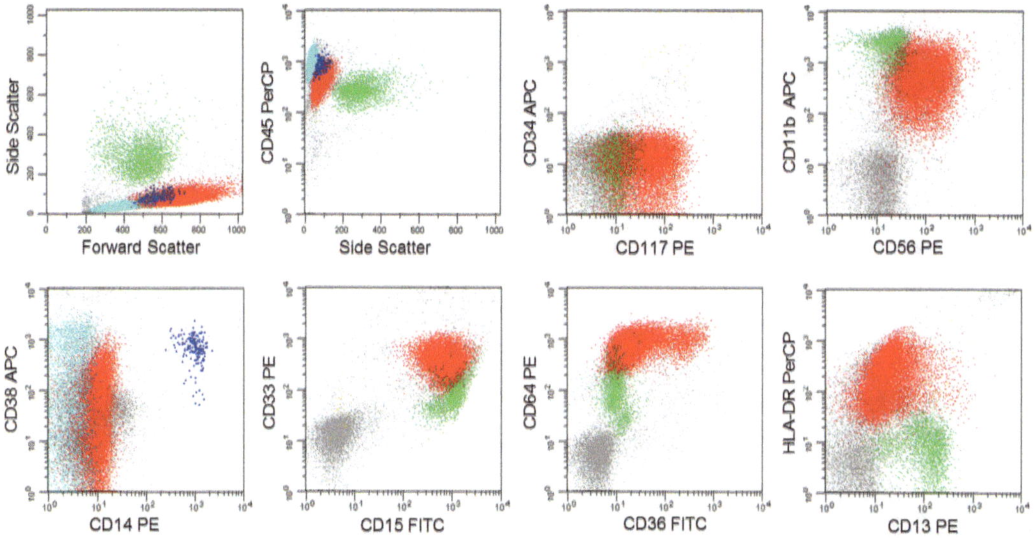

Fig. 8 Acute monoblastic leukemia with t(9;11) (loss of CD14). An example case of acute monoblastic leukemia with t(9;11) in peripheral blood demonstrates a characteristic immunophenotype, similar to previous case: significant downregulation to completely loss of CD14, but retention of CD15(*bright*), CD33, CD36, and CD64 in leukemic cells. Loss of CD14 and bright CD15 are the clue to the immaturity of monocytic cells. Granulocytes are painted in *green*, mature normal monocytes in *dark blue*, lymphocytes in *light blue*

expression of CD14. This discrepancy indicates the presence of an expanded population of CD14(−) immature monocytic cells (cells in circle in Fig. 7), which is confirmed through morphologic examination of the specimen.

Case 5: Acute Monoblastic Leukemia with t(9;11) (Loss of CD14)

This case illustrates one of the common features in acute monoblastic leukemia, significant downregulation to completely loss of CD14, but retention of CD15(bright), CD33, CD36, and CD64. This combined immunophenotype is suggestive of the presence of a large population of CD14(−) immature monocytic cells (Fig. 8). Similar to the previous case in Fig. 7, loss of CD14 and bright CD15 are the immunophenotypic clues to the monocytic immaturity.

Case 6: Acute Monoblastic Leukemia with t(8;16) (Retention of CD14)

This is an unusual case of acute monoblastic leukemia with t(8;16) in which CD14 is largely retained in immature monocytic cells (Fig. 9). This retention of CD14 could be a potential pitfall leading to overlooking the leukemia if this population is relatively small. Interestingly, CD15, similar to the previous case, is brightly expressed, and CD11b is underexpressed, which are potential clues to identifying immaturity in monocytic cells. Careful morphologic

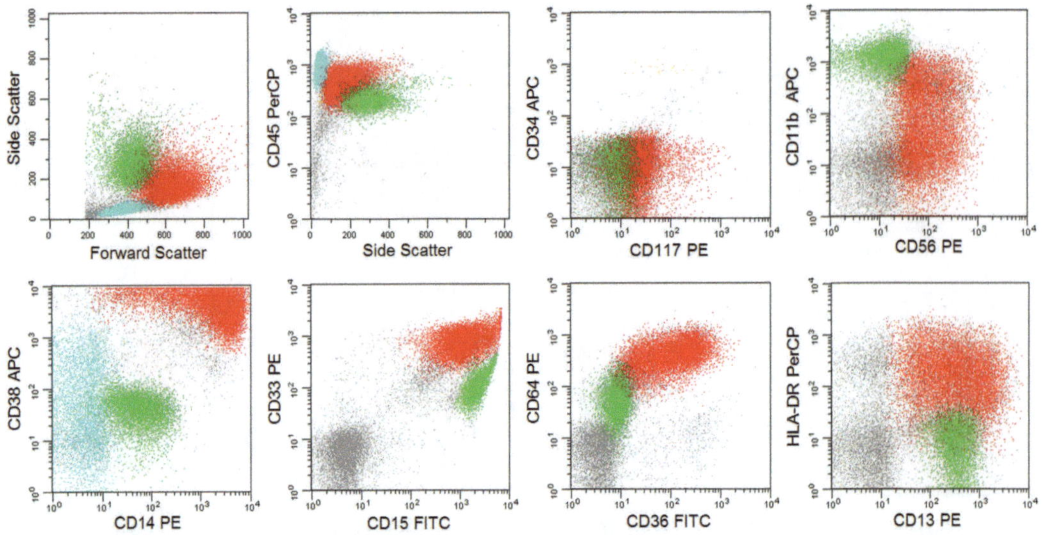

Fig. 9 Acute monoblastic leukemia with t(8;16) (retention of CD14). This is an unusual case of acute monoblastic leukemia with t(8;16) in peripheral blood in which CD14 is largely retained in immature monocytic cells. Bright CD15 expression and underexpression of CD11b may be the clue to the immaturity of monocytic cells. Granulocytes are painted in *green*, lymphocytes in *light blue*

correlation and awareness of this phenomenon are essential to confirm immaturity of the leukemic cells and reach the correct diagnosis.

Case 7: Acute Megakaryoblastic Leukemia

In this example case of adult acute megakaryoblastic leukemia with complex karyotypic abnormalities, myeloid blasts are composed of CD34(+)/CD117(+) myeloblasts (in red) and CD34(dim+)/CD117(−) megakaryoblasts (in blue) (Fig. 10). The clue to megakaryocytic or erythroid differentiation is the expression of CD36 in the absence of CD64 in blasts that fall into the broad CD45 (dim+) blast region [31, 32]. A reflex study further confirms the megakaryocytic lineage differentiation by virtue of a typical immunophenotypic profile: CD41(+), CD61(+), CD71(partial +), and glycophorin A(−) (*see* **Note 8**).

Case 8: Acute Pure Erythroid Leukemia

In this example case of pure erythroid leukemia, there is a predominant population of erythroblasts (>80%) with a high and widely variable SSC (likely related to cytoplasmic vacuolization) (Fig. 11). The clue to megakaryocytic or erythroid leukemia is the expression of CD36 in the absence of CD64 in blasts that fall into the CD45(−) blast region. A reflex study further confirms the erythroid lineage differentiation by virtue of a typical immunophenotypic profile: CD41(−), CD61(−), CD71(strong +), and

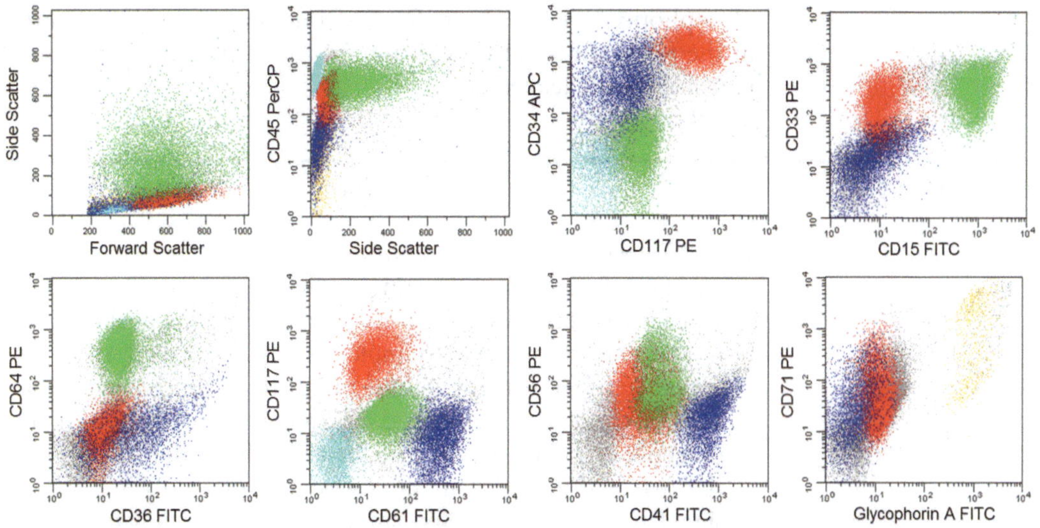

Fig. 10 Acute megakaryoblastic leukemia. An example case of acute megakaryoblastic leukemia in bone marrow demonstrates a characteristic immunophenotype: myeloid blasts composed of CD34(+)/CD117(+) myeloblasts (in *red*) and CD34(dim+)/CD117(–) megakaryoblasts (in *blue*). Megakaryoblasts are CD36(+), CD41(+), CD61(+), CD64(–), CD71(partial +), and glycophorin A (–). Granulocytes are painted in *green*, lymphocytes in *light blue*, erythroids in *yellow*

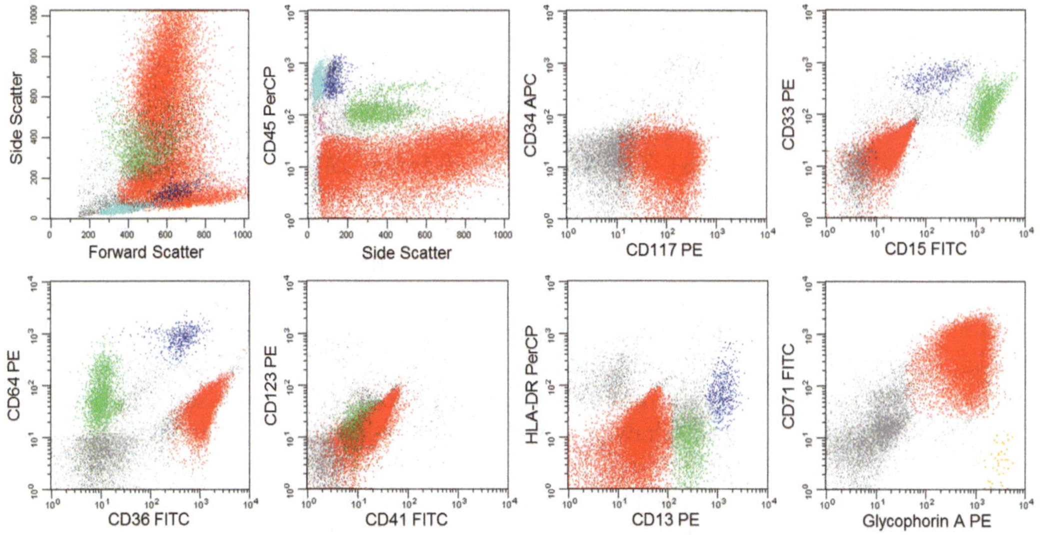

Fig. 11 Acute pure erythroid leukemia. An example case of pure erythroid leukemia in bone marrow demonstrates a characteristic immunophenotype. Erythroblasts are CD36(+), CD41(–), CD61(–), CD64(–), CD71(strong+), and glycophorin A(+). Other markers are widely variable SSC, CD13(–), CD15(–), CD33(–), CD34(–), CD117(+), and HLA-DR(–). Granulocytes are painted in *green*, normal monocytes in *dark blue*, lymphocytes in *light blue*, normal erythroids in *yellow*

glycophorin A (+) (*see* **Note 9**). The immunophenotype obtained in the reflex study is thus opposite to that in the previous case of megakaryocytic leukemia.

4 Notes

1. *Antibody titration and cocktail preparation:* Prior to preparing a cocktail of antibodies, it is imperative to titer antibodies individually for optimal signal-to-noise ratio using the final total volume of the cocktail. For example, adding sufficient PAB to give a total delivered reagent volume of 20–40 μL for routine 4-color antibody tests. For surface and intracellular antigen titration, the objective is to identify an amount of antibody that will provide the maximal intensity at the lowest background (i.e., optimal signal to noise ratio). Special caution should be exercised in titration of intracellular antigen. It may not be possible to demonstrate apparent saturation, as there is a high level of nonspecific binding to cytoplasmic antigens (due to complexity of the intracellular environment and potential abundant binding sites). The prepared cocktails should be tested on representative PB and BM cases to ensure expected antibody reactivity, to detect any unexpected interactions, and to determine cocktail stability.
2. *Specimen processing (up-front bulk lysis* versus *stain-lyse-wash):* Up-front bulk lysis is better suited for samples with low nucleated cell counts (such as cerebrospinal fluid (CSF) and scanty tissue biopsy specimens or fine-needle aspiration (FNA) samples). The additional advantage of this method is to allow for using a single processing protocol that is virtually suitable for all types of panels including surface light chain staining in lymphoma work-up. Moreover, this method preserves cell suspension for up to 1 week, facilitating additional staining if needed for an accurate diagnosis. The antibodies are fixed to the cells by 1% paraformaldehyde after staining to stabilize antigen–antibody interactions and to preserve the light scatter properties. The drawback of the up-front lysis is the potential to lyse some leukocytes. Notably, many laboratories use an alternative protocol, staining first followed by lysis. In this so-called stain-lyse-wash (SLW) protocol, antibodies are incubated with the cells in the presence of erythrocytes. The erythrocytes are lysed (using lysing solution with low level of fixative), and bound antibodies are fixed to the cells to preserve the light scatter properties. These two methods, up-front bulk lysis and stain-lyse-wash, are largely comparable.
3. *Volume of 5% NCS:* Because the cell suspension's final cell count is determined, the amount of 5% NCS added is not critical.

4. *Pitfalls in interpretation of the immature cell markers*: There are a few pitfalls in interpretation of the proposed *immature* cell markers. First, CD117 expression in isolation is not specific for immaturity. CD117 is normally expressed on proerythroblasts, promyelocytes, and mast cells (with a bright pattern) [22]. Second, rare acute monoblastic leukemia, especially cases with t(8;16), may not downregulate CD14 (as illustrated in example Case 6) [33]. In this scenario, the presence of a large population of neoplastic cells by FC and morphologic findings of blasts may be the most important clue to the presence of a leukemic population. Lastly, dim to negative CD14 expression in monocytic cells may be a hint to the presence of unsuspected paroxysmal nocturnal hemoglobinuria (PNH). If clinically appropriate, this should trigger a specific PNH analysis by FC in PB sample for a confirmation.
5. *Caution in interpretation of Glycophorin A:* Glycophorin A is expressed at a high level on erythrocytes. Therefore, it is critical that staining of this antigen should be performed after red cell lysis to avoid false positive result.
6. *CD7 expression in myeloblasts:* CD7 may be expressed on normal myeloblasts at very early stage of maturation. In our experience, it tends to express on a small subset of CD13(dim+) myeloblasts.
7. *Caution in interpretation of antigen expression in acute promyelocytic leukemia:* Leukemic blasts in this entity tend to have a high level of nonspecific fluorescence resulted from nonspecific binding of antibody and autofluorescence, which is likely related to cytoplasmic complexity. Therefore, it is essential to carefully compare the level of antigen expression in leukemia cells to the level of fluorescence on the *same* leukemic population from an isotype control or internal negative control in order to avoid erroneous interpretation of antigen expression.
8. *Caution in interpretation of CD36, CD41, and CD61:* Caution should be exercised in the interpretation of CD36, CD41, and CD61 in myeloid blasts due to adherence of platelets to the blasts. To limit this false positivity, CD36, CD41, and CD61 in blasts are only considered positive if the granulocytes lack positive staining. Alternatively, CD42b can assist in determining whether the staining is due to platelet satellitism, as CD42b is expressed by platelets but is absent from megakaryoblasts.
9. *Caution in assessment of erythroid leukemia:* Erythroid leukemia blasts with less evidence of maturation may lack glycophorin A. Moderate CD71 expression is non-lineage specific, but bright CD71 expression is considered a marker for erythroid differentiation [31]. The clue to erythroid leukemia is expression of CD36 (in the absence of CD64) and CD71 (bright) in the blast population.

Acknowledgments

Dr. Franklin Fuda is gratefully acknowledged for critical reading and commenting the content of this chapter. The authors also thank the medical technologists in the Clinical Flow Cytometry laboratory at the University of Texas Southwestern Medical Center for their technical assistance.

References

1. Swerdlow SH, Campo E, Harrris NL et al (eds) (2008) World Health Organization classification of tumors of haematopoietic and lymphoid tissues, 4th edn. WHO Press, Geneva, Switzerland
2. Craig FE, Foon KA (2008) Flow cytometric immunophenotyping for hematologic neoplasms. Blood 111:3941–3967
3. Kaleem Z, Crawford E, Pathan MH et al (2003) Flow cytometric analysis of acute leukemias. Diagnostic utility and critical analysis of data. Arch Pathol Lab Med 127:42–48
4. Gorczyca W, Sun ZY, Cronin W et al (2011) Immunophenotypic pattern of myeloid populations by flow cytometry analysis. Methods Cell Biol 103:221–266
5. Khoury H, Dalal BI, Nantel SH et al (2004) Correlation between karyotype and quantitative immunophenotype in acute myelogenous leukemia with t(8;21). Mod Pathol 17:1211–1216
6. Kita K, Nakase K, Miwa H et al (1992) Phenotypical characteristics of acute myelocytic leukemia associated with the t(8;21)(q22;q22) chromosomal abnormality: frequent expression of immature B-cell antigen CD19 together with stem cell antigen CD34. Blood 80:470–477
7. Paietta E, Goloubeva O, Neuberg D et al (2004) A surrogate marker profile for PML/RAR alpha expressing acute promyelocytic leukemia and the association of immunophenotypic markers with morphologic and molecular subtypes. Cytometry B Clin Cytom 59:1–9
8. Lin P, Hao S, Medeiros LJ et al (2004) Expression of CD2 in acute promyelocytic leukemia correlates with short form of PML-RARalpha transcripts and poorer prognosis. Am J Clin Pathol 121:402–407
9. Kern W, Voskova D, Schoch C et al (2004) Determination of relapse risk based on assessment of minimal residual disease during complete remission by multiparameter flow cytometry in unselected patients with acute myeloid leukemia. Blood 104:3078–3085
10. San Miguel JF, Vidriales MB, Lopez-Berges C et al (2001) Early immunophenotypical evaluation of minimal residual disease in acute myeloid leukemia identifies different patient risk groups and may contribute to postinduction treatment stratification. Blood 98: 1746–1751
11. Campana D, Coustan-Smith E (1999) Detection of minimal residual disease in acute leukemia by flow cytometry. Cytometry 38:139–152
12. Borowitz MJ, Devidas M, Hunger SP et al (2008) Clinical significance of minimal residual disease in childhood acute lymphoblastic leukemia and its relationship to other prognostic factors: a Children's oncology group study. Blood 111:5477–5485
13. Borowitz MJ, Wood BL, Devidas M et al (2015) Prognostic significance of minimal residual disease in high risk B-ALL: a report from Children's oncology group study AALL0232. Blood 126:964–971
14. Araki D, Wood BL, Othus M et al (2015) Allogeneic hematopoietic cell transplantation for acute myeloid leukemia: time to move toward a minimal residual disease-based definition of complete remission? J Clin Oncol 34:329–336
15. Buccisano F, Maurillo L, Spagnoli A et al (2010) Cytogenetic and molecular diagnostic characterization combined to postconsolidation minimal residual disease assessment by flow cytometry improves risk stratification in adult acute myeloid leukemia. Blood 116:2295–2303
16. Kalina T, Flores-Montero J, van der Velden VH et al (2012) EuroFlow standardization of flow cytometer instrument settings and immunophenotyping protocols. Leukemia 26:1986–2010
17. Wood B (2006) 9-color and 10-color flow cytometry in the clinical laboratory. Arch Pathol Lab Med 130:680–690
18. Stelzer GT, Shults KE, Loken MR (1993) CD45 gating for routine flow cytometric analysis of human bone marrow specimens. Ann N Y Acad Sci 677:265–280

19. Borowitz MJ, Guenther KL, Shults KE et al (1993) Immunophenotyping of acute leukemia by flow cytometric analysis. Use of CD45 and right-angle light scatter to gate on leukemic blasts in three-color analysis. Am J Clin Pathol 100:534–540
20. Harrington AM, Olteanu H, Kroft SH (2012) A dissection of the CD45/side scatter "blast gate". Am J Clin Pathol 137:800–804
21. Xu Y, McKenna RW, Wilson KS et al (2006) Immunophenotypic identification of acute myeloid leukemia with monocytic differentiation. Leukemia 20:1321–1324
22. Wood BL (2003) Myeloid malignancies: myelodysplastic syndromes, myeloproliferative disorders, and acute myeloid leukemia. Clin Lab Med 27:551–575
23. Kussick SJ, Wood BL (2003) Using 4-color flow cytometry to identify abnormal myeloid populations. Arch Pathol Lab Med 127:1140–1147
24. Fuda F, Chen W (2014) Lineage determination in mixed phenotype acute leukemia: response to Marcondes et al. Cytometry B Clin Cytom 86:150–151
25. Al-Mawali A, Gillis D, Lewis I (2009) The role of multiparameter flow cytometry for detection of minimal residual disease in acute myeloid leukemia. Am J Clin Pathol 131:16–26
26. Kern W, Haferlach C, Haferlach T et al (2008) Monitoring of minimal residual disease in acute myeloid leukemia. Cancer 112:4–16
27. Chen W, Konoplev S, Medeiros LJ et al (2009) Cuplike nuclei (prominent nuclear invaginations) in acute myeloid leukemia are highly associated with FLT3 internal tandem duplication and NPM1 mutation. Cancer 115:5481–5489
28. Kussick SJ, Stirewalt DL, Yi HS et al (2004) A distinctive nuclear morphology in acute myeloid leukemia is strongly associated with loss of HLA-DR expression and FLT3 internal tandem duplication. Leukemia 18:1591–1598
29. Rakheja D, Konoplev S, Medeiros LJ et al (2012) IDH mutations in acute myeloid leukemia. Hum Pathol 43:1541–1551
30. Yang DT, Greenwood JH, Hartung L et al (2005) Flow cytometric analysis of different CD14 epitopes can help identify immature monocytic populations. Am J Clin Pathol 124:930–936
31. Karandikar NJ, Aquino DB, McKenna RW et al (2001) Transient myeloproliferative disorder and acute myeloid leukemia in down syndrome. An immunophenotypic analysis. Am J Clin Pathol 116:204–210
32. Wang L, Peters JM, Fuda F et al (2015) Acute megakaryoblastic leukemia associated with trisomy 21 demonstrates a distinct immunophenotype. Cytometry B Clin Cytom 88:244–252
33. Haferlach T, Kohlmann A, Klein HU et al (2009) AML with translocation t(8;16)(p11;p13) demonstrates unique cytomorphological, cytogenetic, molecular and prognostic features. Leukemia 23:934–943

Chapter 5

Single-Cell Mass Cytometry of Acute Myeloid Leukemia and Leukemia Stem/Progenitor Cells

Zhihong Zeng, Marina Konopleva, and Michael Andreeff

Abstract

Mass cytometry time-of-flight (CyTOF) empowers us to understand acute myeloid leukemia (AML) biology at the single-cell level. This technology, combined with advanced data-analysis methods, enables identification and characterization of the rare AML stem/progenitor cells that play key roles in drug resistance and AML relapse. Here we provide a protocol for AML sample preparation for CyTOF and keynotes emphasizing critical steps in and troubleshooting strategies for this procedure.

Key words Acute myeloid leukemia, Mass cytometry time-of-flight

1 Introduction

Acute myeloid leukemia (AML) is a heterogeneous disease characterized by the uncontrolled growth of undifferentiated myeloid cells that originate in the bone marrow (BM) [1]. The prognosis for AML is poor owing to a high relapse rate and short overall survival, with some notable exceptions [2]. AML progenitor/stem cells, often called leukemic stem cells (LSCs), constitute a rare population of AML cells that reside in the BM and are responsible for AML relapse [3]. These cells can initiate AML development in immunodeficient NSG and NSGS mice (leukemia-initiating cells) [4]. The presence of more mature leukemic cells that can result in relapse of AML indicates that leukemia-initiating cells are not restricted to the most immature populations of leukemic progenitor/stem cells [5]. Recently, preleukemia stem cells were identified in healthy individuals with some acquired mutations but apparently were not sufficiently abundant to generate leukemia [6]. Phenotypes of these individuals are unknown.

LSCs and hematopoietic stem cells have several features in common, including low cell frequency, heterogeneity, asymmetrical division, and engraftment potential. However, LSCs do not

Paolo Fortina et al. (eds.), *Acute Myeloid Leukemia: Methods and Protocols*, Methods in Molecular Biology, vol. 1633, DOI 10.1007/978-1-4939-7142-8_5, © Springer Science+Business Media LLC 2017

follow the normal differentiation pattern of hematopoiesis. Rather, they remain immature, appear as a subpopulation of AML blasts, and generate daughter LSCs [7]. Current chemotherapeutic regimens are highly effective in eliminating AML blasts but usually not LSCs [8]. Therefore, LSCs play critical roles in leukemogenesis, therapy resistance, and AML persistence. Improved characterization of these cells is essential for development of LSC-targeted therapy and higher cure rates for AML.

Over the past few decades, fluorescence flow cytometry has been used to characterize the phenotypes and functions of AML and LSCs. However, spectral overlap of fluorescent dyes limits the use of this technique to about 17 simultaneous measurements [9, 10]. Given the phenotypic complexity of AML introduced by the discovery of additional surface and intracellular molecules, the increased appreciation of AML's phenotypic diversity, and the development of intracellular markers that characterize signaling pathways and metabolic states, fluorescence methods can no longer meet the need for a high level of multiparametric analysis of AML's heterogeneity.

Mass cytometry by time-of-flight (CyTOF) is an innovative technology that merges single-cell flow cytometry with mass spectrometry [11, 12]. In this technique, transition elements are substituted for fluorophores to label antibodies, allowing for detection and measurement of up to 130 parameters in a single cell with minimal signal overlap. Furthermore, CyTOF uses rare earth elements that are not found in biological systems, thus minimizing the background noise from cellular signals that often makes analysis of fluorescence problematic. Whereas the current generation of CyTOF instruments (e.g., CyTOF2 and Helios; Fluidigm, San Francisco, CA, USA) can determine 135 simultaneous markers to define a cell in a single experiment, the available metal tags restrict the capacity to analyze 54 parameters.

Several computational analytic tools, including SPADE [13] and viSNE [14], have been developed to organize and display the high-dimensional data generated by CyTOF. Using unsupervised algorithms, these tools capture multidimensional cellular relationships and compress them into two dimensions without losing single-cell identities. CyTOF complemented by these data-analysis tools provides a unique opportunity to comprehensively characterize AML at the single-cell level. Moreover, these computational tools allow for the identification of AML phenotypic and intracellular alterations either transient or permanent after various treatments. Most importantly, these tools empower the characterization of single LSCs that survive therapy, determination of the factors that contribute to the development of AML resistance mechanisms, and, perhaps, identification of new therapeutic approaches to eliminating resistant AML [15–17].

We herein present a protocol for AML sample preparation for CyTOF acquisition. We also provide an example of CyTOF data analysis using SPADE and viSNE and denote critical steps and potential sources of variability in CyTOF sample preparation.

2 Materials

2.1 Reagents and Materials

1. Phosphate-buffered saline (PBS).
2. Bovine serum albumin (BSA, Sigma-Aldrich, St. Louis, MO, USA).
3. Fetal bovine serum (FBS, Invitrogen, Carlsbad, CA, USA).
4. MeOH (Thermo Fisher Scientific, Waltham, MA, USA).
5. Cell-ID cisplatin (Fluidigm) or cisplatin (Sigma-Aldrich).
6. Cell-ID Intercalator-Ir (Fluidigm).
7. Cell-ID 127 IdU (Fluidigm; optional).
8. Beads: EQ Four Element Calibration Beads (EQ Beads; catalog #201078) or CyTOF Calibration Beads (Eu Beads; catalog #201073) (Fluidigm).

2.2 Buffers, Solutions, and Medium

1. Wash buffer: 0.5% BSA in PBS.
2. Staining buffer: 1% BSA in PBS.
3. Quenching buffer: 10% FBS in PBS.
4. Fixation buffer: 1.6% paraformaldehyde (PFA) in PBS (16% PFA catalog #15710 [Electron Microscopy Sciences, Hatfield, PA, USA])
5. Permeabilization buffer: 70–80% MeOH (−20 °C; prepared from 100% methanol).
6. Cisplatin staining solution:
   - 5 μM Cell-ID cisplatin (Fluidigm) in PBS;

     Or
   - 25 μM cisplatin (Sigma-Aldrich) in PBS (freshly prepared from 10 mM working solution in PBS (10× dilution of 100 mM stock solution in DMSO [Sigma-Aldrich] in PBS).
7. IdU staining solution: 25 μM IdU in PBS (optional).
8. Last wash solution: 0.1% BSA in Milli-Q water.
9. Heparin stock solution: 2 mg of heparin sodium powder (Alfa Aesar, Haverhill, MA, USA) in 1 mL of PBS sterilized with a 0.22 μM filter (Thermo Fisher Scientific) and stored at 4 °C.
10. DNase I stock solution: 1 mg/mL DNase I (Roche Applied Sciences, Penzberg, Germany) in PBS sterilized with a 0.22 μM filter and stored at −20 °C.

11. $MgSO_4$ stock solution: 200 mM $MgSO_4$ (Sigma-Aldrich) in PBS sterilized with a 0.22 μM filter and stored at −20 °C.
12. 20% FBS RPMI medium.

3 Methods

3.1 Solution Preparation

3.1.1 Antibody Cocktails

Separately prepare antibody cocktails for surface and intracellular antibodies in staining buffer. We recommend preparing the antibody cocktail such that the final volume for each test is 50 μL. The antibody cocktail can be stored for up to 24 h before staining cells. An example of the antibody cocktail used for the experiment displayed in Fig. 1 is provided in Table 1.

3.1.2 Intercalation Solution

Freshly prepare the intercalation solution for each sample by adding Cell-ID.

Intercalator-Ir to a fixation buffer for a final concentration of 125 nM (1000× dilution of the 125 μM stock solution) and mix via vortexing.

3.1.3 Cell-Reviving Solution

Freshly prepare 10 mL of a cell-reviving solution by adding 500 μL of heparin stock solution, 15 μL of DNase I stock solution, and 500 μL of $MgSO_4$ stock solution to 20% FBS RPMI medium. The cell-reviving solution is used for reviving cryopreserved cells.

3.2 Reviving Cryopreserved Cells

1. Take a cryovial containing cells from liquid nitrogen.
2. Place the cryovial in a 37 °C water bath.
3. Thaw the cells in the cryovial completely.
4. Add the cells to 10 mL of 20% FBS RPMI medium.
5. Spin the mixture at 300 × *g* for 5 min.
6. Resuspend the pellet in a cell-reviving solution; incubate for 15–30 min in a 37 °C incubator.
7. Filter the cells through a cell strainer to remove aggregates and debris.
8. Count the viable cells and centrifuge at 300 × *g* for 5 min.
9. Resuspend the pellet for further experiments.

3.3 CyTOF Sample Preparation

1. Stimulate/inhibit/treat either fresh or revived frozen cells according to an experimental protocol (1.0×10^6 to 1.5×10^6 cells per sample).
2. Wash cells with wash buffer twice and centrifuge cells at 300 × *g* for 5 min.
3. Resuspend the pellet, add 5 μM cisplatin staining solution (Fluidigm) (1×10^7 cell/mL) dropwise to the cells, and incubate

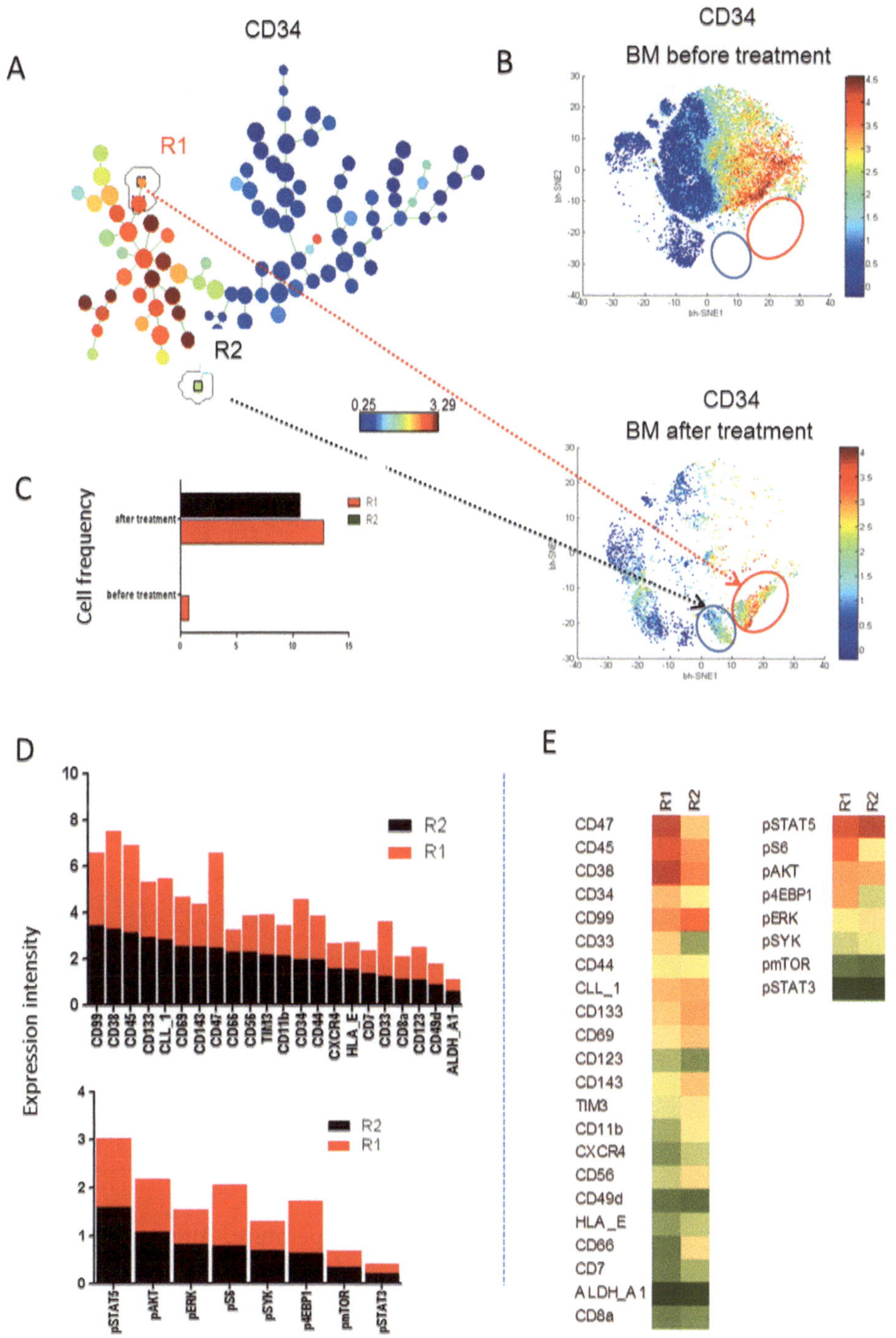

Fig. 1 SPADE- and viSNE-based identification of two treatment-resistant subsets of AML samples. (**a**) SPADE tree displaying the resistant subsets (R1 and R1) and their levels of expression of CD34. (**b**) viSNE plot displaying the locations and geometric shapes of R1 and R2 in the bone marrow (BM) AML samples before (right top) and after (right bottom) treatment. (**c**) Cell frequency of resistant subsets R1 and R2 in the BM samples before and after treatment. (**d** and **e**) Bar graph (D) and heatmap (E) displaying the expression of surface and intracellular markers of R1 and R2 in treated AML cells

Table 1
CyTOF antibody panel

Surface marker panel		Intracellular marker panel	
Antibody	**Metal tag**	**Antibody**	**Metal tag**
CD7	La139	p-4EBP1	Sm147
CD49d	Pr141	p-SYK	Sm149
ALDH1A1	Nd142	p-STAT5	Nd150
CD11b	Nd144	p-STAT3	Sm152
HLA-E	Nd145	p-AKT	Tb159
CD8a	Nd146	p-mTOR	Dy164
CD34	Nd148	p-ERK	Er167
CD123_beads1	Eu151	p-S6	Yb172
CD133_beads2	Eu153		
CD45	Sm154		
TIM-3	Gd156		
CD33	Gd158		
CD69	Dy162		
CD99	Ho165		
CD44	Er166		
CD38	Er168		
CD143	Tm169		
CD47	Er170		
CD66	Yb171		
CLL-1	Yb174		
CXCR4	Lu175		
CD56	Yb176		

them for 5 min at room temperature. Alternatively, add 25 μM cisplatin staining solution (Sigma-Aldrich) (2×10^6 cells/mL) dropwise to the cells and incubate them for 1 min at room temperature.

4. Add 2 mL of quenching buffer to stop the cisplatin reaction and centrifuge cells at 300 × *g* for 5 min.
5. Wash cells with 2 mL of wash buffer and centrifuge them at 300 × *g* for 5 min.
6. Incubate cells with 1 mL of IdU staining solution for 15 min at 37 °C (optional).

7. Add 1.5 mL of wash buffer to the cells and centrifuge them at 300 × *g* for 5 min.
8. Wash cells with 2 mL of a wash buffer twice and centrifuge them at 300 × *g* for 5 min.
9. Surface staining: the surface antibody cocktail in the staining buffer added should be made at a 4× to 5× stock concentration (so that 12.5 or 10.0 μL of the antibody cocktail can be added). Cells should be stained in a total volume of 50 μL (exactly). The volume of residual liquid and cell pellet should be determined with a pipette and enough staining buffer added to make the total volume of the solution 50 μL minus the antibody cocktail volume. Thus, adding the staining buffer will bring the total volume to 50 μL and ensure that the antibody concentration is equivalent in all samples. Incubate cells for 30 min at room temperature.
10. Add 2 mL of wash buffer to the cells and centrifuge them at 300 × *g* for 5 min.; repeat twice.
11. Add 0.5 mL of fixation buffer to cells and fix cells for 10 min at room temperature (in the dark); add 1.5 mL of wash buffer to cells and centrifuge them at 1000 × *g* for 10 min.
12. Wash cells with 2 mL of wash buffer and centrifuge them at 1000 × *g* for 10 min; repeat once.
13. Add 1 mL of permeabilization buffer (−20 °C) dropwise to cells, vortex the mixture to resuspend the cells, permeabilize cells for 10 min on ice, and store them at −20 °C overnight.
14. Add 1.5 mL of wash buffer to cells and centrifuge them at 1000 × *g* for 10 min.
15. Wash cells with 2 mL of wash buffer and centrifuge them at 1000 × *g* for 10 min; repeat once.
16. Intracellular staining: the intracellular antibody cocktail in staining buffer added should be made at a 4× to 5× stock concentration (so that 12.5 or 10.0 μL of the antibody cocktail can be added). Cells should be stained in a total volume of 50 μL (exactly). The volume of residual liquid and cell pellet should be determined with a pipette and enough staining buffer added to make the total volume of the solution 50 μL minus the antibody cocktail volume. Thus, adding the staining buffer will bring the total volume to 50 μL and ensure that the antibody concentration is equivalent in all samples. Incubate the cells for 1 h at room temperature.
17. Add 2 mL of wash buffer to cells and centrifuge them at 1000 × *g* for 10 min; repeat twice.
18. Add 0.5 mL of fixation buffer to cells and fix cells for 10 min at room temperature (in the dark). Then add 1.5 mL of wash buffer to cells and centrifuge them at 1000 × *g* for 10 min.

19. Wash cells with 2 mL of wash buffer and centrifuge cells at 1000 × *g* for 10 min; repeat once.
20. Add 0.5 mL of intercalation solution to cells and incubate the mixture for 20 min at room temperature (in the dark).
21. Add 1.5 mL of wash buffer to cells and centrifuge them at 1000 × *g* for 10 min.
22. Wash cells with 2 mL of wash buffer and centrifuge them at 1000 × *g* for 10 min; repeat once.
23. Resuspend cells in 1 mL of the last wash solution, filter the cells through a cell strainer into a new tube, and count the cells (*see* Subheading 4.1.5 below).
24. Centrifuge cells at 1000 × *g* for 10 min.
25. Save the pellet for use in a CyTOF machine.
26. Before CyTOF, resuspend the pellet in deionized water at concentration of 0.5 × 10^6 cells/50 μL, and add 50 μL beads (final concentration ~30,000 beads/mL) (*see* Subheading 4.1.5 below).

3.4 CyTOF Data Analysis

We provide here an example of CyTOF data analysis that we used to identify treatment-resistant subsets in primary AML samples.

CyTOF data were normalized using a MATLAB-based software program called bead normalization [18]. Normalized data were analyzed using FlowJo software (version 10) to generate clean data by eliminating beads, cisplatin-positive events, background noise, and doubles. The clean data were then exported to SPADE to build a tree of 100 nodes using surface markers clustered by the k-mean clustering algorithm and branched by the minimal spanning tree algorithm. The subsets of AML identified using SPADE were confirmed using viSNE. Results of the analysis are displayed in Fig. 1.

4 Notes

4.1 Critical Steps and Troubleshooting Strategies

4.1.1 Background Signal

Signal overlap from metal tags into other channels generates background signals in CyTOF. However, signal overlap in mass cytometry is much smaller than that in fluorescence flow cytometry. Potential sources for generation of background signals are oxides in mass+16 channels, metal isotope impurities, and sample and/or reagent contamination. Most of these can be minimized or prevented.

1. The isotopes lanthanum, cerium, praseodymium, and neodymium, which have strong oxides, produce a background signals in mass+16 channels. This background noise cannot be prevented but can be reduced by optimizing the plasma temperature, which is part of the CyTOF instrument-tuning procedure.

2. Isotope impurities cause signal overlap in the mass+1 and mass-1 channels, and some signal overlap may not be strictly in mass proximity. This is often seen with the isotopes neodymium-144, neodymium-145, and neodymium-146 and lanthanum-139. The purity of each isotope is determined at the time of its production. This signal overlap can be reduced or prevented by using markers of mutually exclusive lineages such as T-cell markers followed by B-cell markers or dumping the channels that contain the most contaminated isotopes.
3. Environmental contamination causes CyTOF background noise in mass channels.
   (a) Reagents: PFA, MeOH, and argon gas impurities cause background noise with the isotopes of samarium.
   (b) Primary samples generate background noise with isotopes of iodine and platinum.
   (c) Dish soap, detergents, and syringes may generate background noise with isotopes of barium and lead.

   Background noise can be detected in iridium (Ir)-only samples (unstained samples: cells not stained with any antibodies) and need to be gated out before further analysis. Reagent contamination can be avoided by using different product lots.

4.1.2 Cell Quality

Staining of fresh live cells that are 95% viable is always ideal for CyTOF assays. Frozen cells should be revived using a cell-reviving solution (described above) to prevent cell aggregation and death. In experiments in which frozen cells need to be stimulated or inhibited, revived cells should be counted to determine cell viability and number before performing experiments.

4.1.3 Fixation/Permeabilization of Reagent Concentrations

The concentrations of fixation and permeabilization reagents vary in CyTOF assays and depend on the surface and intracellular molecules detected in the cells. Certain cell-surface epitopes can be damaged by high concentrations of fixation and permeabilization solutions. On the other hand, certain intracellular molecules, such as the STAT protein family, need to be permeabilized twice or at high concentrations for better detection. Therefore, it is necessary to titrate the concentrations of fixation and permeabilization solutions once the panel of antibodies is selected. Optimized concentrations are effective for intracellular molecular staining with minimal damage of cell-surface epitopes. Alternatively, replacement of methanol with a gentle detergent such as saponin or Triton X-100 as the permeabilization solution may be considered to preserve surface epitopes.

4.1.4 Loss of Cells during CyTOF Sample Preparation

The number of cells lost after the fixation/permeabilization and wash steps in CyTOF sample preparation can be reduced by adding BSA to 1× PBS wash buffer at concentrations ranging from 0.1 to 2.0%

(w/v), increasing the centrifuge speed to 1000 × *g* and centrifuge time or reducing wash steps.

4.1.5 Filtering Samples in the Last Step of CyTOF Sample Preparation

To minimize buildup of salt residue in the CyTOF instrument, the final wash in CyTOF sample preparation should be performed with the last wash solution (0.1% BSA in Milli-Q water [Subheading 3.3, **step 23**]) and filtered through a cell strainer to remove aggregates, and the cells should be counted before centrifugation at 1000 × *g* for 10 min. The cell pellet then should be resuspended in deionized water at a concentration of 0.5×10^6/50 μL (*See* Subheading 3.3 **step 26**).

4.1.6 Signal Decay and Adding Beads in Samples

The purpose of adding beads in all cell samples in CyTOF is normalization of signal strength decay when acquisition of multiple samples in an experiment. Fluidigm produces two types of beads: (1) EQ Four Element Calibration Beads (EQ Beads; catalog #201078), which contain a natural abundance of cerium (140/142), europium-151/153 (^{151}Eu/^{153}Eu), holmium-165, and lutetium-175/176, and (2) CyTOF Calibration Beads (Eu Beads; catalog #201073), which have a natural abundance of ^{151}Eu/^{153}Eu. EQ Beads contain multiple elements, including cerium, an element that is not available in CyTOF antibody panel design. This ensures that such beads are readily discriminated from the cells in samples. In using Eu beads, all samples must be labeled with iridium (Ir), which enables discrimination of Ir-Eu+ beads from Ir+Eu- cells in samples.

4.1.7 Bead-Normalization Methods

Currently, two methods using different algorithms can be employed to normalize data for signal decay in CyTOF assays. First, the Fluidigm method requires CyTOF software version 6.0.626 and above. This method normalizes data according to a global standard that is determined by each lot of manufactured EQ Beads. Second, the MATLAB-based method, developed by Finck and colleagues [18], requires a software program available from a Stanford University website (http://www.cytobank.org/nolanlab). In this method, data is normalized to the median bead intensity determined by the experimental data file. This method requires collection of the Ir channel even if the sample is not stained with Ir.

4.1.8 Blocking Antibody

The use of a blocking antibody is optional in CyTOF sample staining, but one should be included if cells have high levels expression of Fc receptors, which will contribute to nonspecific antibody binding. This can be prevented by adding 100 μL of Fc block to each sample of cells before surface marker staining (Fc block diluted in a staining buffer; final concentration between 0.5 μg and 1 μg/10^6 cells), incubating the mixture on ice for 20 min, centrifuging at 300 × *g* for 5 min at 4 °C, and discarding the supernatant.

4.1.9 Titrating Antibodies

When using customer-conjugated antibodies in a CyTOF assay, the optimal staining concentration for each antibody should be determined in a titration experiment with an appropriate positive and negative control (e.g., cells with and without the expression of the antibody-target epitopes). If conjugation is performed using Maxpar labeling kits (Fluidigm), the testing concentrations should range from 250 to 8000 ng/mL. Also, the five steps of a threefold serial dilution of the antibody concentration are recommended.

4.1.10 Determination of the Cutoff to Define Positive and Negative Expressions of Surface or Intracellular Molecules

Biological knowledge is often used to set the cutoffs for positive and negative expressions of surface and intracellular molecules in CyTOF sample analysis. However, some stained samples have higher background noise on all channels (even samples of cells biologically negative for expression of certain molecules) than do unstained samples. In such cases, an unstained sample (control) is not ideal for setting the background. A metal-minus-one (MMO) or metal-minus-multiple (MMM) channel(s) is a better control for setting up the cutoff for the background. Another strategy for identifying expression of a molecule in CyTOF sample analysis is to identify a stained cell population (within the sample or another sample being tested) that is biologically known to be negative for expression of the relevant molecule and set the cutoff so that the sample is clearly negative and then count anything above the cutoff as being positive for expression of the molecule. In addition, the mass+1 and mass+16 spillover from very bright channels results in false-positive populations. This can be corrected by using dimmer antibodies in these channels.

4.2 A Newly Developed Barcoding Method for CyTOF Assay and the CyTOF Analytic Program

Recently, Nolan's group [19, 20] and later Fluidigm developed palladium-based cell barcoding methods for CyTOF assays. Barcoded samples can be combined and then stained and examined as one multiplexed sample to prevent sample-specific staining and data-collection variation. Both methods include debarcoding software programs that facilitate sample deconvolution and debarcoding for downstream analysis of the individual component samples. Also, Fluidigm produces a barcoding kit for CyTOF assays (Cell-ID 20-Plex Pd Barcoding Kit [catalog #201060]).

In addition to SPADE and viSNE, Wanderlust [21] and PhenoGraph [17] are advanced analytical programs for high-dimensional CyTOF data analysis. Also, Cytobank (http://www.cytobank.org) is a web-based analytical tool for flow and mass cytometry data analysis. The premium and enterprise versions of Cytobank feature SPADE and viSNE and other software.

4.3 Limitations of CyTOF Technology

Live cells cannot be recovered for sorting and further experimentation in CyTOF. Additionally, CyTOF requires the presence of purified metal isotopes to detect cells. Therefore, a metal-chelating DNA intercalator must be used to ensure detection of all cells. Also, CyTOF has low transmission efficiency (25%). A large starting number of cells are often required to detect rare cell populations. CyTOF also has a slow maximum cell-acquisition rate (~1000 cells/s). Therefore, each sample takes longer to run using CyTOF than it would to run a comparable flow cytometry experiment.

References

1. Estey E, Dohner H (2006) Acute myeloid leukaemia. Lancet 368:1894–1907
2. Szer J (2012) The prevalent predicament of relapsed acute myeloid leukemia. Hematology Am Soc Hematol Am Soc Hematol Educ Program 2012:43–48
3. Konopleva MY, Jordan CT (2011) Leukemia stem cells and microenvironment: biology and therapeutic targeting. J Clin Oncol 29:591–599
4. Lapidot T, Sirard C, Vormoor J et al (1994) A cell initiating human acute myeloid leukaemia after transplantation into SCID mice. Nature 367:645–648
5. Hope KJ, Jin L, Dick JE (2004) Acute myeloid leukemia originates from a hierarchy of leukemic stem cell classes that differ in self-renewal capacity. Nat Immunol 5:738–743
6. Shlush LI, Zandi S, Mitchell A et al (2014) Identification of pre-leukaemic haematopoietic stem cells in acute leukaemia. Nature 506:328–333
7. Hope KJ, Jin L, Dick JE (2003) Human acute myeloid leukemia stem cells. Arch Med Res 34:507–514
8. Dombret H, Gardin C (2016) An update of current treatments for adult acute myeloid leukemia. Blood 127:53–61
9. Chattopadhyay PK, Perfetto SP, Roederer M (2004) The colorful future of cell analysis by flow cytometry. Discov Med 4:255–262
10. Perfetto SP, Chattopadhyay PK, Roederer M (2004) Seventeen-colour flow cytometry: unravelling the immune system. Nat Rev Immunol 4:648–655
11. Bandura DR, Baranov VI, Ornatsky OI et al (2009) Mass cytometry: technique for real time single cell multitarget immunoassay based on inductively coupled plasma time-of-flight mass spectrometry. Anal Chem 81:6813–6822
12. Ornatsky O, Bandura D, Baranov V, Nitz M, Winnik MA, Tanner S (2010) Highly multiparametric analysis by mass cytometry. J Immunol Methods 361:1–20
13. Qiu P, Simonds EF, Bendall SC et al (2011) Extracting a cellular hierarchy from high-dimensional cytometry data with SPADE. Nat Biotechnol 29:886–U181
14. Amir el AD, Davis KL, Tadmor MD et al (2013) viSNE enables visualization of high dimensional single-cell data and reveals phenotypic heterogeneity of leukemia. Nat Biotechnol 31:545–552
15. Behbehani GK, Samusik N, Bjornson ZB, Fantl WJ, Medeiros BC, Nolan GP (2015) Mass cytometric functional profiling of acute myeloid leukemia defines cell-cycle and immunophenotypic properties that correlate with known responses to therapy. Cancer Discov 5:988–1003
16. Han L, Qiu P, Zeng Z et al (2015) Single-cell mass cytometry reveals intracellular survival/proliferative signaling in FLT3-ITD-mutated AML stem/progenitor cells. Cytometry A 87:346–356
17. Levine JH, Simonds EF, Bendall SC et al (2015) Data-driven phenotypic dissection of AML reveals progenitor-like cells that correlate with prognosis. Cell 162:184–197
18. Finck R, Simonds EF, Jager A et al (2013) Normalization of mass cytometry data with bead standards. Cytometry A 83:483–494
19. Fienberg HG, Simonds EF, Fantl WJ, Nolan GP, Bodenmiller B (2012) A platinum-based covalent viability reagent for single-cell mass cytometry. Cytometry A 81:467–475
20. Zunder ER, Finck R, Behbehani GK et al (2015) Palladium-based mass tag cell barcoding with a doublet-filtering scheme and single-cell deconvolution algorithm. Nat Protoc 10:316–333
21. Bendall SC, Davis KL, Amir el AD et al (2014) Single-cell trajectory detection uncovers progression and regulatory coordination in human B cell development. Cell 157:714–725

Chapter 6

Design and Application of Multiplex PCR Seq for the Detection of Somatic Mutations Associated with Myeloid Malignancies

Naomi Park and George Vassiliou

Abstract

Targeted sequencing, in which only a selected set of genomic loci are sequenced, enables a much higher coverage of each target than what is obtained using whole genome or exome sequencing. Multiplex PCR offers a simple and affordable technique for specific capture of target regions and can be easily adapted to generate next-generation sequencing (NGS)-ready amplicons. Here we describe a multiplex PCR (MxPCR) approach for capturing 13 leukemia-associated mutation hotspots followed by MiSeq sequencing that enables robust detection of mutations with a variant allele fraction (VAF) as low as 0.8% (0.008) in blood DNA.

Key words Clonal hemopoiesis, Leukemia, Multiplex PCR, Targeted sequencing

1 Introduction

There is an ever-increasing range of commercial options available for the targeted capture of genomic regions for analysis by NGS, particularly for whole exome and for disease panels [1]. Although highly suited and cost-effective for genome-scale applications, these approaches are prohibitively expensive and slow for re-sequencing of small numbers of hotspot locations as are required for molecular diagnostic applications. Additionally, genome-scale approaches deliver lower sequence coverage depths of hotspot regions leading to reduced power for the detection of low sub-clonal variants. By contrast, MxPCR is capable of simultaneously capturing multiple target regions in a single reaction whilst also incorporating adaptor sequences to generate NGS-ready amplicons [2] without the need for expensive equipment and with the ability to tackle large numbers of samples rapidly and at low cost.

Paolo Fortina et al. (eds.), *Acute Myeloid Leukemia: Methods and Protocols*, Methods in Molecular Biology, vol. 1633, DOI 10.1007/978-1-4939-7142-8_6, © Springer Science+Business Media LLC 2017

1.1 Protocol Outline

In this chapter, we describe a multiplex PCR protocol for the amplification and sequencing of regions known to be recurrently mutated in myeloid malignancies, but the same approach can be applied to any set of target loci. Amplicons included in the two-step PCR protocol described below were designed to capture a narrow size range (190–250 bp) to complement the sequencing length of the MiSeq instrument (Illumina San Diego, CA). The protocol has been validated using the KAPA HiFi HotStart high-fidelity polymerase selected for its capability of amplifying inserts of a wide range of GC compositions [3], but other polymerases with similar characteristics can be tried instead. The first PCR reaction involves a limited number of PCR cycles during which genomic primer annealing takes place during a stepwise reduction in temperature. This enables the gene-specific primers, containing common forward and reverse 5′-tail sequences, to simultaneously anneal every PCR cycle, whilst limited cycle number minimises amplification bias between the different amplicons [2]. The second PCR step involves no additional reagents or cleanup after the first PCR, aside from the addition of a single primer pair that anneals to and extends from the common tails introduced by the first-round PCR primers. During the 19 cycles of second-round PCR, unique sample barcodes are incorporated into the amplicon sequence to enable up to 384-level multiplexing of the sequencing run [4]. A schematic overview of multiplex PCR seq is presented in Fig. 1. The multiplex PCR described in this chapter was designed using the **Hiplex** and **mprimer** primer design tools [2, 5]. The first version of the multiplex was designed using Hiplex, but due to mprimer's more sophisticated design algorithms, additional hotspot primers were designed using mprimer and the final multiplex evaluated with MFEprimer. MFEprimer is a program for checking the specificity of PCR primers against the background DNA [6]. All further in-house MxPCR designs utilised **mprimer** and MFEprimer alone. Primers were synthesised to include a single 2′-*O*-Methyl base substitution, one base from the 3′-end to reduce primer dimer formation. Primer dimers forming in the first round of PCR are particularly problematic if not adequately removed prior to Illumina sequencing, due to the preferential clustering of short fragments containing the sequencing motifs. Here we present the methodology for interrogating 13 leukemia-associated mutation hotspots using multiplex PCR, an approach that was used to detect clonal haemopoiesis in people aged 17–98 years old [7]. Hematological malignancies develop through the serial acquisition of somatic mutations in a process that can take many years or even decades [8–10]. Also, it is clear that the presence of hemopoietic cells carrying leukemia-associated mutations is only followed by the onset of hematological malignancies in a minority of cases [11–15]. In order to understand the incidence and clonal dynamics of pre-leukemic clonal hemopoiesis, we applied the described methodology to ultra-deep sequencing of each hotspot [7].

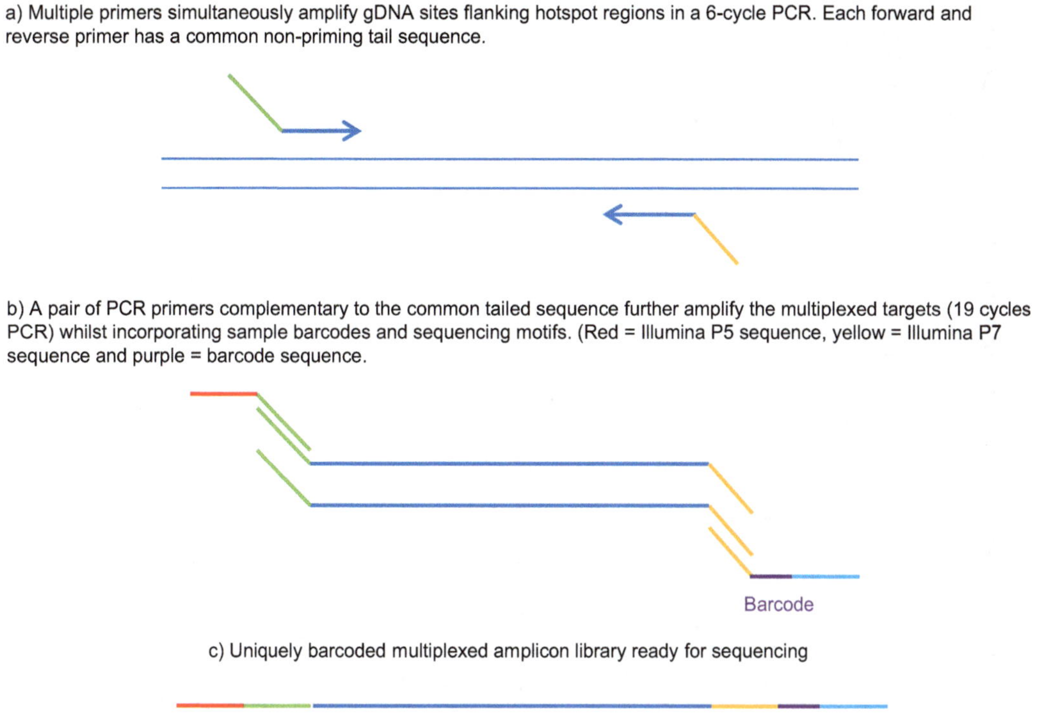

Fig. 1 Multiplex PCR sequencing-ready library workflow

2 Materials

The use of a high-fidelity polymerase capable of amplification of a range of GC contents is important in order to generate adequate coverage of all target hotspots at a representative allele fraction. In order to avoid false variant calls due to PCR product contamination of starting material, it is vital to have dedicated laboratory areas for each processing step, ideally as physically separate locations with their own dedicated equipment for DNA sample preparation, pre-PCR and post-PCR handling steps. All reagents and laboratory equipment associated with each step should be dedicated to a single area and not transferred between areas, other than in the workflow direction (i.e. sample prep to pre-PCR to post-PCR).

2.1 Oligonucleotides

1. Oligonucleotides: Oligonucleotides used in the MxPCR are listed in Table 1. Note that many manufacturers only offer the 2′-*O*-Methyl modification for synthesis scales of 100 nmole or greater (*see* **Note 1**). No further purification above standard desalting is necessary. Centrifuge and resuspend freeze-dried oligonucleotides to 500 μM in T0.1E buffer (10 mM Tris, 0.1 mM EDTA, pH 8.0) or similar. When not in use, primers should be stored at −20 °C. Before use, primers should be defrosted, pulse centrifuged and gently vortexed.

Table 1
Oligonucleotide sequences used in the MxPCR protocol. Volumes of each primer pair vary to enable even amplification of each PCR in the mutiplex [19]

Primer Name	Chromosome	Start Coordinate (GRCh37)	Sequence	Concentration (μM)	Volume (μL)
DNMT3A_p.R882_F	2	25,457,060	ACACTCTTTCCCTACACGACGCTCTTCC GATCTCCTCATGTTCTTGGTGTTTTmAT	500	5.29
DNMT3A_p.R882_R	2	25,457,302	TCGGCATTCCTGCTGAACCGCTCTTCCG ATCTTTTTCTCCCCCAGGGTMTTmUG	500	5.29
IDH1_p.R132H_1_F	2	209,112,927	ACACTCTTTCCCTACACGACGCTCTTCCG ATCTTAAATGTGTGTAAATATACAGTTmAT	500	4.80
IDH1_p.R132H_1_R	2	209,113,173	TCGGCATTCCTGCTGAACCGCTCTTC CGATCTRTTATCTGCAAAAATATCYCmCC	500	4.80
IDH2_p.R140_R172_F	15	90,631,745	ACACTCTTTCCCTACACGACGCTCTT CCGATCTAAGARGATGKCTAGGYGAGmGA	500	16.61
IDH2_p.R140_R172_R	15	90,631,986	TCGGCATTCCTGCTGAACCGCTCTTC CGATCTCTCAMAGAGTTCAAGCTGAmAG	500	16.61
SRSF2_p.P95_F	17	74,732,797	ACACTCTTTCCCTACACGACGCTCTTCC GATCTTGCTTCGCCGCGGACCTTTmGT	500	4.72
SRSF2_p.P95_R	17	74,733,038	TCGGCATTCCTGCTGAACCGCTCTTCC GATCTGAGGACGCTATGGATGCCAmUG	500	4.72
SF3B1_p.K700_F	2	198,266,642	ACACTCTTTCCCTACACGACGCTCTTCCG ATCTTAGTAATTTAGATTTATGTCGmCC	500	5.17
SF3B1_p.K700_R	2	198,266,886	TCGGCATTCCTGCTGAACCGCTCTTCCG ATCTGGCATAGTTAAAACCTGTGTmUT	500	5.17
SF3B1_p.K666_F	2	198,267,228	ACACTCTTTCCCTACACGACGCTCTTCCG ATCTACCCTGTCTCCTAAAGAAAAmAA	500	6.21

SF3B1_p.K666_R	2	198,267,470	TCGGCATTCCTGCTGAACCGCTCTTCCGA TCTTAGAGCTTTTGCTGTTGTAmGC	500	6.21
NPM1_p.L287fsX_F	5	170,837,352	ACACTCTTTCCCTACACGACGCTCTTCCGA TCTTGTTTGGAATTAAATTACATCTmGA	500	11.00
NPM1_p.L287fsX_R	5	170,837,602	TCGGCATTCCTGCTGAACCGCTCTTCCGAT CTAAAATTTTTTAACAAATTGTTTAAAmCT	500	11.00
JAK2V617_F	9	5,073,696	ACACTCTTTCCCTACACGACGCTCTTCCG ATCTAGTCTTTCTTTGAAGCAGCAmAG	500	3.36
JAK2V617_R	9	5,073,887	TCGGCATTCCTGCTGAACCGCTCTTCCG ATCTAGTTTACACTGACACCTAGCmUG	500	3.36
KIT_exon17_F	4	55,599,207	ACACTCTTTCCCTACACGACGCTCTTCC GATCTTGGTTTTCTTTTCTCCTCCAmAC	500	4.85
KIT_exon17_R	4	55,599,396	TCGGCATTCCTGCTGAACCGCTCTTCCG ATCTTCCTTTGCAGGACWGTCAmAG	500	4.85
KRAS_G12_F	12	25,398,214	ACACTCTTTCCCTACACGACGCTCTTC CGATCTTGTTSGATCATATTCRTCCAmCA	500	4.20
KRAS_G12_R	12	25,398,416	TCGGCATTCCTGCTGAACCGCTCTTCC GATCTAAGGTACTGGTGGAGTATTTmGA	500	4.20
602911NRAS_G12_F	1	115,258,606	ACACTCTTTCCCTACACGACGCTCTTCCG ATCTATGGGTAAAGATGATCCGACmAA	500	1.88
NRAS_G12_R	1	115,258,831	TCGGCATTCCTGCTGAACCGCTCTTCCG ATCTCGCCAATTAACCCTGATTACmUG	500	1.88
NRAS_Q61_F	1	115,256,340	ACACTCTTTCCCTACACGACGCTCTTCCGA TCTCCCTAGTGTGGTAACCTCATmUT	500	14.66
NRAS_Q61_R	1	115,256,573	TCGGCATTCCTGCTGAACCGCTCTTCCG ATCTAGATGGTGAAACCTGTTTGTmUR	500	14.66

(continued)

Table 1
(continued)

Primer Name	Chromosome	Start Coordinate (GRCh37)	Sequence	Concentration (μM)	Volume (μL)
FLT3_D835_F	13	28,592,585	ACACTCTTTCCCTACACGACGCTCTTCC GATCTTAGGAAATAGCAGCCTCACAmUT	500	3.60
FLT3_D835_R	13	28,592,819	TCGGCATTCCTGCTGAACCGCTCTTCCGA TCTGGTACCTCCTACTGAAGTTGmAG	500	3.60
				Total volume (μL)	172.69
				Effective concentration of each primer (μM)	14.48
				Dilution factor to 0.4 μM	36.19

2. Oligonucleotide pool: Pipette volumes of each primer according to Table 1 into a 1.5 mL Eppendorf to generate a pool containing an effective concentration of 14.48 μM of each primer. Briefly vortex and pulse centrifuge. Combine 10 μL of this pool with 351.9 μL EB (10 mM Tris–Cl, pH 8.5) for a working concentration of 0.4 μM of each primer. Store at −20 °C in aliquots to reduce the event of multiple freeze-thaw cycles.

2.2 PCR Components

1. Oligonucleotide pool (*see* Subheading 2.1).
2. T0.1E buffer (10 mM Tris, 0.1 mM EDTA, pH 8.0).
3. Elution buffer (10 mM Tris–Cl, pH 8.5) (Qiagen).
4. gDNA normalised to 10 μL at 20 ng/μL (*see* **Note 2**).
5. 96-well skirted PCR plate, 0.2 mL polypropylene or 0.2 mL PCR tubes.
6. KAPA HiFi HotStart ReadyMix 2X (Kapa Biosystems).
7. Nuclease-free water.
8. Reagent reservoir.
9. Adhesive PCR Plate Seals (such as Thermo Fisher AB-0558).
10. Vortexer.
11. Plate centrifuge: Ideally with a refrigeration capability.
12. PCR thermocycler with heated lid capability.
13. Second round PCR primers and PE1.0: Dispense 1 μL (at 10 μM) of each into a PCR plate. Make multiple copies of single use plates, seal and store at −20 °C. (*see* **Note 3** and ref. 16).
14. Multichannel pipette (8 or 12 channels).

2.3 PCR Product QC and Cleanup

1. Agencourt AMPure XP (Beckman Coulter, Inc).
2. Dynal magnetic rack suitable for 1.5 mL Eppendorf tubes.
3. 80% Ethanol: Combine 80 mL of absolute ethanol with 20 mL of water (*see* **Note 4**).
4. Elution buffer (10 mM Tris–Cl, pH 8.5) (Qiagen).
5. Agilent 2100 Bioanalyzer System (*see* **Note 5**).
6. Agilent DNA 1000 Kit.
7. Agilent High Sensitivity DNA Kit.
8. qPCR Instrument such as StepOne™ Real-Time PCR Systems (Applied Biosystems).
9. Kapa Library Quantification Kit for Illumina platforms.
10. Multichannel pipette (8 or 12 channels).

2.4 Illumina Miseq Sequencing

1. MiSeq Reagent Kit v2 (500 cycle).
2. Freshly diluted 0.2 N NaOH.

3. Long-reach pipette tip 100/200 μL
4. iPCRtag sequencing primer (PAGE purified): AAGAGCGGTTCAGCAGGAATGCCGAGACCGATCTC

3 Methods

3.1 PCR

Defrost all components at room temperature and place on ice prior to use.

1. Dispense 10 μL of gDNA (20 ng/μL) to 96-well PCR plate(s).
2. Prepare a PCR master mix sufficient for the number of samples (N) plus a 10% excess. Combine:

   1.1 × N × 12.5 μL KAPA HiFi HotStart ReadyMix.

   1.1 × N × 0.5 μL AML pool (0.4 μM).

   Vortex, pulse centrifuge and transfer to a reagent reservoir. Keep on ice until ready for use. With a multichannel P20 pipette, dispense 13 μL of master mix to each PCR plate well containing DNA. Apply an adhesive plate seal, taking care to apply sufficient pressure to seal all wells. Gently vortex and centrifuge at 1200 *g* for 1 min. If possible, set the centrifuge to 4 °C for **step 4**.
3. Transfer to a thermocycler and run the following program (with heated lid set to a constant 100 °C): 95 °C for 3 min, (98 °C for 20 s, 65 °C for 60 s, 60 °C for 60 s, 55 °C for 60 s, 50 °C for 60 s, 70 °C for 60 s) × 6 cycles. Hold at 4 °C.
4. Centrifuge at 1200 *g* for 1 min (ideally at 4 °C) and place on ice. Defrost and spin down a prealiquoted plate containing indexing primers and PE1.0 primers as prepared in Subheading 2.2, **step 11**. Place on ice.
5. Carefully remove seals from both plates, taking extra care not to splash any liquid—temporarily remove plates from the ice to facilitate the ease of this. Using a multichannel pipette and fresh tips for each sample, transfer the entire volume of PCR products, one row at a time, to the plate containing the second round primers. Keep both plates on ice throughout the transfer step (*see* **Note 6**).
6. Seal with a plate seal, taking care to apply sufficient pressure to ensure every well is sealed. Centrifuge at 1200 *g* for 1 min (ideally at 4 °C).
7. On ice, transfer the plate to a dedicated post-PCR thermocycler and run the following program (with heated lid set to a constant 100 °C): (98 °C for 20 s, 62 °C for 15 s, 72 °C for 30 s) × 19 cycles and 72 °C 60 s. Hold at 4 °C.

3.2 PCR Product QC, Pooling and Cleanup

1. Assess the PCR products by directly running a 12 sample subset on an Agilent Bioanalyzer using an Agilent DNA 1000 Kit (Fig. 2) (*see* **Note 7**).
2. Using a P10 multichannel pipette and fresh tips for each sample, take a 5 μL aliquot of each row, dispensing into a reagent reservoir in-between rows. Up to 384 samples may be pooled, each having a different barcode incorporated during the second PCR. With a single-channel P200 pipette set to 200 μL, thoroughly mix the pooled samples by aspirating and dispensing across the reservoir. Transfer pooled sample to a fresh 1.5 mL Eppendorf.
3. Alternatively, if only a few samples require pooling, combine in a 1.5 mL Eppendorf with a single-channel pipette.
4. Using a P100, accurately transfer 100 μL of pooled PCR sample into a labelled fresh 1.5 mL Eppendorf. If there is less than 100 μL of pooled amplicon, make up to volume with EB. Add exactly 55 μL of room temperature SPRI beads, briefly vortex to mix and pulse centrifuge to collect all liquid at the bottom of the tube without disturbing the bead suspension.
5. Incubate at room temperature for 5 min before transferring to a magnetic rack. Wait until supernatant is clear and all beads are collected at the side of the magnet before collecting ~155 μL

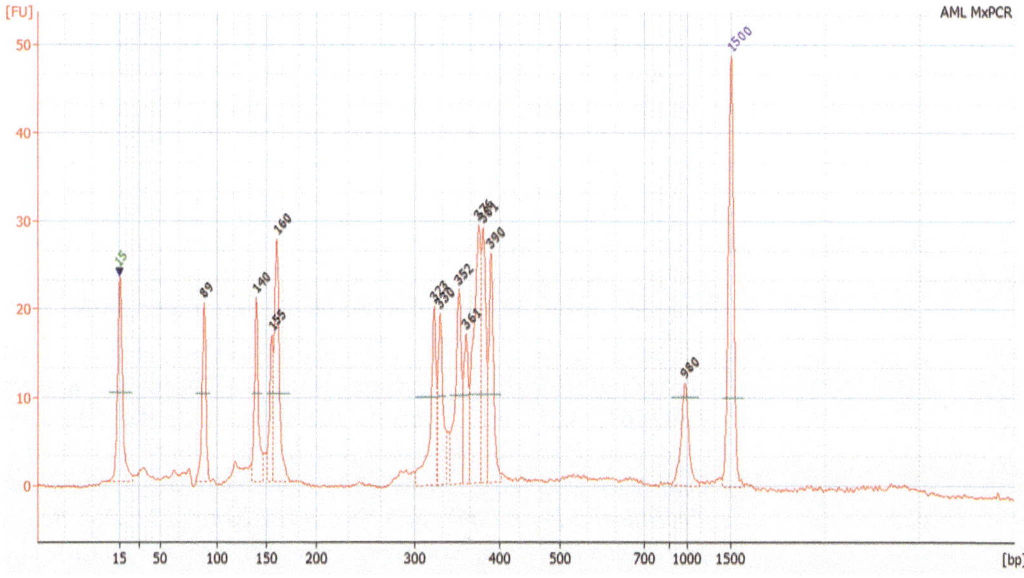

Fig. 2 A typical profile obtained of an AML MxPCR runs directly (without any Ampure SPRI purification) on an Agilent Bioanalyzer DNA1000 chip. Peaks <170 bp are due to unincorporated primers and primer dimers, peaks 300–400 bp are from on target products and a larger peak at ~950 bp is due to amplification across two adjacent products

supernatant and transferring to a labelled fresh 1.5 mL Eppendorf tube. (*see* **Note 8**).

6. Using a P20, add a further 20 μL of room temperature SPRI beads to the supernatant from **step 4**, vortex and pulse centrifuge.
7. Incubate at room temperature for 5 min before transferring to a magnetic rack. Once the supernatant is clear and all beads are captured on the side of the magnet, remove and discard the supernatant (*see* **Note 9**).
8. Wash by adding 700 μL of 80% ethanol, being careful not to disturb the beads captured on the magnet. After 30 s, remove and discard the ethanol. Repeat for a total of two washes.
9. Pulse centrifuge to draw residual ethanol to the bottom of the tube and remove with a P10 pipette. Air dry at room temperature for approximately 2 min, until beads have a "wet paint" appearance (*see* **Note 10**).
10. With a P20 pipette, re-suspend beads in 20 μl of EB and incubate off the magnet for 5 min to release the target product into solution.
11. Transfer to the magnetic rack. Once the supernatant is clear and beads are captured on the magnet, transfer supernatant containing the purified pool to a labelled fresh Eppendorf tube.
12. Make a 1 in 10 dilution of 1 μL of the purified pool for analysis with an Agilent Bioanalyzer High Sensitivity DNA Kit (Fig. 3) (*see* **Note 11**).
13. For accurate quantification, required to enable optimal cluster density during MiSeq sequencing, use a KAPA SYBR FAST qPCR complete kit or similar compatible with your qPCR instrument. Dilute library to 4 nM with EB, ready for Miseq sequencing.

3.3 Illumina Miseq Sequencing

1. Prepare 8 pM denatured libraries for loading onto the 500-cycle MiSeq cartridge according to "Preparing Libraries for Sequencing on the MiSeq®" (Illumina Part number 15039740).
2. Sequence as a 250, 11, 250 paired-end single-index read according to "MiSeq® System Guide" (Document number 15027617 v01) using default chemistry, with the following exception: *Pierce the foil seal at port 13 and, using a P100 with a long-reach pipette tip, remove 100 μL. Transfer to a clean 1.5 mL Eppendorf tube and spike in 3.5 μL of iPCRtag (100 μM). Briefly pipette mix and transfer the entire contents back into port 13.* The addition of the custom index sequencing primer into the default index sequencing primer cartridge location enables the standard "default" chemistry option to be selected on the MiSeq

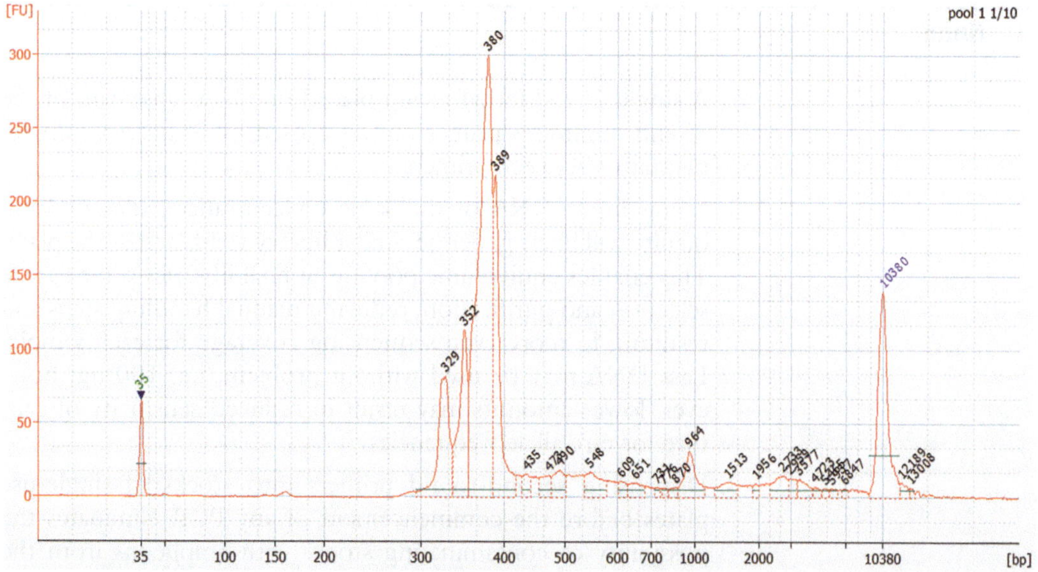

Fig. 3 A typical profile obtained of an Ampure SPRI size selected AML MxPCR, run on an Agilent Bioanalyzer High Sensitivity DNA chip. Note remaining peak at ~160 bp, a result of primer dimers between first-round genomic PCR primers. Due to their size, these will preferentially cluster during sequencing and result in data loss. Aim to remove all peak of this size by repeating a X0.75 SPRI until not visible by bioanalyzer analysis. A remaining peak at ~950 bp is not of concern

sample sheet. Only the complementary custom index primer will successfully anneal and extend during the index read.

3.4 Data Analysis

A number of different approaches can be used for data analysis, depending on the required sensitivity for variant allele detection. The method described here was used by McKerrell et al. [7] to reliably detect variant alleles with VAFs as low as 0.8% (0.008): Sequencing data are aligned to the human reference genome (hg19) using BWA. Subsequently, the SAMTOOLS pileup command is used to generate pileup files from the generated bam files (version 0.1.8; http://samtools.sourceforge.net [17]). The flexible in-house Perl script MIDAS generated by our group [18] was modified in order to interrogate only the hotspot nucleotide positions of interest on the pileup file, considering only those reads with a sequence quality higher than 25 and a mapping quality higher than 15. For each sample, the numbers of reads reporting the reference and variant alleles at each position were extracted. VAFs were derived by dividing the number of reads reporting the most frequent variant nucleotide to the total. In order to detect NPM1 mutations with high sensitivity, the bespoke tool described by McKerrell et al. can be used [7].

4 Notes

1. A single 2′-*O*-Methyl group placed one base upstream of the 3′-end minimises primer dimers caused by 3′-hetero complementarity between primers.
2. Using input DNA of the same concentration, quantity and quality will likely generate similar library yields across the plate. This enables equivolume pooling of final libraries prior to size selection and purification, reducing manual handling steps and resulting in more even sequencing coverage for each sample. Less DNA may be used without problem, i.e. 100 ng; however, lower amounts may result in reduced sensitivity of capture for rare allele frequencies.
3. Dispensing second-round primers into stocks of single-use plates before the commencement of any PCR eliminates the possibility of contaminating stocks with amplicons from the first PCR step. It also simplifies combining first-round products with second-round primers, reducing the potential for mispipetting and sample to sample mix-ups.
4. 80% ethanol is hygroscopic. When opened, overtime the ethanol will both evaporate and absorb water. Despite the % ethanol decreasing, the solution remains usable for at least 2 weeks, as 70% ethanol is also suitable for washing DNA-bound SPRI beads. Note that because of miscibility of ethanol with water, measuring 80 mL ethanol and 20 mL water separately, and then combining them will generate ~95 mL of 80% ethanol. Do not top up to 100 mL.
5. Alternative methods for evaluating the size range of amplicons may be used, such as agarose gel electrophoresis.
6. KAPA HiFi HotStart DNA Polymerase was activated in the first PCR and therefore should be kept on ice to inhibit any undesirable polymerase and exonuclease activity prior to the second round PCR.
7. Peaks between ~300 and 400 bp represent the desired (on-target) Illumina sequencing-ready amplicons. A larger peak at ~921 bp is the amplification across two adjacent products and does not require absolute removal prior to sequencing. Peaks around ~150 bp are a result of primer dimers formed in the first PCR cycles and must be removed prior to sequencing. These shorter products will preferentially cluster during MiSeq sequencing and may result in reduced sequencing quality and yield.
8. During the X0.55 Ampure SPRI incubation, a large proportion of products >500 bp will precipitate onto the magnetic beads, leaving smaller fragments in solution. By retaining the

supernatant for the addition of further Ampure SPRI beads, an upper size selection is performed in this step.

9. Adding an additional 20 μL of beads to the supernatant (~155 μL) from the previous step is equivalent to a X0.75 Ampure SPRI. Small primer dimers and unincorporated primers <170 bp will remain in the supernatant whilst desired amplicons precipitate onto the beads.
10. Excessive drying of beads at room temperature or on a heat block will make the DNA difficult to resuspend into elution buffer which may result in a reduced yield.
11. For optimal sequencing results, repeat X0.75 Ampure SPRI if a peak remains at ~160 bp.

References

1. Kozarewa I et al (2015) Overview of target enrichment strategies. In: Current protocols in molecular biology. Wiley, Hoboken
2. Nguyen-Dumont T et al (2013) A high-plex PCR approach for massively parallel sequencing. Biotechniques 55(2):69–74
3. Quail MA et al (2011) Optimal enzymes for amplifying sequencing libraries. Nat Methods 9:10–11
4. Quail MA et al (2014) SASI-Seq: sample assurance Spike-Ins, and highly differentiating 384 barcoding for Illumina sequencing. BMC Genomics 15(1):1–13
5. Shen Z et al (2010) MPprimer: a program for reliable multiplex PCR primer design. BMC Bioinformatics 11(1):1–7
6. Qu W, Zhang C (2015) Selecting specific PCR primers with MFEprimer. Methods Mol Biol 1275:201–213
7. McKerrell T et al (2015) Leukemia-associated somatic mutations drive distinct patterns of age-related clonal hemopoiesis. Cell Rep 10(8):1239–1245
8. Ford AM et al (1998) Fetal origins of the TEL-AML1 fusion gene in identical twins with leukemia. Proc Natl Acad Sci U S A 95(8):4584–4588
9. Kyle RA et al (2002) A long-term study of prognosis in monoclonal gammopathy of undetermined significance. N Engl J Med 346(8):564–569
10. Grove CS, Vassiliou GS (2014) Acute myeloid leukaemia: a paradigm for the clonal evolution of cancer? Dis Model Mech 7(8):941–951
11. Busque L et al (2012) Recurrent somatic TET2 mutations in normal elderly individuals with clonal hematopoiesis. Nat Genet 44(11): 1179–1181
12. Genovese G et al (2014) Clonal hematopoiesis and blood-cancer risk inferred from blood DNA sequence. N Engl J Med 371(26): 2477–2487
13. Jacobs KB et al (2012) Detectable clonal mosaicism and its relationship to aging and cancer. Nat Genet 44(6):651–658
14. Jaiswal S et al (2014) Age-related clonal hematopoiesis associated with adverse outcomes. N Engl J Med 371(26):2488–2498
15. Laurie CC et al (2012) Detectable clonal mosaicism from birth to old age and its relationship to cancer. Nat Genet 44(6): 642–650
16. Quail MA et al (2014) SASI-Seq: sample assurance Spike-Ins, and highly differentiating 384 barcoding for Illumina sequencing. BMC Genomics 15:110
17. Li H et al (2009) The sequence alignment/map format and SAMtools. Bioinformatics 25(16):2078–2079
18. Conte N et al (2013) Detailed molecular characterisation of acute myeloid leukaemia with a normal karyotype using targeted DNA capture. Leukemia 27(9):1820–1825
19. Nguyen-Dumont T et al (2013) Cross-platform compatibility of Hi-Plex, a streamlined approach for targeted massively parallel sequencing. Anal Biochem 442(2):127–129

Chapter 7

AMLprofiler: A Diagnostic and Prognostic Microarray for Acute Myeloid Leukemia

Marco Alessandrini, Sharon S. Kappala, and Michael S. Pepper

Abstract

Acute myeloid leukemia is characterized by the proliferation and accumulation of immature hematopoietic cells of the myeloid lineage in the bone marrow. The disease is typified by diverse genetic abnormalities and marked heterogeneity both with regard to response to treatment and survival. The AMLprofiler is a qualitative in vitro diagnostic microarray developed by SkylineDx for use with Affymetrix technology. The AMLprofiler makes use of RNA chemistry and incorporates seven separate assays based on three different technologies—cytogenetics, mutation, and expression analysis—to predict post-therapy survival rates in patients with acute myeloid leukemia. The assay has been validated for processing of bone marrow samples from which RNA is isolated within 48 h. The samples are subsequently processed using Affymetrix GeneChip reagent kits and analyzed on the Affymetrix GeneChip 3000Dx v2 system. The scanned AMLprofiler data is sent to a centralized server of SkylineDx via a secured Internet connection, and a diagnostic report is generated within 15 min. We have performed several AMLprofiler assays in our laboratory and found the data generated via this assay to be consistent with standard modalities.

Key words Acute myeloid leukemia, AMLprofiler, SkylineDx, Microarray

1 Introduction

In the United States of America alone, over 20,000 diagnoses and 10,000 deaths occur due to acute myeloid leukemia (AML) annually [1]. The disease is characterized by the proliferation and accumulation in the bone marrow of immature hematopoietic cells of myeloid lineage. AML is further typified by diverse genetic abnormalities and marked heterogeneity both with regard to response to treatment and survival.

Laboratory diagnosis of AML requires a multidisciplinary and often time-consuming approach, which encompasses a range of tests based on cell morphology, immunophenotyping, and specific genetic markers. The AMLprofiler is a microarray-based assay that utilizes RNA chemistry to detect specific chromosomal aberrations, mutations, and gene expression patterns relevant to the diagnosis and prognosis of AML. More specifically, the AMLprofiler

Paolo Fortina et al. (eds.), *Acute Myeloid Leukemia: Methods and Protocols*, Methods in Molecular Biology, vol. 1633, DOI 10.1007/978-1-4939-7142-8_7, © Springer Science+Business Media LLC 2017

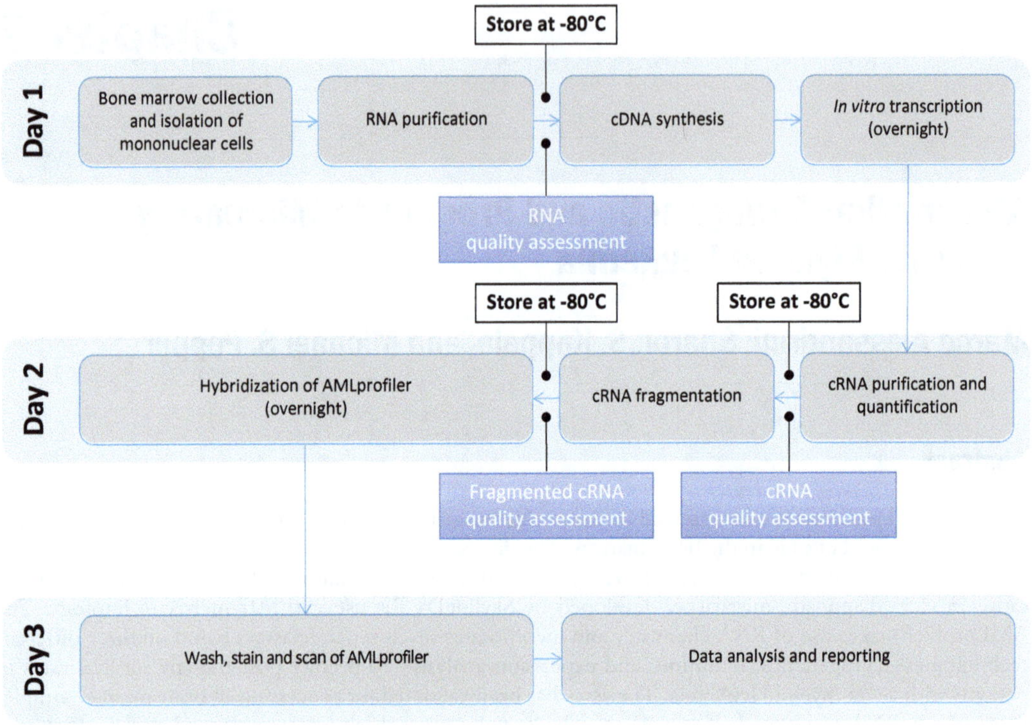

Fig. 1 Overview of methodology used for AMLprofiler analysis. Visual representation of the day-to-day processing of AMLprofiler microarrays. Adapted from [2]

replaces seven separate assays that are routinely used for the detection of favorable prognostic markers, including t(16;16)/inv.(16), t(8;21), t(15;17), CEBPA double mutations, NPM1 type A/B/D mutations, "low BAALC" expression, and expression of the "very poor" prognostic marker, EVI1.

The AMLprofiler assay is performed on the Affymetrix GeneChip 3000Dx v.2 system and is hence designed for in vitro diagnostic use. Following scanning of the AMLprofiler chip, data generated in the laboratory setting is automatically sent via a secured Internet connection to the centralized server of SkylineDx, and the diagnostic report is generated in under 15 min, thus making it a valuable and efficient tool for diagnostic purposes. The AMLprofiler workflow and methodology [2], as described in this chapter, are outlined broadly in Fig. 1.

2 Materials

2.1 Equipment

1. Affymetrix GeneChip 3000Dx v2 Instrument system, which includes an Affymetrix FS450Dx v2 Fluidics Station, Affymetrix GeneChip 3000Dx v2 Scanner, Affymetrix GeneChip Hybridization Oven 645, and an Affymetrix GeneChip 3000Dx v2 workstation with AMDS operating software.

2. Thermocycler (e.g., GeneAmp PCR System 9700, Thermo Fisher Scientific, USA).
3. Thermoblock (e.g., AccuBlock Digital Dry Bath, Labnet International, USA).
4. Vacuum concentrator (e.g., Savant SpeedVac, Thermo Fisher Scientific, USA).
5. Micro-centrifuge (for 0.2, 0.5, 0.6, and 1.5 mL tubes), capable of reaching 15,000 × *g* (e.g., Sorvall Legend Microcentrifuge, Thermo Fisher Scientific, USA).
6. Brayer or soft rubber microplate sealer (e.g., Mylar Plate Sealer, Thermo Fisher Scientific, USA).
7. Centrifuge with rotors/swing buckets for 15 mL tubes and 96-well plates (e.g., Heraeus Multifuge, Thermo Fisher Scientific, USA).
8. Vortex (e.g., Vortex Genie 2, Scientific Industries, USA).
9. Compression pad for thermocycling with 96-well PCR plates (e.g., Axygen, USA).
10. Benchtop cooler (−20 °C) (Thermo Fisher Scientific, USA).
11. Plastic rack for 96-well PCR plates.
12. Pipettes for volumes between 1 μL and 1000 μL.
13. Magnetic stand for 96-well plates.
14. Electrophoresis system for RNA/cRNA quality control (e.g., TapeStation 2200, Agilent Technologies, USA).
15. Spectrophotometric system for RNA/cRNA quality control (e.g., NanoDrop, Thermo Fisher Scientific, USA).

2.2 Reagents

1. Histopaque-1077 (Sigma-Aldrich, USA).
2. RNA isolation kit (AllPrep DNA/RNA Mini Kit, Qiagen, Germany).
3. Affymetrix GeneChip reagent kits (*see* Table 1).

2.3 Consumables

1. 96-well PCR plates (compatible for use with the sealing film and compression pad).
2. Aluminum adhesive foil for PCR or cold storage (in case PCR plates are used).
3. 96-well U-bottom plate compatible with the magnetic stand.
4. 0.2 mL, 0.5 mL, or 0.6 mL thin-walled PCR tubes.
5. Powder-free gloves.
6. Nuclease-free 1.5 mL nonstick tubes, without lid.
7. Nuclease-free 15 mL nonstick tubes.
8. Pipette tips with aerosol-resistant filters, RNase-free.

Table 1
Affymetrix reagent kits required for AMLprofiler analysis

Affymetrix kit	Components
GeneChip® 3′ IVT PLUS Reagent Kit (P/N 902416)	3′ IVT PLUS Amplification Kit—Module 1 1. 3′ first-strand enzyme 2. 3′ first-strand buffer 3. 3′ second-strand enzyme 4. 3′ second-strand buffer 5. 3′ IVT enzyme 6. 3′ IVT buffer 7. 3′ IVT biotin label 8. Nuclease-free water 3′ IVT PLUS Amplification Kit—Module 2 9. Purification beads 10. 3′ fragmentation buffer GeneChip® Hybridization Control Kit 11. 20× hybridization controls 12. 3 nM control Oligo B2
GeneChip® Hybridization, Wash, and Stain Kit (P/N 900720 Kit)	Hybridization module 13. Pre-hybridization mix 14. 2× hybridization mix 15. DMSO 16. Nuclease-free water Stain module 17. Stain cocktail 1 18. Stain cocktail 2 19. Array holding buffer Wash buffers 20. Wash buffer A 21. Wash buffer B

9. Crushed ice.
10. Tough-spots (3/8 in.).
11. RNase-free micro-centrifuge tubes (sterile, amber, 1.5 mL).
12. RNase-free micro-centrifuge tubes (sterile, 1.5 mL).

2.4 Chemicals

1. Deionized water.
2. Certified nuclease-free water.
3. 100% ethanol for molecular biology.

3 Methods

The AMLprofiler workflow includes many steps and typically takes place over a period of 3 days (Fig. 1). Please refer to **Notes 1–4** for general principles to adhere to throughout the workflow. Each step is described in detail in the subsections to follow.

3.1 Bone Marrow Collection and Isolation of Mononuclear Cells

It is recommended that a minimum of 1 mL bone marrow aspirate is collected in either an EDTA (ethylenediaminetetraacetic acid) or heparin tube. This is sampled by the clinician according to standard operating procedures used for diagnostics and transported to the laboratory at ambient temperature, i.e., the collected sample should not be refrigerated, frozen, or exposed to temperatures exceeding 37 °C (*see* **Note 5**).

Isolation of mononuclear cells from collected bone marrow samples should be performed within 48 h of collection in order to allow for enrichment of the blast cells. The number of white blood cells is usually determined prior to RNA isolation. It is recommended that a WBC count of at least 5×10^6 is required to proceed to further processing.

Several approaches can be used for the enrichment of blasts, but the most commonly used method is a manual protocol involving a Ficoll-based separation, which is included as a gold standard in many diagnostic laboratories. The step-by-step protocol followed in our laboratory is described below:

1. Add 2 mL of Histopaque-1077 to a 15 mL conical centrifuge tube, and allow for up to 30 min to settle at room temperature (*see* **Note 6**).
2. Dilute the 1 mL of bone marrow aspirate with 3 mL of phosphate-buffered saline (PBS).
3. Gently layer the above 4 mL of diluted bone marrow on top of the Histopaque-1077.
4. Centrifuge for 20 min at 300 × *g* at room temperature.
5. Carefully remove the white intermediate layer containing the enriched blasts with a pipette, and transfer it to a new 15 mL conical centrifuge tube.
6. Wash the cells by filling the tube to 15 mL with PBS, resuspend gently, and centrifuge for 5 min at 300 × *g*.
7. Remove the PBS without disturbing the pellet at the bottom of the tube, and resuspend the washed pellet in 1 mL PBS before transferring to a 1.5 mL microfuge tube.

3.2 RNA Purification and Quality Assessment

Isolate mRNA (messenger RNA) from the enriched blast cells according to the laboratory's current procedure. MicroRNA extraction procedures should not be used.

3.2.1 Quality Assessment of Purified mRNA

Once isolated, the RNA should be assessed for both concentration and integrity/quality. The former should be performed via a spectrophotometric method. RNA concentration (in ng/μL) should be determined by 260 nm absorbance. The purity of the RNA is determined by the 260 nm (A260) and 280 nm (A280) ratio (A260/A280). The RNA purity should preferably be between ratios of 1.6 and 2.0.

RNA quality is an important parameter to be assessed in any microarray protocol. This is typically determined via an electrophoretic method. For the AMLprofiler assay, quality analysis is performed at three definitive points during the protocol, namely, (1) after RNA isolation from mononuclear cells, (2) after the in vitro transcription reaction, and (3) after fragmentation of cRNA (*see* Fig. 1).

To prepare RNA samples for analysis, the recommended protocol provided by the manufacturer is usually followed depending on the type of instrument used. A molecular ladder that allows for fragments of between 200 and 4000 nucleotides to be viewed should be included in every assay run. Once completed, and confirmation is obtained that the assay was adequately performed (i.e., the ladder is comparable to its specifications, and the markers indicate completeness of electrophoresis), the quality of the isolated mRNA can be assessed according to the expected electrophoretic profile illustrated in Fig. 2.

It is critical that only good quality RNA be used for the AMLprofiler analysis, which will avoid any downstream complications and also possible failure of the assay. One must proceed to cDNA synthesis only when the recommended criteria are met for RNA concentration, purity, and integrity.

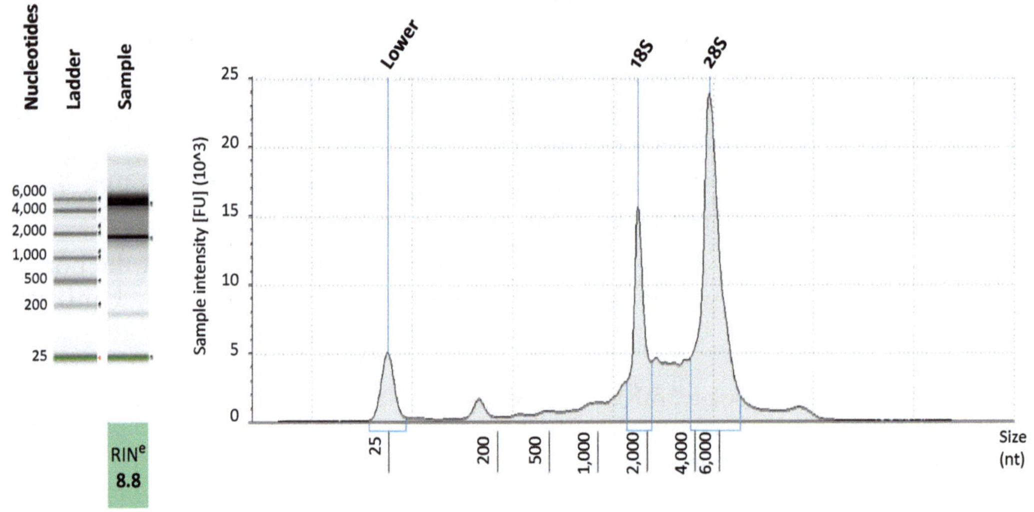

Fig. 2 Expected electrophoretic profile for isolated RNA. RNA purified from mononuclear cells, demonstrating the presence of 18S and 28S ribosomal RNA (rRNA) fragments, as generated in our laboratory using the TapeStation 2200 (Agilent Technologies). Electrophoretic peaks of 28S fragments should be at least 1.9 times that of the 18S peak. This is also reflected in the RNA integrity number (RIN) which is greater than 8.0 and hence indicative of good quality RNA. The "lower" fragment at 25 nucleotides is included in every assay for alignment purposes

3.3 cDNA Synthesis

The synthesis of complementary DNA (cDNA) is performed in two reactions, namely, first-strand and second-strand cDNA syntheses. If more than one sample is assayed at a time, reactions can be performed in a 96-well PCR plate or in individual nuclease-free PCR tubes.

The starting RNA concentration required for the cDNA synthesis reaction is 100 ng/μL, which is to be prepared to a final volume of 6 μL. An algorithm illustrating a simplified approach to achieve this is presented in Fig. 3.

3.3.1 First-Strand cDNA Synthesis

Reagents for the first-strand cDNA synthesis reaction should be prepared on ice, and if more than one sample is being analyzed at a time, it is recommended that a master mix be prepared in a nuclease-free nonstick tube. Reaction contents and reagent volumes for the first-strand cDNA synthesis are listed in Table 2.

1. Once thawed, mix the first-strand buffer by vortexing briefly, and then pulse-spin to collect the contents at the bottom of the tube.
2. Pulse-spin the first-strand enzyme and place in a benchtop cooler (or on ice).
3. Prepare the master mix (Mix1) according to the number of samples being assayed. As a general rule, volumes of 1.1 times of each reagent listed in Table 2 should be added for the master mix.
4. Resuspend the final master mix and pulse-spin to collect contents at the bottom of the tube.
5. Immediately transfer 5 μL of Mix1 to the bottom of the appropriate wells of the 96-well PCR plate or PCR tubes, and keep on ice.

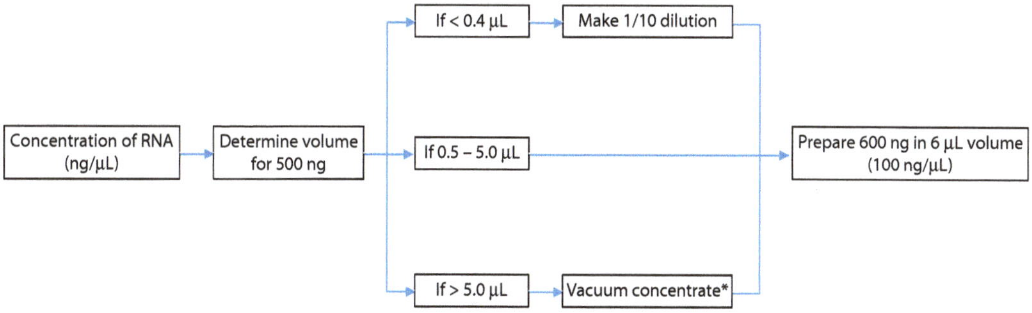

Fig. 3 Algorithm for preparation of RNA concentration for cDNA synthesis. (*asterisk*) Vacuum concentrate at 30 °C, while regularly checking the volume, evaporate to approximately 7 μL. In case the sample is (or becomes) <7 μL, add nuclease-free water to a total volume of 7 μL. Check the RNA concentration (ng/μL) and the purity again using a spectrophotometric method. The undiluted RNA concentration should be ≥100 ng/μL. The RNA purity should preferably be between 1.6 and 2.0

Table 2
Reagents and volumes for the first-strand synthesis

Pipetting sequence	Reagent	Volume per reaction (μL)
1	First-strand buffer	4
2	First-strand enzyme	1
	Total volume	**5**

If preparing a master mix, use 1.1 times the reagent volumes listed in the table

Table 3
Temperature cycling for the first-strand cDNA synthesis

Method and program name	Temperatures and duration
First-strand cDNA synthesis—"first strand"	42 °C for 2 h, followed by 4 °C for 10 min, and 4 °C hold

6. While keeping on ice, add 5 μL (500 ng) of the RNA sample to the 5 μL of Mix1 in the appropriate wells of the 96-well plate or nuclease-free PCR tubes. Gently mix by resuspending three times.
7. Close the tubes or seal the PCR plate with aluminum adhesive foil using a brayer.
8. Pulse-spin the final reaction contents if using PCR tubes. If using 96-well PCR plates, centrifuge 300 × *g* in a centrifuge with buckets for 96-well plates for no more than 10 s at room temperature to collect the solution at the bottom of the wells.
9. Place the PCR tubes or 96-well PCR plate in a thermocycler and run the "first-strand" program provided in Table 3. Perform reaction with the lid of the thermocycler closed (105 °C if it can be programmed), and enter a total volume of 10 μL if required for the thermocycler.
10. To prepare for the second-strand synthesis reaction, remove the second-strand buffer from its storage location, and place on ice to allow it to thaw.
11. Remove the PCR tubes or 96-well plate from the thermocycler after at least 2 min but within 10 min of completion of the 42 °C incubation.
12. Pulse-spin the PCR tubes or centrifuge the 96-well PCR plates for no more than 10 s at 300 × *g* to collect the contents at the bottom of the wells.
13. Immediately place on ice and proceed to the second-strand cDNA synthesis.

3.3.2 Second-Strand cDNA Synthesis

The second-strand synthesis reaction should be initiated immediately, since holding the first-strand cDNA synthesis reaction for longer than 10 min may significantly reduce copy RNA (cRNA) yield.

1. Pre-cool the thermocycler block to 16 °C.
2. Briefly vortex and pulse-spin the second-strand buffer and keep on ice.
3. Pulse-spin the second-strand enzyme and place in a benchtop cooler (or on ice).
4. If assaying more than one sample at a time, prepare the second-strand master mix (Mix2) according to contents listed in Table 4.
5. Vortex the reaction or master mix thoroughly and pulse-spin to collect the contents at the bottom of the tube.
6. Ensure that the PCR tubes or 96-well PCR plate have been cooled on ice for at least 2 min before adding Mix2.
7. Transfer 20 μL of Mix2 to the side wall of each PCR tube or appropriate wells of the 96-well plate containing the 10 μL of first-strand reaction. Mix by resuspending three times.
8. Close the PCR tubes properly or cover the 96-well plate with a new aluminum foil cover and carefully seal with a brayer.
9. Pulse-spin the final reaction contents if using PCR tubes. If using 96-well PCR plates, centrifuge 300 × *g* in a centrifuge with buckets for 96-well plates for no more than 10 s at room temperature to collect the solution at the bottom of the wells.
10. Place the PCR tubes or 96-well PCR plate in a thermocycler and run the "second-strand" program provided in Table 5. Perform reaction **without closing the lid** of the thermocycler, and enter a total volume of 30 μL if required for the thermocycler.

Table 4
Reagents and volumes for the second-strand synthesis

Pipetting sequence	Reagent	Volume per reaction (μL)
1	Nuclease-free water	13
2	Second-strand buffer	5
3	Second-strand enzyme	2
	Total volume	**20**

If preparing a master mix, use 1.1 times the reagent volumes listed in the table

Table 5
Temperature cycling for the second-strand cDNA synthesis

Method and program name	Temperatures and duration
Second-strand cDNA synthesis—"second strand"	16 °C for 1 h, followed by 65 °C for 10 min, 4 °C for 10 min, and 4 °C hold

11. To prepare for the in vitro transcription (IVT) reaction, place the IVT buffer on ice and the RNA biotin label at room temperature.
12. Remove the plate from the thermocycler following the 65 °C incubation, after at least 2 min and within 10 min at 4 °C.
13. Pulse-spin the PCR tubes or centrifuge the 96-well PCR plates for no more than 10 s at 300 × *g* to collect the contents at the bottom of the wells.
14. Proceed immediately to the in vitro transcription reaction.

3.4 In Vitro Transcription

In the in vitro transcription reaction, biotinylated cRNA is synthesized.

1. Remove the IVT enzyme from its storage location and place in a benchtop cooler (or on ice).
2. Once the IVT buffer is thawed completely on ice, place it at room temperature for at least 10 min before proceeding with the reaction. Vortex briefly and pulse-spin to collect the buffer at the bottom of the tube.
3. Prepare the IVT reaction at room temperature, and if assaying more than one sample at a time, prepare the IVT master mix (Mix3) according to the contents listed in Table 6.
4. Vortex thoroughly and collect the reagents or Mix3 at the bottom by pulse-spinning.
5. After at least 5 min at room temperature, open the PCR tube(s) or carefully remove the aluminum adhesive foil from the PCR plate containing the cDNA, and add 30 μL of Mix3 to the side walls. Mix directly by pipetting up and down three times.
6. Close the PCR tubes properly or cover the 96-well plate with a new aluminum foil cover and carefully seal with a brayer.
7. Pulse-spin the final reaction contents if using PCR tubes. If using 96-well PCR plates, centrifuge at 300 × *g* in a centrifuge with buckets for 96-well plates for no more than 10 s at room temperature to collect the solution at the bottom of the wells.
8. Place in a thermocycler and run the "IVT" program provided in Table 7. Perform reaction with the lid of the thermocycler

Table 6
Reagents and volumes for in vitro transcription

Pipetting sequence	Reagent	Volume per reaction (μL)
1	IVT biotin label	4
2	IVT buffer	20
3	IVT enzyme	6
	Total volume	**30**

If preparing a master mix, use 1.1 times the reagent volumes listed in the table

Table 7
Temperature cycling for in vitro transcription

Method and program name	Temperatures and duration
In vitro transcription—"IVT"	40 °C for 4 h, followed by a 4 °C hold

Program can run overnight and samples removed within 20 h of starting the IVT reaction

closed (105 °C if it can be programmed), and enter a total volume of 60 μL if required for the thermocycler.

9. After no longer than 20 h from starting the IVT reaction, remove the PCR tubes or 96-well PCR plate from the thermocycler.
10. Pulse-spin the PCR tubes or centrifuge the 96-well PCR plates for no more 10 s at 300 × *g* to collect the contents at the bottom of the wells.
11. Place on ice and proceed to purification of the labeled cRNA.

3.5 cRNA Purification and Quantification

Purification of cRNA is performed by means of a magnetic bead separation technique, following which the purified cRNA is quantified to determine the total amount. A detailed outline of the procedure is provided below, which is performed at room temperature.

3.5.1 cRNA Purification

1. Aliquot 50 μL per sample of nuclease-free water into a nuclease-free 1.5 mL tube.
2. Preheat the nuclease-free water at 65 °C for at least 10 min in a heating block or incubator.
3. Prepare fresh dilutions of 80% ethanol wash solution each time from 100% ethanol (molecular biology grade or equivalent) and nuclease-free water. A total of 650 μL for each reaction should be prepared.

4. Open the PCR tubes or remove the aluminum foil from the 96-well plate containing the cRNA.
5. Mix the purification beads container by briefly vortexing.
6. Pipette the magnetic bead suspension up and down three times, and then add 100 μL into each 60 μL IVT reaction mixture. Resuspend gently and transfer the samples to a U-bottom 96-well plate.
7. Mix well by pipetting up and down ten times, and incubate for 10 min at room temperature.
8. Place the U-bottom plate on a magnetic stand to capture the purification beads, and allow the beads to pellet for 5–10 min until the solution is clear (*see* **Note 7**).
9. Keep the plate on the magnetic stand, and carefully aspirate and discard the supernatant without disturbing the beads.
10. Mix the 80% ethanol wash solution by inversion, and while keeping the plate on the magnetic stand, wash each sample with 80% ethanol two times as follows:
    (a) Take 200 μL of 80% ethanol wash solution and add to the side wall of each sample well without disturbing the beads. Incubate for 30–50 s at room temperature.
    (b) Slowly aspirate and discard the supernatant without disturbing the beads.
11. Repeat these wash steps twice for a total of three washes. For the last wash, ensure that all the supernatant is removed without disturbing the beads.
12. Air-dry the plate for approximately 5 min while keeping the plate on the magnetic stand until no liquid is visible and the pellet appears shiny. Do not cover the plate and do not over dry the beads. An overdried pellet is recognizable by a dull appearance and apparent "surface cracks." This will reduce elution efficiency.
13. Remove the plate from the magnetic stand.
14. Remove the nuclease-free water from the 65 °C heat block. Aspirate 27 μL and discard. Aspirate 27 μL per sample and add to each sample well. Do not use the last 27 μL of the nuclease-free water.
15. Incubate for 1 min on the lab bench at room temperature, and then mix well by pipetting up and down approximately ten times.
16. Check that the pellet of beads is fully dispersed. If the pellet is not fully dispersed, pipette up and down ten times to fully disrupt the pellet.

17. Move the plate to the magnetic stand again and allow beads to settle for approximately 5 min. The solution must be clear and all the beads pelleted against the magnet.
18. Only once the solution is transparent and the beads have settled, very carefully remove the supernatant without disturbing the pellet. Transfer the supernatant containing the eluted cRNA to a new 96-well plate or individual tubes while measuring the elution volumes for each sample. This can be performed easily by aspirating decreasing volumes until the elution volume is established.
19. Immediately proceed to measure the cRNA concentration.

3.5.2 cRNA Quantification

1. Make a 1/10 dilution of the cRNA with nuclease-free water in a new PCR tube.
2. Determine the concentration in ng/μL using a spectrophotometric method.
3. The A260/A280 ratio is also to be recorded in order to determine the purity of the cRNA product. This ratio should preferably be between 2.03 and 2.07.
4. Calculate the cRNA yield from the concentration based on the following equation:

$$\left(\left[\frac{\text{Conc. of cRNA in } \frac{\text{ng}}{\mu\text{L}}}{1000}\right] \times x(\mu\text{L}) \times 10\right) = \text{cRNA yield}(\mu g)$$

"x" is derived from the volume of eluted cRNA collected in Subheading 3.5.1.

5. The cRNA yield should be ≥12.7 μg. If less, do not proceed further with sample processing (*see* **Note 8**).
6. An aliquot of 1.3 μL of the diluted cRNA sample(s) should be stored for quality analysis by means of an electrophoretic method (*see* **Note 8**).
7. Proceed immediately to cRNA fragmentation or store the cRNA sample at −20 °C for intermediate storage or −80 °C for long-term storage.

3.6 cRNA Fragmentation and Quality Assessment

Fragmentation of the cRNA is the final step in preparing the sample for hybridization to the AMLprofiler microarrays. Efficient fragmentation (and confirmation thereof) is an important aspect that contributes to the success of hybridization.

1. Calculate the Volume of Undiluted cRNA Sample that Contains 7.5 μg cRNA According to the Following Equation

$$\frac{7.5\mu g}{\text{cRNA yield in}\mu g / x\mu L} = y\text{in}\mu L$$

"x" is the volume of eluted cRNA collected in Subsection 3.5.1, while "y" represents the volume required to obtain 7.5 µg cRNA.

2. Prepare the fragmentation reaction for each sample in a 0.5 mL PCR tube, and label each tube with the respective sample ID.
3. Prepare the fragmentation reaction on ice and according to the contents in Table 8.
4. Mix each tube thoroughly by vortexing, and pulse-spin to collect the fragmentation reaction at the bottom of the tube.
5. Place in a thermocycler and run the "Fragmentation" program provided in Table 9. Perform reaction with the lid of the thermocycler closed (105 °C if it can be programmed), and enter a total volume of 20 µL if required for the thermocycler.
6. Remove the plate from the thermocycler after at least 2 min at 4 °C, but within 10 min of completion of the 94 °C incubation.
7. Pulse-spin the fragmented cRNA to collect the contents at the bottom of the tube, and place the samples on ice.

Table 8
Reagents and volumes for cRNA fragmentation

Pipetting sequence	Reagent	Volume per reaction (µL)
1	cRNA (7.5 µg)	*y*
2	Nuclease-free water	16-*y*
3	3′ fragmentation buffer	4
	Total volume	**20**

If preparing a master mix, use 1.1 times the reagent volumes listed in the table

Table 9
Temperature cycling for cRNA fragmentation

Method and program name	Temperatures and duration
cRNA fragmentation—"Fragmentation"	94 °C for 35 min, followed by 4 °C for 10 min and a 4 °C hold

8. Aliquot 1.3 μL of the fragmented cRNA sample(s) into separate PCR tubes or a 96-well plate, and proceed to quality analysis by means of an electrophoretic method.
9. The fragmented cRNA can be stored at −20 °C (intermediate storage) or at −80 °C for long term.

3.6.1 Quality Assessment of cRNA and Fragmented cRNA

Quality assessment of intact and fragmented cRNA is performed via an electrophoretic method. Following the recommended procedures and confirming that the assay was adequately performed (i.e., the ladder is comparable to its specifications, and the markers indicate completeness of electrophoresis), the quality of the RNA can be assessed according to the expected electrophoretic profile illustrated in Fig. 4.

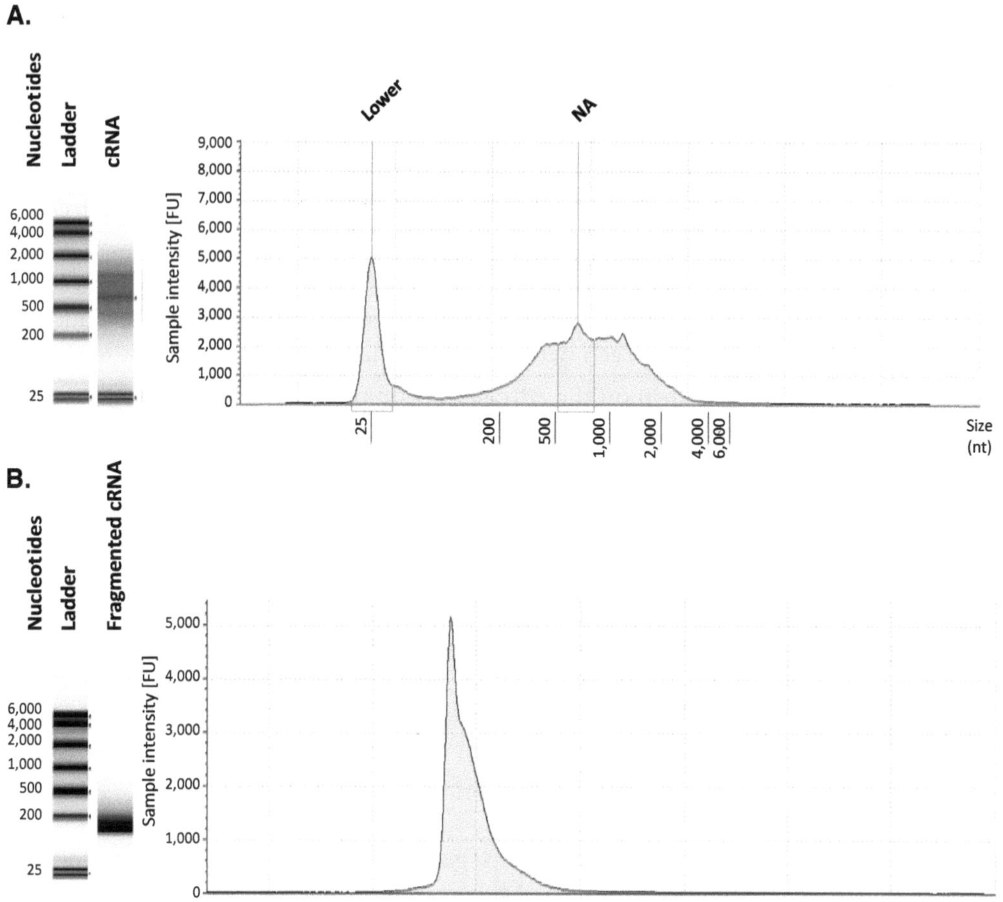

Fig. 4 Expected electrophoretic results for intact and fragmented cRNA. (**a**) Electrophoretic profile expected after cDNA synthesis and in vitro transcription, as generated in our laboratory using the TapeStation 2200 (Agilent Technologies). The gel smear reflects a broad range of cDNA amplification and conversion to cRNA. Occasionally distinct fragments are visible around 1000 nucleotides. This has no impact as long as a "smear" between 200 and 4000 nucleotides is still present. (**b**) Fragmented cRNA is typically observed as an intense range of fragments between 50 and 150 nucleotides

If the cRNA and fragmented cRNA meet the expected quality criteria and reflect similar electrophoretic profiles as demonstrated in Fig. 4, then proceed to hybridization of the AMLprofiler.

3.7 Hybridization of AMLprofiler Microarrays

The most important step in the processing of the AMLprofiler involves hybridization of the fragmented cRNA to the AMLprofiler chips. In the hybridization steps of the protocol, the fragmented cRNA is hybridized to the AMLprofiler microarrays. Details for preparation of the hybridization cocktail, pre-hybridization of AMLprofilers, and hybridization of the arrays are described below.

3.7.1 Preparation for Hybridization

1. Remove the AMLprofiler microarray from the refrigerator, verify that the pouch is still intact (otherwise take a new array), and allow it to equilibrate (unopened) to room temperature for at least 30 min. This is very important as the rubber septa may be prone to cracking, and hence leaking might occur if used cold.
2. Remove the Oligo B2, 20× hybridization control, 2× hybridization mix, DMSO, and pre-hybridization buffer from their respective storage conditions, and allow them to thaw at room temperature.
3. Turn on the hybridization oven, set the temperature to 45 °C, and set the rotation speed to 60 rpm.
4. Once the AMLprofiler array(s) have equilibrated to room temperature (after 30 min), remove them from the pouch and label each with the sample numbers to be assayed.
5. Turn on the Affymetrix computer and login.
6. Click on the **Active Worklist** button on the left panel and then on **Create** to create a new test request. Enter a **Specimen ID** and select the AMLprofiler **Assay Name** for each sample to be assayed, and click on **Submit**.
7. Navigate to the **Registration** page (button on the left panel). Click on the hyperlinked specimen ID, and enter the sample particulars in the pop-up screen. **Save and Close** and scan the corresponding AMLprofiler microarray barcode with the Affymetrix barcode scanner. Repeat this for each sample to be assayed, and click on the **Complete Step** button.
8. Proceed to pre-hybridization.

3.7.2 Pre-hybridization

1. Insert a pipette tip (generally a 20 μL tip) gently into the upper right septum of the array until you feel it penetrate the rubber septum (*see* Fig. 5). This allows for venting of the array.
2. Hold the array up vertically in the orientation shown in Fig. 5.
3. Wet the array with 80 μL of pre-hybridization mix by filling it through the bottom left septum of the array. Also gently penetrate the rubber septum first before dispensing the pre-hybridization mix.

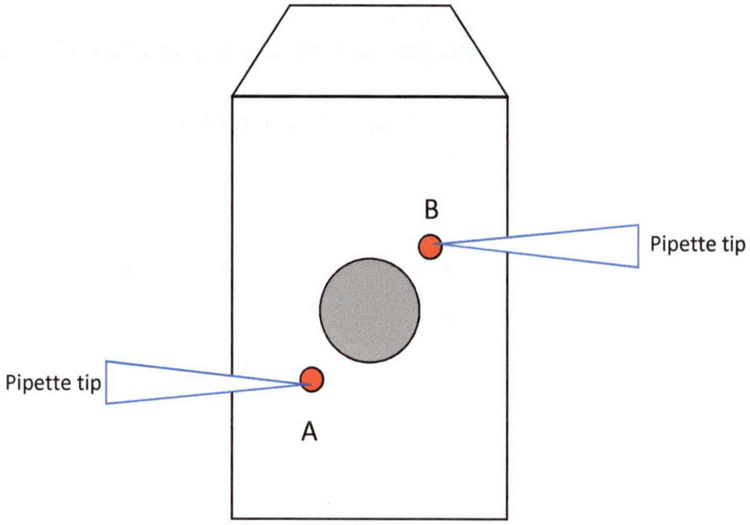

Fig. 5 Adding and removing fluids to the AMLprofiler microarray. Image adapted from [2]

Table 10
Preheating of 20× hybridization control

Method and program name	Temperatures and duration
Pre-hybridization—"Pre-hyb"	65 °C for 5 min

4. Remove the pipette tip from the upper right septum of the array, and incubate the array in the hybridization oven for 10–30 min at 45 °C and 60 rpm rotation.

3.7.3 Hybridization

1. Once all reagents are thawed to room temperature, vortex briefly (2 s at 80 × *g*), and pulse-spin to collect them at the bottom of their respective tubes.
2. Preheat an aliquot of 5.6 μL per microarray of the 20× hybridization control at 65 °C for 5 min on a thermocycler according to the program in Table 10.
3. Prepare the hybridization reaction mix at room temperature according to the reagents listed in Table 11, and if multiple samples are being assayed at the same time, prepare a master mix (Mix4) in a nuclease-free 1.5 mL microfuge tube.
4. Mix thoroughly by vortexing (2 s at 80 × *g*), and pulse-spin to collect the contents at the bottom of the tube(s).
5. Aliquot 13.3 μL of the fragmented cRNA sample(s) into new nuclease-free PCR tube(s).

Table 11
Reagents and volumes for preparation of the hybridization reaction (Mix4)

Pipetting sequence	Reagent	Volume per reaction (μL)
1	Oligonucleotide B2	1.7
2	20× hybridization controls	5
3	2× hybridization mix	50
4	DMSO	10
5	Nuclease-free water	20
	Total volume	**86.7**

If preparing a master mix, use 1.1 times the reagent volumes listed in the table

Table 12
Reagents and volumes for preparation of the hybridization cocktail

Pipetting sequence	Reagent	Volume per reaction (μL)
1	Fragmented cRNA (5 μg)*	13.3
5	Hybridization mix (Mix4)	86.7
	Total volume	**100**

*cRNA is labeled and the equivalent of 5 μg is used, based on the standardization performed under Subheading 3.6

Table 13
Heating of the hybridization cocktail

Method and program name	Temperatures and duration
Hybridization cocktail—"hybcocktail"	99 °C for 5 min, followed by 45 °C for 5 min

6. Add 86.7 μL of the hybridization reaction mix (Mix4) to the fragmented cRNA to prepare the hybridization cocktail (*see* Table 12).
7. Mix thoroughly by vortexing (2 s at 80 × *g*), and pulse-spin to collect the contents at the bottom of the tube.
8. Place the hybridization cocktail in the thermocycler and run the "hybcocktail" program provided in Table 13.
9. Centrifuge the hybridization cocktail at 13,000 × *g* for 5 min at room temperature.

10. Remove the pre-hybridized AMLprofiler array(s) from the hybridization oven.
11. Insert a pipette tip into the upper right septum to vent the array (Fig. 5).
12. Hold the array up vertically and remove the pre-hybridization mix with a 200 μL pipette tip via the bottom left septum and discard it.
13. Fill the AMLprofiler array(s) with 80 μL (all but the insoluble matter on the bottom) of the matching hybridization cocktail(s).
14. Store the remainder of the cocktail (~20 μL) at −20 °C for intermediate (overnight) storage or at −80 °C for long-term storage.
15. Close both of the septa of the AMLprofiler array with tough-spot stickers, and place the AMLprofiler arrays(s) back into the hybridization oven.
16. Login to the Affymetrix computer and navigate to the **Hybridization Oven** menu (on left-hand side panel). Highlight the sample(s) to be hybridized and click on **Start**.
17. Hybridization of the AMLprofilers will initiate, and the program will run overnight for 17 ± 1 h at 45 °C and 60 rpm in the hybridization oven.

3.8 Washing, Staining, and Scanning AMLprofiler Arrays

Prior to initiating the following steps, ensure that the Affymetrix Fluidics Station is in good order and adequately cleaned (*see* **Note 9**).

3.8.1 Priming of the Affymetrix Fluidics Station

1. Remove buffer A and buffer B from the refrigerator and allow them to equilibrate to room temperature (approximately 1 h or the previous evening).
2. Connect bottles with at least 250 mL of buffers A and B, and deionized (DI) water to the Fluidics Station, as indicated on the right-hand side of the instrument.
3. Load three empty 1.5 mL microfuge tubes in the sample holders of each module to be primed.
4. Login on the Affymetrix computer and click on the **Fluidics** icon button on the left panel.
5. Click on the **Station Setup** button.
6. Select the **Station #**, the **Assay**, and the **Modules** to be primed (i.e., only those to be used in the AMLprofiler processing that follows).
7. Click the **Prime** button and follow the instructions provided on the digital display of the Fluidics Station.

8. The Fluidics Station will enter into the priming protocol, which will continue for approximately 15–20 min.
9. Once completed, a "Priming Done" message will appear on the display of each of the modules primed.
10. Click on the **Close Station Setup** button to return to the Fluidics screen.

3.8.2 Washing and Staining the AMLprofiler Arrays

1. Remove the AMLprofiler(s) from the hybridization oven after approximately 17 h of hybridization in the oven.
2. Click on the **Complete Step** button in the **Hybridization Oven** tab, and continue to scanning of the AMLprofiler(s).
3. Remove the tough-spot stickers from the AMLprofiler and vent the array by inserting a clean pipette tip into the upper right septum (Fig. 5). Extract the hybridization cocktail with the pipette through the lower left septum of the AMLprofiler array while holding it in a vertical orientation.
4. Add the hybridization cocktail back to the sample tube containing the remainder of the hybridization cocktail, and store at −20 °C for intermediate (overnight) storage or at −80 °C for long-term storage.
5. Fill the AMLprofiler array entirely (>100 μL) with buffer A.
6. If any AMLprofiler arrays are not to be processed immediately on the Fluidics Station, these can be stored in the refrigerator (5 ± 3 °C) for up to 24 h.
7. Prepare and aliquot the staining reagents for each AMLprofiler array, as indicated in Table 14 below.
8. Pulse-spin all tubes to remove any air bubbles.
9. For each module on the Fluidics Station to be used:
   (a) Place stain cocktail 1 tube in sample holder 1 of the Fluidics Station.
   (b) Place stain cocktail 2 tube in sample holder 2 of the Fluidics Station.
   (c) Place array holding buffer tube in sample holder 3 of the Fluidics Station.

Table 14
Preparation of stain reagents for each AMLprofiler array

Stain reagent	Volume and tube
Stain cocktail 1 (light sensitive)	600 μL in amber 1.5 mL microfuge tube
Stain cocktail 2	600 μL in clear 1.5 mL microfuge tube
Array holding buffer	800 μL in clear 1.5 mL microfuge tube

10. Place the AMLprofiler arrays to be processed in each of the allocated modules of the Fluidics Station (without lowering the needle lever yet).
11. Login on the AMLprofiler computer and click on the **Fluidics** button on the left-hand side panel.
12. Click **Start** and allow the wash and stain program to run, which takes approximately 1 h and 15 min to complete.
13. Once completed, the "Eject and Inspect Cartridge" message will be displayed on each module of the Fluidics Station.
14. Check the glass window on the front of the AMLprofiler and verify that no large air bubble(s) are present. If there are any, then vent the upper septum (Fig. 5), remove all the liquid from the array, and fill it completely with fresh array holding buffer (>105 μL).
15. Clean any excess fluid from around the septa and seal them with tough-spots.
16. Login on the Affymetrix computer and click on the **Complete Step** button in the **Fluidics** tab, and proceed immediately to scanning of the AMLprofiler(s).

3.8.3 Scanning the AMLprofiler Arrays

1. Switch on the Affymetrix GeneChip Scanner 3000 and allow it to warm up (approximately 15 min before scanning).
2. When the scanner status is reflected as ready, insert the AMLprofiler arrays randomly into the scanning tray. The autoloader functionality will read the barcodes and automatically assign the microarrays to the corresponding specimen IDs.
3. Login to the Affymetrix computer and navigate to the Scanner tab on the left panel.
4. Highlight the arrays to be scanned and click **Start**.
5. Each array will be scanned, and when completed, click **Complete Step**.

3.9 Data Analysis and Reporting

Once the scanning of AMLprofilers is completed, the data is sent via a secured Internet connection to SkylineDx for analysis and reporting. A test result report is generated for each array and returned to the DX2 Affymetrix system automatically within 15 min. This report displays the two QC parameters of the assay: % Present and R^2 for the hybridization controls, as well as the AMLprofiler marker results. If these QC criteria are not met, INVALID comments are automatically returned.

4 Notes

In our experience, we have found that the aspects listed below are critical for successful processing of the AMLprofiler microarrays. Even the slightest deviation in timing, temperature, and storage conditions might result in the failure of the assay or give intermediate products of low yield and quality. An excellent and detailed protocol is provided by SkylineDx, which is to be followed at all times throughout the processing of samples.

1. *Time management for processing of reagents*: Please ensure to maintain the exact time interval between the subsequent reactions throughout the processing of AMLprofiler microarrays. The protocol provided by the manufacturer should be strictly followed for setting up reactions to maintain the same recommended time conditions. This includes the time intervals between each reaction, the time required to take out the final product from the thermocycler, and also the time at which the next reaction should be started.
2. *Temperature maintenance for setting up each reaction*: Please ensure to maintain the reactions at the exact recommended temperatures in the thermocycler for the required period of time. In the detailed protocol provided by the manufacturer, there are stages where the thermocycler should also be set to a certain temperature prior to placing the reaction tubes inside.
3. *Temperature maintenance for storage of reagents*: Please ensure that the AMLprofiler reagents are stored at the right temperatures, including 4 °C, 20 °C, and −80 °C, as recommended by the manufacturer.
4. *Storage of intermediate products*: Throughout the processing of AMLprofiler, the intermediate products can be stored at certain temperatures in order to continue the processing at a later stage. Please maintain these intermediate products at the recommended temperatures in order to prevent the total failure of the reaction, low yield, and low quality of products.
5. *Sample collection (Subheading 3.1)*: Most people tend to place the bone marrow sample on ice or at 4 °C prior to isolation of the mononuclear cells. This should be avoided, and the sample should be maintained at room temperature.
6. *Isolation of mononuclear cells (Subheading 3.1)*: Be sure to equilibrate the Histopaque®-1077 to room temperature prior to isolation of the mononuclear cells. In addition, the entire isolation protocol should be performed at room temperature, including the centrifugation steps. The tendency is often to keep the sample chilled or at 4 °C.

7. *cRNA purification (Subheading 3.5.1)*: One should be highly attentive during the purification of cRNA while using the magnetic plate for separation of cRNA using the magnetic beads solution. Wait until the solution is totally clear after separation and don't leave the wells to dry longer than recommended.
8. *cRNA yield and quality assessment (Subheading 3.5.2)*: The processing of AMLprofiler cannot be continued if the yield and the quality of cRNA does not meet the requirements of the manufacturer's protocol.
9. *Bleach protocol and replacement of tubingin the Affymetrix Fluidics System (Subheading 3.8)*: The Affymetrix Fluidics Station requires regular cleaning via a bleach protocol (weekly) and changing of the peristaltic silicone tubing (monthly). Ensure that these aspects are attended to regularly (according to the Affymetrix guidelines) and hence that the Fluidics Station is free from contamination prior to proceeding with the processing of the AMLprofiler arrays. This can take up to 3 h and one should bear this in mind when preparing for the final day of AMLprofiler processing.

References

1. Siegel R, Miller R, Jemal A (2015) Cancer statistics, 2015. CA Cancer J Clin 65:21254
2. SkylineDx (2015) AMLprofiler Assay: Instructions For Use.

Chapter 8

Microsphere-Based Assessment of DNA Methylation for AML Prognosis

Gerald B.W. Wertheim, Marlise R. Luskin, Martin Carroll, and Stephen R. Master

Abstract

Epigenetic dysregulation, including aberrant methylation of cytosine residues in DNA, is a hallmark of cancer and clearly results in oncogenic cellular alterations such as transcriptional attenuation of tumor suppressors and genomic instability. A number of studies have examined DNA methylation alterations in patients with acute myeloid leukemia (AML) and have shown that analysis of multilocus methylation patterns can identify biologically distinct AML subclasses and can predict patient prognosis. In order to utilize the prognostic capability of methylation analysis in a clinical setting, we have developed a microsphere-based HpaII tiny fragment enrichment by ligation-mediated PCR (xMELP) assay to interrogate the methylation state of genomic multiple loci along with a random forest-based classification algorithm that correlates DNA methylation status with patient prognosis. These tools can be easily implemented in a clinical molecular pathology laboratory and can be utilized for more accurate risk stratification of AML patients.

Key words Methylation, Help, xMELP, Acute myeloid leukemia, M-score, Random forest

1 Introduction

Aberrant cytosine methylation at CpG dinucleotides is a recurrent feature of many tumors, including acute myeloid leukemia (AML) [1–3]. The importance of cytosine methylation in AML pathogenesis is highlighted by the fact that multiple recurrent mutations in AML are within genes that regulate methylation, and mice that harbor targeted mutations in these genes can develop AML [4–7]. A number of studies have analyzed the global pattern of DNA methylation in AML [2–8]. Not only have these demonstrated that patterns in AML are distinct from normal hematopoietic precursors, but they have shown that AML can be subclassified into biologically and clinically relevant categories simply by their cytosine methylation profiles. Additionally, patient outcomes can be predicted from the methylation profiles. Indeed, we and others have shown that analysis of DNA methylation at a restricted number of

Paolo Fortina et al. (eds.), *Acute Myeloid Leukemia: Methods and Protocols*, Methods in Molecular Biology, vol. 1633,
DOI 10.1007/978-1-4939-7142-8_8, © Springer Science+Business Media LLC 2017

loci can stratify patients with AML into significantly distinct risk groups, and that this stratification is independent of other commonly used markers of AML prognosis [2, 8–10]. Thus, clinical assessment of multilocus or even global DNA methylation allows for proper patient classification and can aid with therapeutic decisions.

Many methods to assess DNA methylation on a global level have been developed. These include enzymatic methods that utilize the differential sensitivity of restriction enzymes to cytosine methylation, DNA pull down assays that use antibodies or proteins to bind and precipitate methylated DNA, and bisulfite treatment methodologies that convert unmethylated cytosine to uracil [11, 12]. Analysis of the digested, precipitated, or bisulfite converted DNA can then be performed on various platforms such as array hybridization, mass spectrometry, and next generation sequencing. Of note, although each technique assesses cytosine methylation, they are distinct and can yield distinct patterns of methylation. Thus, comparing global methylation results across platforms should be done with extreme caution.

One of the initial techniques used to assess global DNA methylation in AML samples was the *H*paII tiny fragment *e*nrichment by *l*igation-mediated *P*CR (HELP) assay [13]. This method relies on the differential sensitivity of the restriction enzyme isoschizomers HpaII and MspI—both of which recognize and digest the tetranucleotide CCGG sequence after the first C—to cytosine methylation. HpaII does not digest methylated sequences, whereas MspI retains activity regardless of methylation status. Thus, after isolation, genomic DNA is divided into two aliquots and digested with either MspI or HpaII. Using the CG overhang for annealing specificity, oligonucleotide linkers are ligated to the digested DNA and linker-specific PCR with Taq polymerase is performed. Since Taq polymerase inefficiently amplifies fragments >2 kb, only relatively small fragments will be amplified. Analysis of the relative amounts of amplified regions, which in the original HELP assay is done by hybridization of fluorescently labeled products to custom-made solid oligonucleotide arrays, reflects the level of methylation of the flanking cytosines (Fig. 1). Using this technique, Figueroa et al. demonstrated that the DNA methylation pattern of 18 loci could predict outcome of AML patients independently of known prognostic factors such as patient age, cytogenetics, and recurrent mutations in FLT3 and NPM1 [2].

Since HELP-derived DNA methylation data predicted outcome of patients with AML, and since the laboratory techniques used for HELP (i.e., restriction enzyme digestion, ligation, and PCR) are commonplace in clinical molecular pathology laboratories, we developed a revised version of the HELP assay (termed xMELP for e*x*pedited *m*icrosphere H*ELP*) with the specific intent of multilocus methylation profiling in a clinical setting [9, 10]. For

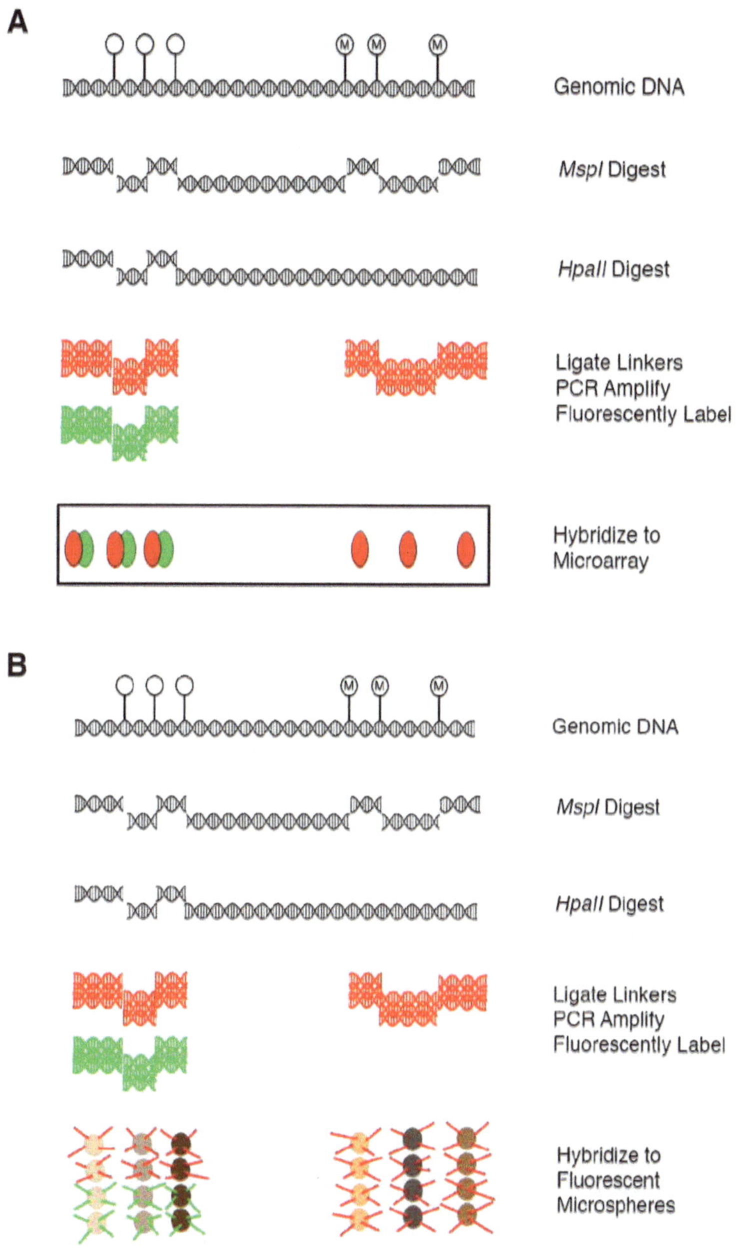

Fig. 1 Schematic diagram of HELP (A) and xMELP (B). Genomic DNA is shown with either unmethylated (open circles) or methylated (circles with M) regions. The DNA is digested with either MspI or HpaII into fragments shown. Linkers are ligated, and PCR with linker-specific primers is carried out. Small fragments are preferentially amplified. For HELP (A), after labeling and hybridization to solid phase microarrays, the relative signals of amplicons from MspI and HpaII reactions reflect levels of methylation. For xMELP (B), amplicon identity is determined by hybridization to oligonucleotide-coupled fluorescent microspheres. As with HELP, the ratio of amplicon signal from MspI and HpaII reactions reflect level of methylation (figure originally published in [9], used by permission)

the most part, xMELP is identical to HELP, yet differs in at least two important ways. First, the linker primers for xMELP have been modified from the original HELP assay and allow digestion and ligation to be performed simultaneously. Second, xMELP detection of methylated regions is through a branched DNA hybridization of products onto fluorescent microspheres rather than onto custom-made solid arrays. This modification allows the assay to be done in a highly reproducible and cost-effective manner, as many clinical laboratories currently possess the instrumentation to perform xMELP.

In the course of assay modification, we also identified additional prognostic loci and developed a more robust algorithm for methylation-based risk assessment than was originally utilized by Figueroa et al. [2]. Specifically, we used a random forest machine learning algorithm (based on building an ensemble of decision trees) that predicts AML survival using variations in methylation at 17 loci that have been normalized to 3 loci previously shown to exhibit constant methylation across a wide set of AML samples [9, 10]. These 17 normalized loci are combined into a single score that predicts risk (low score corresponds to low risk/favorable prognosis, while high score corresponds to high risk/unfavorable prognosis), and we have designed this the M-Score (methylation score). We have previously published the data and software necessary to perform the M-Score calculation, and a standalone script for the R statistical program is available [14]. Additionally, we have created a web-accessible application that allows investigators to determine the M-Score based on their own data [14].

Here we describe both our laboratory method of xMELP, as well as the analytic algorithm we use to assess the methylation data obtained by xMELP in relation to patient prognosis.

2 Materials

2.1 Genomic DNA Extraction, Digestion/Ligation, and Amplification of Tiny Fragments

1. Qiagen Gentra Puregene Blood DNA isolation kit (Qiagen, Hilden, Germany).
2. Primer JHpa12xxxx (HPLC purified), 5′-CG**C**CTGTTCATG-3, resuspend at 12 OD/mL. The first two bases (underlined) in this primer hybridize to the genomic DNA to allow for specific ligation. The third base (in bold) is modified from the original JHpa12 primer to remove the MspI/HpaII site in the ligated product to allow for simultaneous ligation.
3. Primer JHpa24xxxx (HPLC purified), 5′-CGACGTCGACTATCCATGAACAG**G**-3′, resuspend at 6 OD/mL. The last base (in bold) is modified from the original JHpa12 primer to remove the MspI/HpaII site in the ligated product to allow for simultaneous ligation.

4. Preannealed primers. Mix equal volumes of JHpa12xxxx and JHpa24xxxx. Place in heat block at 98 °C. Remove block from heat source and let cool on bench. Annealed linkers can be stored at −20 °C.
5. HpaII restriction enzyme, supplied with 10× CutSmart buffer (NEB, Ipswich, MA).
6. MspI restriction enzyme, supplied with 10× CutSmart buffer (NEB).
7. 100 mM ATP, pH 7 (Roche, Basel, Switzerland).
8. T4 DNA ligase (Thermo Fisher Scientific, Waltham, MA, USA).
9. dNTP mix, 10 mM each (Thermo Fisher Scientific).
10. Native Taq polymerase (Thermo Fisher Scientific), supplied with 10× Buffer and 50 mM magnesium chloride.
11. Thermocycler.

2.2 Amplicon Hybridization to Microspheres and Fluorescence Detection

1. Luminex FlexMAP 3D system with xPONENT software (*see* **Note 1**).
2. Hand-held magnetic plate for 96-well plate (Affymetrix #EPX-55555-000) (*see* **Note 2**).
3. VorTemp 56 shaker incubator (*see* **Note 3**).
4. Tabletop centrifuge with plate adaptors.
5. QuantigenePlex 2.0 Microsphere Assay (*see* **Note 4**).
6. QuantigenePlex DNA Assay Kit (Affymetrix #QPD1010). Kit contains Pre-Amplifier probe and diluent, amplifier probe, label probe and diluent, streptavidin-PE (SAPE), wash buffer components, SAPE wash, blocking reagent, Proteinase K, Lysis mixture, Neutralization buffer, 96-well plates (hybridization and magnetic separation), plate seals.
7. 1 N sodium hydroxide.

3 Methods

Since both HELP and xMELP rely on differential Taq amplification of large and small fragments, intact genomic DNA must be isolated and digested to completion. We recommend evaluation of extracted DNA by gel electrophoresis (or equivalent method) and overnight digestion. Additionally, we advise against use of FFPE samples (e.g., aspirate clot sections) as DNA undergoes fragmentation with sample processing. We also recommend evaluation of PCR amplicons by electrophoresis prior to microsphere hybridization. To control for genomic integrity, the restriction enzyme can be eliminated from the digestion/ligation reaction.

3.1 Extraction and Amplification

1. Pellet 1–3 million cells at room temperature in a 15 mL conical at 300 × *g* for 5 min. Remove supernatant, resuspend in 5 mL of PBS, and pellet again at 300 × *g*.
2. Extract DNA using Qiagen Gentra Puregene kit (*see* **Note 5**). Resuspend the cell pellet in 200 μL of 10 mM Tris pH 8.0. This may require overnight incubation at room temperature or an increase in the resuspension volume for large quantities of DNA.
3. Quantitate DNA and run 1–5 μL on a 0.8% agarose gel to check quality. Unsheared genomic DNA should run at >10 kb.
4. Prepare the digestion/ligation mix as follows (*see* **Notes 6–8**):
   (a) 250–500 ng of genomic DNA.
   (b) 5 μL 10x NEB CutSmart buffer (supplied with restriction enzymes).
   (c) 7.5 μL Annealed JHpa12xxxx and JHpa24xxxx oligonucleotides.
   (d) 0.5 μL 100 mM ATP.
   (e) 2 μL HpaII or MspI.
   (f) 2 μL T4 DNA ligase.
   (g) ddH_2O to 50 μL total reaction volume.
5. Incubate reaction mixture in thermocycler set at 25 °C for at least 12 h (*see* **Note 9**).
6. Add 450 μL of ddH_2O to the reaction mixture.
7. Prepare PCR mix as follows
   (a) 10 μL diluted digested/ligated DNA.
   (b) 1 μL dNTPs.
   (c) 1.5 μL $MgCl_2$.
   (d) 5 μL 10× PCR buffer.
   (e) 1 μL JHpa24xxxx primer.
   (f) 0.5 μL Taq polymerase.
   (g) 31 μL ddH_2O.
8. Run PCR cycling as follows (*see* **Notes 9** and **10**):
   (a) 72 °C for 5 min.
   (b) 20 cycles of
      - 95 °C for 30 s.
      - 72 °C for 3 min.
   (c) 72 °C for 10 min.
   (d) 4 °C hold.
9. Run 5 μL of the PCR products on a 1.5% gel to assess amplification. Most products should appear between 100 bp and 2 kb. If the products are appropriate, proceed to the hybridization steps.

3.2 Amplicon Hybridization to Microspheres and Fluorescence Detection (See Note 11)

1. Prewarm lysis mixture buffer to 37 °C. Then mix the following reagents (*see* **Note 12**)
   (a) 8 μL PCR product.
   (b) 18 μL Lysis mixture buffer.
   (c) 12.5 μL 1 N sodium hydroxide.
   (d) 5 μL probeset.
   (e) 24.5 μL ddH_2O.
2. Incubate the mixture at room temperature for 30 min.
3. During this incubation, prepare the microsphere mix by mixing (*see* **Note 12**)
   (a) 15 μL.
   (b) 0.2 μL Proteinase K.
   (c) 2 μL blocking reagent.
   (d) 1 μL beadset.
   (e) 1.8 μL ddH_2O.
4. If a master mix was made, aliquot 20 μL of this latter mix into wells of the hybridization plate.
5. After incubation of the probeset mix, add 12 μL of neutralization buffer to the probeset mix, pipette up and down, and add the entire 80 μL to the beadset mix in the hybridization plate.
6. Seal the plate with the pressure seal, place in the VorTemp incubator, and incubate for at least 12 h at 54 °C with shaking at 600 rpm (*see* **Note 13**).
7. Place amplifier diluent in 37 °C water bath.
8. Make enough wash buffer with wash buffer components (amount sufficient for remaining steps). Wash buffer components are included in DNA assay kit. To make buffer mix
   (a) 100 μL wash buffer component 1.
   (b) 1.6 mL wash buffer component 2.
   (c) 31.6 ddH_2O.
9. After incubation, spin plate for 30 s in the tabletop centrifuge to collect the liquid in each well. Transfer reactions to the magnetic separation plate.
10. Place the magnetic separation plate on the magnetic washer and let stand for 1 min. Invert the plate on a paper towel to remove liquid. Wash three times with 100 μL wash buffer per well, inverting plate on paper towel each time to remove liquid.
11. Dilute 6 μL preamplifier in 1.9 mL prewarmed amplifier diluent (*see* **Note 14**). Mix well. Add 100 μL to each well with magnetic microspheres. Seal the plate with the plate sealer,

place in the VorTemp incubator, and incubate 1 h at 50 °C with shaking at 600 rpm.

12. Place the magnetic separation plate on the magnetic washer and let stand for 1 min. Invert the plate on a paper towel to remove liquid. Wash three times with 100 μL wash buffer per well, inverting plate on paper towel each time to remove liquid.
13. Dilute 6 μL amplifier in 1.9 mL amplifier diluent. Mix well. Add 100 μL to each well with magnetic microspheres. Seal the plate with the plate sealer, place in the VorTemp incubator, and incubate 1 h at 50 °C with shaking at 600 rpm.
14. Place the magnetic separation plate on the magnetic washer and let stand for 1 min. Invert the plate on a paper towel to remove liquid. Wash three times with 100 μL wash buffer per well, inverting plate on paper towel each time to remove liquid.
15. Dilute 6 μL label probe in 1.9 mL label probe diluent. Mix well. Add 100 μL to each well with magnetic microspheres. Seal the plate with the plate sealer, place in the VorTemp incubator, and incubate 1 h at 50 °C with shaking at 600 rpm.
16. Place the magnetic separation plate on the magnetic washer and let stand for 1 min. Invert the plate on a paper towel to remove liquid. Wash three times with 100 μL wash buffer per well, inverting plate on paper towel each time to remove liquid.
17. Turn the VorTemp to 25 °C and place a bag of ice in the VorTemp (*see* **Note 15**).
18. Dilute 6 μL SAPE in 1.9 mL SAPE diluent. Mix well. Add 100 μL to each well with magnetic microspheres. Seal the plate with the plate sealer, place in the VorTemp incubator, and incubate 30 min at 25 °C with shaking at 600 `.
19. Place the magnetic separation plate on the magnetic washer and let stand for 1 min. Invert the plate on a paper towel to remove liquid. Wash three times with 100 μL SAPE wash buffer per well, inverting plate on paper towel each time to remove liquid.
20. Add 100 μL SAPE wash buffer to each well.
21. Analyze microspheres from each well on FlexMAP 3D instrument running XPONENT software (*see* **Notes 16** and **17**).

3.3 Data Processing and M-Score Calculation

1. To utilize xMELP for AML prognosis, detection reagents for the 17 test loci and 3 control loci previously described must first be obtained from the manufacturer.
2. In order to use the standalone software available electronically in the supplementary materials, the R statistical software program (www.r-project.org) must first be installed along with appropriate libraries (including the randomForestSRC package

version 1.4). Because of the additional technical challenges associated with this installation, a web-accessible program is also available at https://labapps.shinyapps.io/MScore/.

3. To correctly use the provided software or web-accessible application to calculate M-Score, samples should be named with a unique identifier that is preceded by "H" (HpaII digests) or "M" (MspI digests). For example, for material processed from subject 1234, the respective samples should be named H1234 and M1234 in order to allow the software to automatically pair these samples. The individual probes (listed as separate columns) may occur in any order, but they should match the previously published locus names (e.g., "MSPI0406S00011246").
4. Data files from the FlexMAP 3D instrument should be saved in CSV (comma-separated values) format.
5. Using the web application, the CSV file may be loaded into the M-score calculator. Upon loading, the full file is shown along with a subset representing median count data (to manually ensure that the data file has been correctly interpreted). Selecting the "Process" function will calculate M-Scores for all matched (HpaII and MspI both present) samples.
6. A quality control cutoff (which may be altered in the web application or by editing the source code of the standalone program) is provided as a minimum value for the median counts. Previously published work has established 100 as a reasonable default [10]. Samples that do not reach the necessary level of signal are omitted from the results. Low signal of a single enzyme (HpaII or MspI) sample suggests an amplification failure, while low signal in both samples suggests an issue with DNA quality.

4 Notes

1. Alternative instruments, such as the significantly less expensive Luminex 100/200 systems with associated software, can be used.
2. Numerous magnetic plates that are compatible with 96-well pates are available. We use the one listed since it has clamps that prevent the 96-well plate from dislodging from the magnet when inverted. We have found that placing a strip of magnetic tape on the underside of the 96-well plate also prevents dislodging. Automatic magnetic plate washers may also be used.
3. As communicated by Affymetrix, optimal mixing occurs in the VorTemp 56 incubator. We have not attempted the assay in other shaker incubators.

4. The assay employing the 17 prognostic loci and 3 control loci is listed as Affymetrix # 411816–120. The list loci used in the AML xMELP assay can be found in Wertheim et al. [15]. Custom-made microsphere assays are available from Affymetrix.
5. We use the Qiagen Gentra Puregene kit as this was recommended by Figueroa et al. [13] and we were specifically advised to avoid silica column binding (ME Figueroa, personal communication). However, we have successfully performed xMELP on purified DNA from other investigators who have used alternative methods of DNA extraction, including silica adsorption. IMPORTANTLY, in at least one case we have identified a Puregene kit that resulted in uniformly poor HpaII digestion in all samples and artifactually high M-scores. DNA "cleanup" methods on this DNA do NOT correct the inappropriate M-scores. We suggest, therefore, multiple samples with known M-scores should be re-extracted as a quality control each time a new Puregene kit is used.
6. Master mixes can be used for this reaction and the following PCR step. For these mixes, we calculate amounts for at least one additional reaction in order to account for pipetting error.
7. The ligation reaction requires ATP, not dATP.
8. These reactions can proceed at room temperature on the benchtop; however, temperature standardization in a water bath or thermocycler is recommended.
9. Given large number of amplifiable fragments in the starting DNA pool, the PCR reaches saturation between 10 and 20 cycles. Increasing the number of cycles beyond 20 does not increase the assay sensitivity.
10. The first extension prior to the cycling is critical. The ligation only ligates the JHpa24xxxx primer to the genomic DNA through the 5′ phosphate retained on the genomic DNA. The JHpa12xxxx primer does not ligate since it lacks a 5′ phosphate. The initial 72 °C incubation allows extension of sequence that is complementary to JHpa24xxxx and is required for the subsequent PCR cycles to proceed.
11. The method used was developed by Affymetrix and additional details can be found at http://cdn.panomics.com/downloads/UM17353_QGP_DNAMagSep_UserManual_RevA_091105.pdf.
12. Master mixes can be used for the probeset mix and the microsphere mix. For these mixes, we calculate amounts for at least one additional reaction in order to account for pipetting error. For large sample numbers, we generally calculate amounts for two or three additional reactions. For larger numbers of samples, n + 2 or even n + 3 reactions should be made.

13. The proper plate and seal combination must be used to ensure that the seal remains intact during the incubation. Improper sealing can result in sample contamination and evaporation.
14. This is essentially a master mix. Reagent amounts needed for this and subsequent hybridization steps can be calculated using the 6 μL reagent to 1.9 mL diluent ratio.
15. The VorTemp incubator will not start if the temperature is too high. We place a bag of ice in the incubator while performing the previous washes in order to cool rapidly. If the SAPE reaction is prepared prior to incubator cooling, it can be kept at room temperature wrapped in aluminum foil.
16. As indicated in the description of equipment, the alternative instruments and software can be used to analyze the microspheres. All Luminex instruments require calibration and validation microspheres, and instructions for use of the instrument should be consulted prior to performing experiments. Microsphere regions for PE analysis (i.e., Luminex bead numbers) are provided with the probeset order. These should be entered into the analysis software prior to performing the experiment. Other instrument parameters are provided by Affymetrix.
17. During instrument setup, the plate should remain shaking to prevent microsphere clumping. If we are running more than 48 samples, we will pause the analysis half way through the run, shake for 2 min, and resume the analysis.

Acknowledgments

M. Luskin, NIH T32 cancer epidemiology grant CA 09679-22; G. Wertheim, pilot project grant from the Perelman School of Medicine Hematologic Malignancies Translational Center of Excellence, grant IRG-78-002-35 from the American Cancer Society, and National Institutes of Health (1R21CA185365-01); M. Carroll, National Institutes of Health (1R21CA185365-01, 1R01CA149566-01A1, and 5R21CA185365-02), Veterans Affairs Administration (1I01BX000918-01); S.R. Master, National Institutes of Health (1R21CA185365-01). This project was supported in part by the UPenn Institute for Translational Medicine and Therapeutics (ITMAT) through a grant from the National Center for Research Resources, Grant UL1RR024134 (now at the National Center for Advancing Translational Sciences, Grant UL1TR000003).

References

1. Baylin SB, Jones PA (2011) A decade of exploring the cancer epigenome—biological and translational implications. Nat Rev Cancer 11(10):726–734
2. Figueroa ME, Lugthart S, Erpelinck-Verscheuren C et al (2010) DNA methylation signatures identify biologically distinct subtypes in acute myeloid leukemia. Cancer Cell 17(1):13–27
3. Hanahan D, Weinberg RA (2011) Hallmarks of cancer: the next generation. Cell 144(5):646–674
4. An J, Gonzales-Avalos E, Chawla A et al (2015) Acute loss of TET function results in aggressive myeloid cancer in mice. Nat Commun 6:10071
5. Cancer Genome Atlas Research, N (2013) Genomic and epigenomic landscapes of adult de novo acute myeloid leukemia. N Engl J Med 368(22):2059–2074
6. Ogawara Y, Katsumoto T, Aikawa Y et al (2015) IDH2 and NPM1 mutations cooperate to activate Hoxa9/Meis1 and hypoxia pathways in acute myeloid leukemia. Cancer Res 75(10):2005–2016
7. Yang L, Rau R, Goodell MA (2015) DNMT3A in haematological malignancies. Nat Rev Cancer 15(3):152–165
8. Bullinger L, Ehrich M, Dohner K et al (2010) Quantitative DNA methylation predicts survival in adult acute myeloid leukemia. Blood 115(3):636–642
9. Wertheim GB, Smith C, Figueroa ME et al (2014) Microsphere-based multiplex analysis of DNA methylation in acute myeloid leukemia. J Mol Diagn 16(2):207–215
10. Wertheim GB, Smith C, Luskin M et al (2015) Validation of DNA methylation to predict outcome in acute myeloid leukemia by use of xMELP. Clin Chem 61(1):249–58
11. Fazzari MJ, Greally JM (2010) Introduction to epigenomics and epigenome-wide analysis. Methods Mol Biol 620:243–265
12. Harris RA, Wang T, Coarfa C et al (2010) Comparison of sequencing-based methods to profile DNA methylation and identification of monoallelic epigenetic modifications. Nat Biotechnol 28(10):1097–1105
13. Figueroa ME, Melnick A, Greally JM (2009) Genome-wide determination of DNA methylation by Hpa II tiny fragment enrichment by ligation-mediated PCR (HELP) for the study of acute leukemias. Methods Mol Biol 538: 395–407
14. AML methylation score (M-Score). https://labapps.shinyapps.io/MScore/
15. Wertheim GBW, Smith C, Luskin M et al (2015) Validation of DNA methylation to predict outcome in acute myeloid leukemia by use of xMELP. Clin Chem 61(1):249–258

Chapter 9

Genome-Wide Analysis of DNA Methylation in Hematopoietic Cells: DNA Methylation Analysis by WGBS

Mira Jeong, Anna G. Guzman, and Margaret A. Goodell

Abstract

DNA methylation is a major epigenetic modification that regulates gene expression, genome imprinting, and development and has a role in diseases including cancer. There are various methods for whole-genome methylation profiling that differ in cost and resolution. Recent advances in high-throughput sequencing technologies coupled with bisulfite treatment enable absolute DNA methylation quantification and genome-wide single-nucleotide resolution analysis. In this chapter, we provide detailed protocols for whole-genome bisulfite sequencing (WGBS), which captures the complete methylome. Using WGBS, we are able to generate a reference DNA methylome for normal or malignant hematopoietic cells.

Key words DNA methylation, CpG islands, Whole-genome bisulfite sequencing, High-throughput sequencing

1 Introduction

DNA methylation is a well-studied, heritable, and reversible epigenetic modification essential for diverse cellular processes. Specifically, DNA methylation is achieved via an enzymatic mechanism in which a methyl group is added to the five-position of cytosine, usually in the context of a CpG dinucleotide (Fig. 1a). CpG is almost invariably methylated, except when CpGs are at high density, in which case methylation tends to be lower or absent altogether. While methylation patterns are fairly stable across cell types, some regions of the genome, such as enhancers, are variable in methylation levels among different cell and tissue types. Aberrant DNA methylation patterns are associated with a number of human diseases such as cancer and neurodevelopmental diseases. While DNA methylation in promoters and enhancers generally is correlated with repression of gene expression, DNA methylation in gene bodies is positively correlated with active transcription. Comprehensive genome-wide DNA methylation maps may shed light on the role of DNA in normal development and diseases.

Paolo Fortina et al. (eds.), *Acute Myeloid Leukemia: Methods and Protocols*, Methods in Molecular Biology, vol. 1633,
DOI 10.1007/978-1-4939-7142-8_9, © Springer Science+Business Media LLC 2017

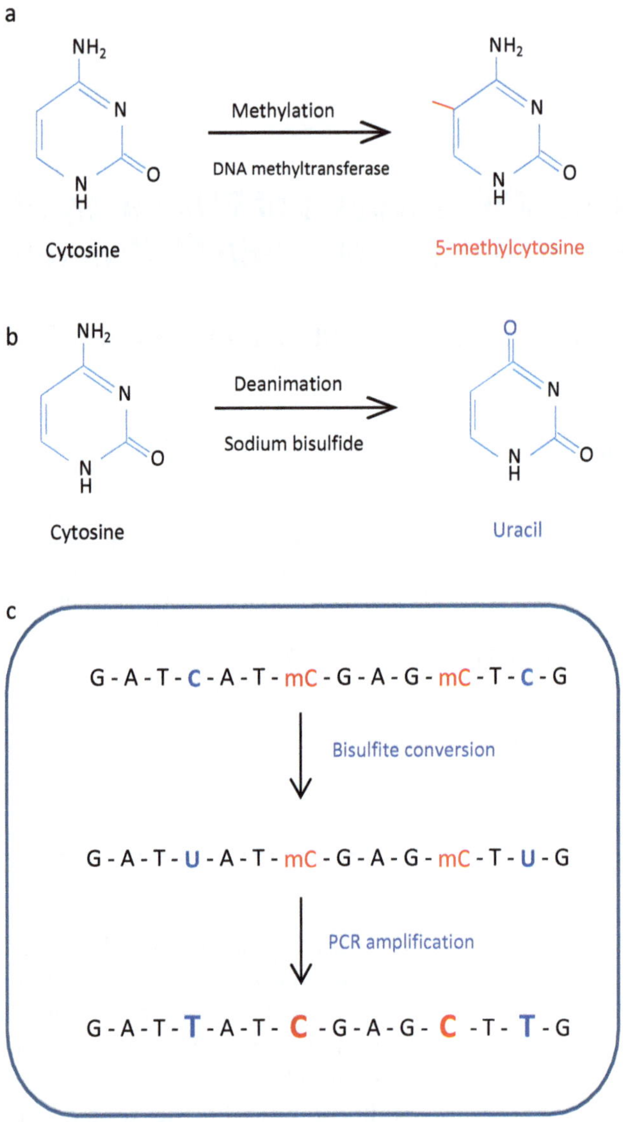

Fig. 1 (**a**) Methylation of cytosine to 5-methylcytosine by DNA methyltransferase. (**b**) Deamination of cytosine by sodium bisulfite conversion. Unmethylated cytosines are converted to uracil. (**c**) DNA sequences following bisulfite conversion and PCR amplification. Unmethylated cytosine will be detected as thymine

Therefore, genome-wide mapping of DNA methylation is of great interest for epigenetic studies.

The development of high-throughput sequencing technology has facilitated genome-wide measurement of DNA methylation. Currently, several methods falling into three major assay types are utilized to study DNA methylation [1]. Bisulfite conversion-based methods, such as whole-genome bisulfite sequencing (WGBS) [2, 3] and reduced representation bisulfite sequencing, (RRBS) are currently the most standard methods [4, 5], but methylation arrays and affinity capture methods are also used to assay methylation differences, particularly in human cells.

In bisulfite sequencing methods, sodium bisulfite is used to convert cytosines into uracils (Fig. 1b), which are then detected as thymines in subsequent PCR and sequencing [6]. In contrast, methylated cytosines and hydroxymethylated cytosines are left unmodified and identified as cytosines during DNA sequencing (Fig. 1c). The bisulfite conversion method has become a very effective approach for detecting genome-wide DNA methylation differences at a single-nucleotide resolution.

Affinity capture-based methods, such as methylated DNA immunoprecipitation sequencing (MeDIP-seq) [7, 8] and hydroxymethylated DNA immunoprecipitation sequencing (hMeDIP-seq) [9], use antibodies that recognize methylcytosines and hydroxymethylcytosines, respectively, to pull down methylated and hydroxymethylated genomic regions. Cytosine 5-methylenesulfonate sequencing (CMS-seq) utilizes both bisulfate conversion and affinity capture methods for 5hmC detection [10] using CMS-specific antiserum. The last approach utilizes enrichment-based methods such as methylation-sensitive restriction enzyme digestion sequencing (MRE-seq) [11].

Affinity capture- and enrichment-based methods are cost-effective and simple; however, they provide lower resolution than bisulfite conversion. Bisulfite conversion-based methods, especially WGBS, provide high resolution and accurate data and are better at detecting differentially methylated regions, particularly with high sequencing coverage. The drawback to these approaches is that they are expensive and have bioinformatic challenges. For example, bisulfite conversion can vary in efficiency and challenges in aligning bisulfite-converted sequences to the reference genome due to the conversion of the many unmethylated Cs to Ts. Each method has its own advantages and disadvantages; therefore, it is important to choose the right method based on the question to be addressed. Here, we provide detailed experimental protocols for WGBS on the Illumina platform.

While we focus below on sample preparation (Fig. 2), sequencing depth should also be considered, as this is a significant factor in the total cost of the procedure. We recommend a minimum average coverage of 10–15-fold. This translates to approximately 200 million reads using the current Illumina HiSeq protocols. However, better resolution and power to detect minor methylation differences can be attained with higher coverage.

Finally, the discovery of 5-hydroxymethylcystosine (5hmC) as a type of DNA methylation with potentially different properties from 5mC has increased interest in detecting this mark. Importantly, bisulfite sequencing methods cannot distinguish between 5mC and 5hmC, as cytosine modified with either mark are protected from

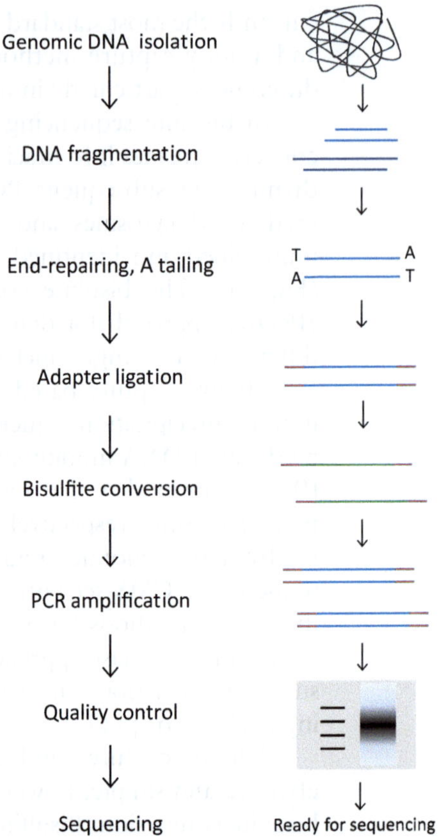

Fig. 2 Overview of the WGBS protocol. Isolated genomic DNA is fragmented to average 350 bp size. Repair the 3′ and 5′ overhangs into blunt ends and add single "A" to the 3′ end of the blunt fragment. After A-tailing, ligate methylated adapters to the A-tailed fragment, and treat with sodium bisulfite. Perform final amplification PCR and check library quality

bisulfite. Therefore, bioinformatics analysis and interpretation must take this into account. Alternative methods such as oxidative bisulfite sequencing (OxBS-seq) [12] or Tet-assisted bisulfite sequencing (TAB-seq) [13] can be used to detect the 5hmC if desired.

2 Materials

2.1 Reagents

1. PureLink Genomic DNA Mini Kit (Invitrogen, Carlsbad, CA, USA).
2. Quant-iT dsDNA Assay Kit, high sensitive (Invitrogen, Carlsbad, CA, USA).
3. Snap-Cap MicroTUBE vials (Covaris, Woburn, MA, USA).
4. 4–20% Criterion™ TBE Gel (Bio-Rad, Hercules, CA, USA).
5. Low-binding DNAse-/RNAse-free microtubes (Ambion, Waltham, MA, USA).

6. TBE buffer, 10×, Molecular Biology Grade (Promega, Madison, WI, USA).
7. Sybr Gold (Invitrogen, Waltham, MA, USA).
8. TruSeq Nano DNA Sample Prep Kit (Illumina, San Diego, CA, USA).
9. EpiTect Bisulfite Kit (Qiagen, Hilden, Germany).
10. AMPure XP beads (Beckman Coulter, Brea, CA, USA).
11. PfuTurbo Cx hotstart DNA polymerase (Agilent Technologies, Santa Clara, CA, USA).
12. 100 mM dNTP mix (25 mM of each dNTP; Agilent Technologies, Santa Clara, CA, USA).
13. EvaGreen (Biotium, Fremont, CA, USA).
14. 100% ethanol.
15. 10× PBS (GenDepot, Katy, TX, USA).
16. Ultrapure DNAse-/RNAse-free water (Thermo Fisher, Waltham, MA, USA).
17. 100 bp DNA Ladder (GenDepot, Katy, TX, USA).
18. 6× DNA loading dye (Promega, Madison, WI, USA).
19. High Sensitivity DNA Kit (Agilent, Santa Clara, CA, USA).

2.2 Equipment

1. Covaris S2 system (Covaris, Woburn, MA, USA).
2. MicroTube holder (Covaris, Woburn, MA, USA).
3. Dark Reader transilluminator (Clare Chemical Research, Dolores, CO, USA).
4. Qubit fluorometer (Invitrogen, Carlsbad, CA, USA).
5. DynaMag-2 magnet (Invitrogen, Carlsbad, CA, USA).
6. Bio-Rad Thermal cycler (Bio-Rad, CFX96 Touch, Hercules, CA, USA).
7. Real-time PCR cycler (Bio-Rad, C1000, Hercules, CA, USA).
8. Criterion cell system (Bio-Rad, Hercules, CA, USA).
9. Heat blocks.
10. Vortex mixer.
11. Bioanalyzer (Santa Clara, CA, USA).
12. Illumina HiSeq 2500 (San Diego, CA, USA).

3 Methods

3.1 Genomic DNA Isolation

1. Resuspend cells into 200 μL of PBS, add 20 μL of proteinase K and 20 μL of RNase from the PureLink Genomic DNA isolation kit, mix thoroughly, and incubate for 2 min at room temperature (*see* **Notes 1–3**).

2. Add 200 μL PureLink Genomic lysis/binding buffer and mix well by vortexing.
3. Incubate at 55 °C for 3 h to overnight (*see* **Note 4**).
4. Add 200 μL of 96–100% ethanol to the lysate. Mix well by vortexing to yield a homogenous solution.
5. Proceed immediately to isolating DNA using a spin column from the PureLink Genomic DNA Kit.
6. Place spin column in a provided collection tube. Transfer 640 μL of reaction mix to the spin column and centrifuge for 30 s at full speed.
7. Wash column with 500 μL of washing buffer and centrifuge for 30 s at full speed.
8. Centrifuge column in the same collection tube for an additional 30 s at full speed to remove remaining buffer.
9. Place column into a clean PCR tube and elute genomic DNA with 50 μL of warm elution buffer from the kit. Perform a second elution to recover more DNA using an additional 50 μL of warm elution buffer.
10. Measure the DNA concentration using Qubit dsDNA HS assay kit according to the manufacturer's instructions.
11. Quantify 100 ng–1 μg of DNA in up to 100 μL of volume. If the DNA volume is <100 μL, add EB buffer to make total volume equal to 100 μL.

3.2 DNA Fragmentation and Cleanup Fragmented DNA

1. Fill the Covaris water bath with deionized water up to the level indicated on the tank. Turn on the cooling system connected to the Covaris to maintain the bath temperature between 6 and 8 °C, and degas the water bath for 30 min prior to use.
2. Set the Covaris at the appropriate operating condition. Covaris conditions for a 350 bp size fragmentation are as follows:

Duty cycle	10%
Intensity	4
Cycle/burst	200
Time	40 s

3. Transfer 100 μL of genomic DNA into the microtube through the presplit septa by slowly releasing sample along the wall of the microtube. Make sure to keep the cap on the tube and avoid the introduction of bubbles.
4. Load the microtube inside the Covaris holder.
5. Start run process (*see* **Note 5**).

6. After process, remove holder and transfer the processed sample to a new 1.5 mL tube.
7. Let AMPure XP beads come to room temperature, and vortex for at least 1 min to ensure even distribution. Add 1.6× AMPure XP beads to sample and pipette entire volume ten times to homogenize.
8. Incubate at room temperature for 5 min.
9. Place sample on a magnetic rack at room temperature for 5 min or until the liquid is clear.
10. Carefully remove and discard all supernatant from the tubes without disturbing the beads.
11. With tubes on magnetic rack, rinse twice with 200 μL of freshly made 80% EtOH.
12. Air-dry the bead pellet on the magnetic stand for 5 min.
13. Resuspend beads with 62.5 μL of resuspension buffer and mix well by pipetting entire volume ten times. Incubate homogenized sample for 2 min at room temperature.
14. Place tubes back on magnetic rack for 5 min.
15. Transfer 60 μL of clear supernatant into a new PCR tube.
16. Quantify DNA concentration by using Qubit dsDNA HS assay kit.

3.3 End-Repair, Poly-a Tailing, and Adaptor Ligation (Illumina Nano DNA Sample Prep kit)

1. Use 100 ng–1 μg of fragmented DNA in up to 60 μL of volume. Add resuspension buffer to bring the total volume to 60 μL.
2. Add 40 μL end-repair mix for a total volume of 100 μL, mix well by pipetting entire volume ten times, and centrifuge for 30 s at full speed.
3. Incubate at 30 °C for 30 min, and then place the samples on ice (*see* **Note 6**).
4. Vortex the sample purification beads from the kit to ensure even distribution. Warm beads to room temperature before use.
5. Dilute 95 μL of sample purification beads in 65 μL nuclease-free water.
6. Add 160 μL of diluted sample purification beads to the end-repair reaction mixture. Pipette the entire volume ten times and incubate at room temperature for 5 min.
7. Place the tubes on a magnetic stand for 5 min.
8. Transfer 250 μL of the supernatant, containing the DNA of interest, from each tube to a new PCR tube. Discard tubes containing beads.

9. Vortex sample purification beads for at least 1 min. Add 30 μL of room temperature undiluted sample purification beads to each sample containing 250 μL of the supernatant with DNA. Pipette the entire volume ten times.
10. Incubate at room temperature for 5 min.
11. Place sample on a magnetic rack at room temperature for 5 min or until liquid is clear.
12. Carefully remove and discard all supernatant from the tubes without disturbing the beads.
13. With tubes on the magnetic rack, rinse twice with 200 μL of freshly made 80% EtOH.
14. Air-dry the bead pellet on the magnetic stand for 5 min.
15. Resuspend beads with 20 μL of resuspension buffer and mix well by pipetting the entire volume ten times. Incubate for 2 min at room temperature.
16. Place tubes on magnetic rack for 5 min.
17. Transfer 17.5 μL of clear supernatant into a new PCR tube.
18. Add 12.5 μL A-tailing mix to 17.5 μL supernatant, and pipette the entire volume of the reaction mixture ten times.
19. Incubate at 37 °C for 30 min and 70 °C for 5 min and hold at 4 °C (*see* **Note 7**).
20. When the thermal cycler temperature has been at 4 °C for 5 min, remove tubes from it. Briefly centrifuge and keep on ice then proceed to the next ligation step.
21. Add 2.5 μL of resuspension buffer, 2.5 μL of Ligation Mix, and 2.5 μL of DNA adaptor index to the reaction mixture.
22. Pipette the entire volume ten times and centrifuge briefly.
23. Incubate at 30 °C for 10 min, and then place on ice.
24. Add 5 μL of Stop Ligation Buffer to the mix and pipette to mix.
25. Add 42.5 μL well-mixed sample purification beads, pipette ten times, and incubate 5 min at room temperature.
26. Place the tubes on a magnetic rack for 5 min.
27. Carefully remove and discard 80 μL of the supernatant without disturbing beads.
28. Wash the beads twice with 200 μL freshly made 80% ethanol. Allow to air-dry at room temperature for 5 min.
29. Remove tubes from the magnetic rack and resuspend the beads in 52.5 μL of resuspension buffer by pipetting ten times. Incubate for 2 min at room temperature.
30. Place tubes on the magnetic rack for 5 min at room temperature.
31. Transfer 50 μL of supernatant to a new PCR tube.

32. Add 50 μL of well-mixed sample purification beads, pipette ten times, and incubate 5 min at room temperature.
33. Carefully remove and discard 100 μL of the supernatant without disturbing beads.
34. Wash the beads twice with 200 μL freshly made 80% ethanol. Allow to air-dry at room temperature for 5 min.
35. Remove tubes from the magnetic rack and resuspend the beads in 27.5 μL resuspension buffer by pipetting ten times. Incubate for 2 min at room temperature.
36. Place tubes on the magnetic rack for 5 min at room temperature.
37. Transfer 25 μL of supernatant to a new PCR tube.
38. Proceed to bisulfite conversion.

3.4 Bisulfite Conversion

1. Set up a bisulfite conversion per the manufacturer's recommendations (EpiTect Bisulfite Kit, Qiagen).

   Bisulfite conversion reaction mix:

Reagents	Volume per reaction (μL)
Ligated DNA library	20
Bisulfite mix (dissolved)	85
DNA protect buffer	35
Total volume	140

2. Perform bisulfite conversion as per manufacturer's recommendations to avoid template degradation and DNA loss during treatment and cleanup, while achieving high bisulfite conversion rates of the DNA. Two consecutive rounds of bisulfite conversion help to achieve ≥99% conversion ratio.
3. PCR conditions.

Stage	Temperature and time
Denaturation	95 °C for 5 min
Incubation	60 °C for 25 min
Denaturation	95 °C for 5 min
Incubation	60 °C for 85 min
Denaturation	99 °C for 5 min
Incubation	60 °C for 175 min
Hold	20 °C forever

4. Once the bisulfite conversion is complete, briefly centrifuge PCR tubes and transfer the complete bisulfite reactions to

clean 1.5 mL tubes (any precipitants in the solution will not affect the performance or yield of the reaction).

5. Make a master mix of 310 μL of freshly prepared buffer BL + 10 μg/mL carrier RNA. Mix the master mix solution by vortex and centrifuge briefly. Add 310 μL of the master mix to each sample.
6. Add 250 μL ethanol, vortex for 15 s, and centrifuge briefly to remove any drops from inside the lid.
7. Place an EpiTect spin column and collection tube in a suitable rack. Transfer the solution from **step 3** into the EpiTect spin column, and centrifuge the column at maximum speed for 30 s. Run the flow-through once more through the column and centrifuge at maximum speed for 1 min. Discard flow-through.
8. Add 500 μL of Buffer BW (wash buffer) to the spin column, and centrifuge at maximum speed for 1 min. Discard flow-through, and place the spin column back into the collection tube.
9. Add 500 μL of Buffer BD (desulfonation buffer) to the spin column and incubate for 15 min at room temperature. Centrifuge column at maximum speed for 1 min, and discard flow-through.
10. Add 500 μL of Buffer BW. Centrifuge at maximum speed for 1 min. Discard flow-through.
11. Repeat **step 7**.
12. Place the spin column into a clean 1.5 mL microcentrifuge tube. Add 20 μL of warm Buffer EB to the center of the column. Elute the purified DNA by centrifugation for 1 min at 15,000 × *g* (12,000 rpm).
13. Add an additional 20 μL of warm Buffer EB to the center of the column, and centrifuge for 1 min at 15,000 × *g* (12,000 rpm) (*see* **Notes 8** and **9**).

3.5 Library PCR Amplification and Bead Purification

1. Prepare a PCR master mix.

Component	Amount (μL)
PfuTurbo Cx DNA polymerase buffer (10×)	10
dNTP (25 mM each, 100 mM)	1
DNA template	20
Primer cocktail	10
Pfu Turbo Cx DNA polymerase	2
EvaGreen	5
Water	57

Add the PCR master mix to each 20 μL bisulfite-converted library. Mix well and divide the reaction into two tubes with 50 μL each (*see* **Note 10**).

2. Amplify the Reaction in Real-Time PCR Cycle.

Stage	Temperature (°C)	Time	Cycles
Denaturation	95	3 min	1
Library amplification	98 60 72	20 s 15 s 30 s	5–15
	4	Hold	1

3. To minimize the bias caused by PCR, monitor the amplification cycles. The optimal PCR cycle is the midpoint of the linear phase of the amplification curves. The red line marks the midpoint of the linear phase of the amplification curves and is used to determine the optimal numbers of amplification cycles (Fig. 3a, *see* **Note 11**).
4. When the PCR is finished, combine each reaction set and purify PCR products using 1× AMPure XP bead.
5. Elute into 20 μL of resuspension buffer.

3.6 Library Quality Control

1. Quantify libraries using Qubit fluorometer. Expected DNA concentration is 10–30 ng/μL.
2. Check the library size distribution by running 1 μL of the final library using Bioanalyzer High Sensitivity DNA Kit. Expected average size of distribution is 300–500 bp (Fig. 3b).

4 Notes

1. Bench, pipettes, and racks used should be thoroughly cleaned with DNA decontamination solution.
2. Use low DNA-binding DNAse-/RNAse-free plastic tubes and filter tips.
3. We recommend starting with a minimum of 50,000 cells for best results. The yield of genomic DNA per hematopoietic cell is around 5–10 pg on average.
4. Avoid DNA degradation and remove cellular RNA and proteins completely. Remaining RNA will affect DNA quantification, and DNA-binding proteins will affect downstream enzyme reactions as well as bisulfate conversion. Intact genomic DNA without degradation and without protein and RNA contamination is important.

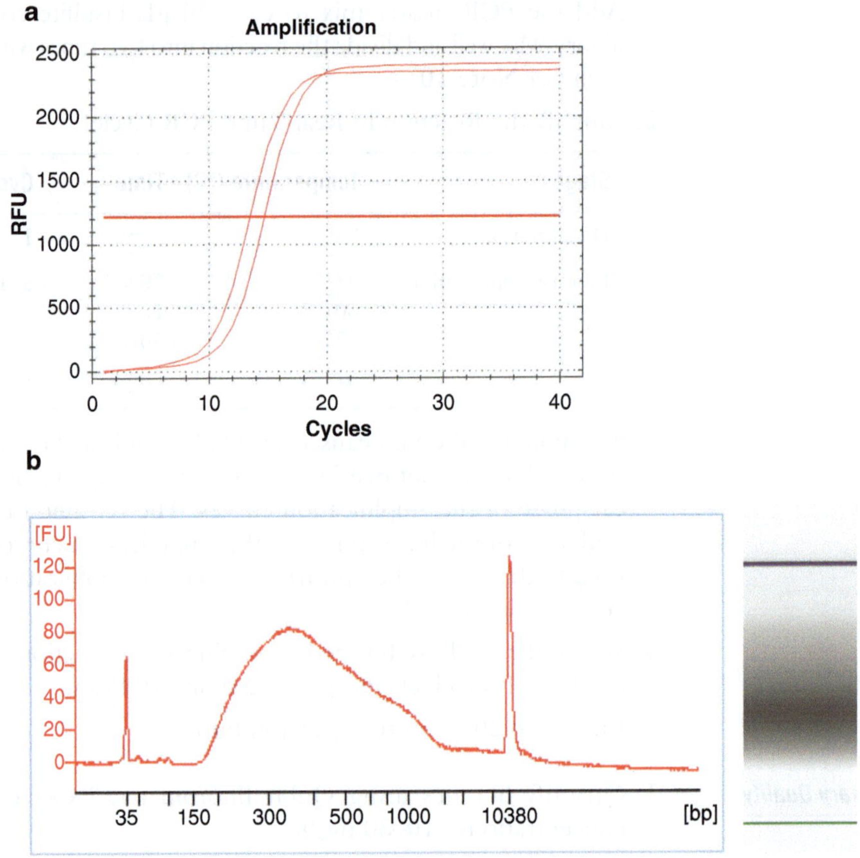

Fig. 3 WGBS library QC. (**a**) Example of real-time analysis of final PCR amplification with fluorescent dye EvaGreen in it. Results were obtained using CFX96 Touch Real-Time PCR Detection systems (Bio-Rad). (**b**) Example for a size distribution of final library analyzed on a Bioanalyzer (Agilent)

5. Covaris shearing generates dsDNA fragment with 3′ or 5′ overhangs.
6. If the thermocycler cannot hold 100 μL volume, divide reaction mix into two tubes or use water bath. In this step, DNA fragments with overhangs are converted to blunt-ended fragments.
7. A single "A" nucleotide is added to the 3′ ends of the blunt fragments to prevent them from ligating to each other during the adapter ligation reaction. A corresponding single "T" nucleotide on the 3′ end of the adapter provides a complementary overhang for ligating the adapter to the fragment. This strategy ensures a low rate of chimera (concatenated template) formation.
8. Bisulfite-converted DNA can be stored at −80 °C for about 6 months. The major sources of sequencing bias and measurement error come from incomplete bisulfite conversion. Confirm bisulfite conversion rate is >99% (Bisulfite conver-

sion rate = Total number of C conversions in non-CpG context divided by total number of Cs in non-CpG context).

9. Bisulfite conversion defects include fC, caC detected as unmethylated C, and 5mC and 5hmC detected as methylated C.
10. PfuTurbo Cx DNA polymerase is a proofreading PCR enzyme that does not stall when it encounters uracil, the product of the bisulfite reaction. Differential PCR efficiency for methylated versus unmethylated sequence is one of the potential sources of biased results.
11. The WGBS method is accurate and reproducible compared with other methods. The major sources of bias and measurement error stem from incomplete bisulfite conversion and differential PCR efficiency for methylated versus unmethylated versions of the sequences.

Acknowledgments

This work was supported by the NIH (DK092883, CA183252, CA125123, P50CA126752, T32DK060445), the Edward P Evans Foundation, the Adrienne Helis Malvin Medical Research Foundation, and by CPRIT (RR140053).

References

1. Laird PW (2010) Principles and challenges of genomewide DNA methylation analysis. Nat Rev Genet 11:191–203
2. Jeong M, Sun D, Luo M et al (2014) Large conserved domains of low DNA methylation maintained by Dnmt3a. Nat Genet 46:17–23
3. Urich MA, Nery JR, Lister R, Schmitz RJ, Ecker JR (2015) MethylC-seq library preparation for base-resolution whole-genome bisulfite sequencing. Nat Protoc 10:475–483
4. Gu H, Smith ZD, Bock C et al (2011) Preparation of reduced representation bisulfite sequencing libraries for genome-scale DNA methylation profiling. Nat Protoc 6:468–481
5. Boyle P, Clement K, Gu H et al (2012) Gel-free multiplexed reduced representation bisulfite sequencing for large-scale DNA methylation profiling. Genome Biol 13:R92
6. Hayatsu H (2008) Discovery of bisulfite-mediated cytosine conversion to uracil, the key reaction for DNA methylation analysis--a personal account. Proc Jpn Acad Ser B Phys Biol Sci 84:321–330
7. Weber M, Davies JJ, Wittig D et al (2005) Chromosome-wide and promoter-specific analyses identify sites of differential DNA methylation in normal and transformed human cells. Nat Genet 37:853–862
8. Jacinto FV, Ballestar E, Esteller M (2008) Methyl-DNA immunoprecipitation (MeDIP): hunting down the DNA methylome. BioTechniques 44:35, 37, 39 passim
9. Tan L, Xiong L, Xu W et al (2013) Genome-wide comparison of DNA hydroxymethylation in mouse embryonic stem cells and neural progenitor cells by a new comparative hMeDIP-seq method. Nucleic Acids Res 41:e84
10. Pastor WA, Pape UJ, Huang Y et al (2011) Genome-wide mapping of 5-hydroxymethylcytosine in embryonic stem cells. Nature 473:394–397
11. Li D, Zhang B, Xing X, Wang T (2015) Combining MeDIP-seq and MRE-seq to investigate genome-wide CpG methylation. Methods 72:29–40
12. Booth MJ, Ost TW, Beraldi D et al (2013) Oxidative bisulfite sequencing of 5-methylcytosine and 5-hydroxymethylcytosine. Nat Protoc 8:1841–1851
13. Yu M, Hon GC, Szulwach KE et al (2012) Tet-assisted bisulfite sequencing of 5-hydroxymethylcytosine. Nat Protoc 7:2159–2170

Chapter 10

Detection and Quantification of Acute Myeloid Leukemia-Associated Fusion Transcripts

Jonathan Schumacher, Philippe Szankasi, and Todd W. Kelley

Abstract

Real-time quantitative reverse transcription polymerase chain reaction (RT-qPCR)-based detection of abnormal fusion transcripts is an important strategy for the diagnosis and monitoring of patients with acute myeloid leukemia (AML) with t(8;21)(q22;q22); *RUNX1-RUNX1T1*, inv(16)(p13.1;q22); *CBFB-MYH11* or t(15;17)(q22;q12); *PML-RARA*. In RT-qPCR assays, patient-derived cDNA is subjected to amplification using PCR primers directed against the fusion transcript of interest as well as a reference gene for normalization. Quantification is typically performed by constructing standard curves for each PCR run using a series of plasmid standards of known concentration that harbor the same fusion transcript or the same reference gene of interest. Fusion transcripts and reference gene copy numbers are then calculated in patient samples using these standard curves. The process of constructing standard curves is laborious and consumes additional reagents. In this chapter, we give the method details for a multiplex RT-qPCR strategy to detect and quantify the acute myeloid leukemia (AML)-associated fusion transcripts *PML-RARA* in patients with t(15;17) without the need for standard curves. This general method can also be applied to other AML-associated fusion transcripts such as *CBFB-MYH11* and *RUNX1-RUNX1T1*.

Key words Acute myeloid leukemia, *PML-RARA*, RT-qPCR, Normalized copy number, Minimal residual disease

1 Introduction

Acute myeloid leukemia (AML) is a genetically heterogeneous group of hematologic malignancies that arise due to acquired chromosomal rearrangements and mutations. Common, recurrent translocations include t(8;21)(q22;q22), t(15;17)(q22;q21), and inv(16)(p13.1;q22) generating *RUNX1-RUNX1T1*, *PML-RARA*, and *CBFB-MYH11* fusion transcripts, respectively [1, 2]. The identification of cytogenetic abnormalities is important for risk stratification and for therapeutic decisions [3, 4].

Expression of *PML-RARA* fusion transcripts is a hallmark of acute promyelocytic leukemia (APL) [5]. This cytogenetic

Paolo Fortina et al. (eds.), *Acute Myeloid Leukemia: Methods and Protocols*, Methods in Molecular Biology, vol. 1633, DOI 10.1007/978-1-4939-7142-8_10, © Springer Science+Business Media LLC 2017

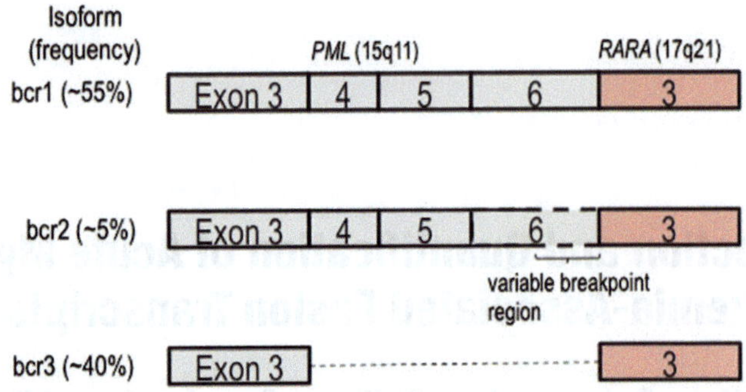

Fig. 1 Illustration of three *PML-RARA* isoforms and involved exons

abnormality confers a favorable prognosis. Patients are treated with a regimen unique to APL utilizing all-trans-retinoic acid (ATRA) and arsenic trioxide (ATO) [6]. Despite the high rate of complete remission, up to 30% of patients eventually relapse [7].

Three *PML-RARA* isoforms exist and differ in the location of the *PML* breakpoint (*see* Fig. 1) [8]. The bcr1 *PML* breakpoint is intronic and forms fusion transcripts between *PML* exon 6 and *RARA* exon 6. The bcr2 breakpoint occurs in variable regions within *PML* exon 6 and fuses to *RARA* exon 6. The bcr3 *PML* breakpoint is also intronic and forms fusion transcripts between *PML* exon 3 and *RARA* exon 6. Other *PML-RARA* isoforms have been described but occur rarely [9].

Real-time reverse transcription quantitative PCR (RT-qPCR) analysis of *PML-RARA* fusion transcripts can be an important component in the monitoring of patients owing to its simplicity and sensitivity. This method also allows for detection of minimal residual disease (MRD) and early relapse [10, 11]. It is possible to target both bcr1 and bcr2 forms with the same primer and hydrolysis probe set because of their similar breakpoints (*see* Fig. 1). The bcr3 forms can be detected with a second primer set and a reference gene with a third. The most common method of quantitation is amplifying a series of plasmid standards of known concentration to generate standard curves. The crossing point (C_p), or point at which fluorescence rises above background during a PCR reaction in patient specimens, is determined for each reaction and used to calculate copy number (CN) by extrapolating from the standard curves. A normalized copy number (NCN) is then generated reflecting the ratio of fusion transcripts to reference transcripts. The NCN value is monitored in follow-up specimens to assess treatment response.

The use of plasmid standards for quantitation has several disadvantages. First, the large number of required plasmid standards increases assay complexity. Second, the plasmid standards are laborious to create or purchase and add to assay costs. Here we describe the method details for a strategy to quantitate

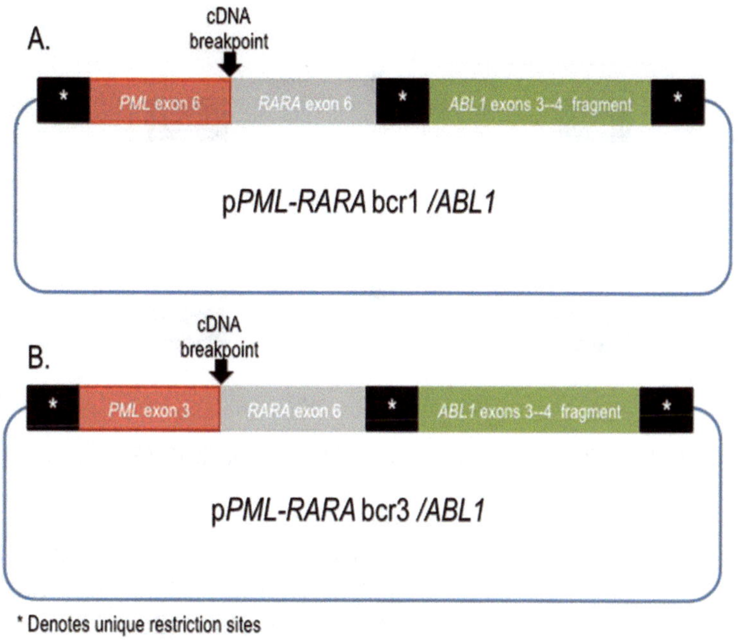

Fig. 2 Design strategy for *PML-RARA* bcr1/*ABL1* (**a**) and bcr3/*ABL1* (**b**) plasmid calibrators

PML-RARA fusion transcripts that does not require the generation of standard curves. The NCN of each fusion and reference is calculated relative to a single plasmid calibrator that contains one copy of the bcr1 or bcr3 cDNA fusion and one copy of the *ABL1* reference on the same plasmid molecule representing a 1:1 ratio of fusion and reference (*see* Fig. 2). The plasmid calibrator is amplified at a single concentration, and the NCN in patient specimens on the same run is calculated by extrapolation using the $\Delta\Delta C_p$ method [12–14].

2 Materials

2.1 PML-RARA bcr1/ABL1 and PML-RARA bcr3/ABL1 Plasmid Calibrators (Integrated DNA Technologies, Coralville, IA)

1. Two plasmid calibrators are synthesized. The bcr1/*ABL1* plasmid consists of a *PML* exon 6-*RARA* exon 3 fusion and a fragment of *ABL1* exons 3–4. The bcr3/*ABL1* plasmid consists of a *PML* exon 3-*RARA* exon 3 fusion and a fragment of *ABL1* exons 3–4. The *PML-RARA* bcr1/*ABL1* or bcr3/*ABL1* plasmid calibrators were designed using the following reference sequences: *PML*-NM_033238.2, *RARA*-NM_000964.3, and *ABL1*-NM_005157.5. The bcr1 calibrator was synthesized with the following elements: *EcoRI* restriction site, *PML* nt positions 1539–1797, *RARA* nt positions 657–805, *HindIII* restriction site, *ABL1* nt positions 426–793, and *BglII* restriction site. The bcr3 calibrator links the following

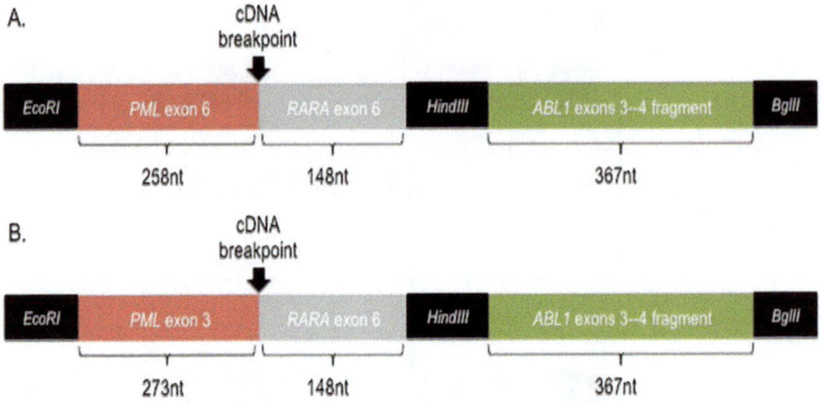

Fig. 3 Illustration of *PML-RARA* bcr1/*ABL1* (**a**) and bcr3/*ABL1* (**b**) target regions included in plasmid calibrators

fragments: *EcoRI* restriction site, *PML* nt positions 1050–1323, *RARA* nt positions 657–805, *HindIII* restriction site, *ABL1* nt positions 426–793, and *BglII* restriction site (*see* Fig. 3). Both fragments were cloned into pIDTSMART (Integrated DNA Technologies) (*see* **Note 1**).

2. 10 mM Tris–HCl, 0.5 mM EDTA, pH = 8.0.

2.2 RNA Isolation

1. Hematology analyzer (*see* **Note 2**).
2. RNA-dedicated biocontainment hood.
3. Maxwell® instrument (Promega, Madison, WI) (*see* **Note 3**).
4. Maxwell 16® LEV simplyRNA Purification Kit (Promega).
5. Centrifuge and vortex.
6. Sterile 15 mL conical tubes.

2.3 Reverse Transcription

1. Ipsogen RT Kit (Qiagen, Valencia, CA) (*see* **Note 4**).
2. Thermocycler.
3. Nuclease-free PCR strip tubes and caps.
4. Nuclease-free water.

2.4 RT-qPCR

1. LightCycler® 480 real-time PCR instrument (Roche, Basel, Switzerland) (*see* **Note 5**).
2. LightCycler® 480 Multiwell Plate 96 (Roche).
3. LightCycler® 480 Multiwell Plate 96 Sealing films (Roche).
5. PerfeCta® Multiplex qPCR ToughMix® (no ROX) (Quanta Biosciences, Gaithersburg, MD).
6. PCR primers and probes (Integrated DNA Technologies) (*see* Table 1 and **Note 6**).
7. PCR primer and probe resuspension calculator (available at http://www.idtdna.com/Calc/resuspension/).

Table 1
Primer and probe sequences

Oligonucleotide	Sequence (5′ – 3′)	Target exon(s)	Target positions
PML-RARA:			
PML bcr1/2 F	ACCTGGATGGACCGCCTAG	6	1702 – 1720
PML bcr3 F	CCGATGGCTTCGACGAGTT	3	1258 – 1276
RARA R	GCTTGTAGATGCGGGGTAGAG	6	737 – 717
RARA P	6-FAM AACTGCTGC/ZEN/ TCTGGGTCTCAATGG[a]	6	680 – 657
ABL1:			
ABL1 F	GCAATGCCGCTGAGTATC	3	593 – 610
ABL1 R	GGGACACACCATAGACAGTG	4	880 – 861
ABL1 P	Cy5 ACACTGCTTCTGATGGCAAGCTCT[b]	3–4	722 – 745

Primers and probes designed based upon the following reference sequences:
PML: NM_033238.2, RARA: NM_000964.3, and ABL1: NM_005157.5
F forward, *R* reverse, and *P* probe
[a]The *RARA* probe is labeled with a 5′ 6-FAM dye and is double-quenched with ZEN™ internal and 3′ Iowa Black® FQ
[b]The *ABL1* probe is labeled with a 5′ Cy5 dye and is single-quenched with 3′ Iowa Black® RQ-SP

3 Methods

Carry out all steps in a dedicated clean laboratory devoid of PCR amplicon and plasmid, unless otherwise specified. Wear gloves and laboratory coat at all times and change gloves often during RNA isolation and reverse transcription or when working with plasmids. Plasmids should be diluted individually to reduce the likelihood of cross-contamination. Maintain all reagents at recommended temperatures.

3.1 Plasmid Calibrator Preparation

1. If lyophilized, centrifuge plasmids at 6000 × *g* for 1 min. Reconstitute plasmids to 50 ng/μL with Tris–EDTA, pH = 8.0. Aliquot plasmids into multiple tubes can be stored at −20 °C for long term.
2. Dilute plasmids to a 1:10,000 working stock in Tris–EDTA, pH = 8.0, and store at −20 °C.

3.2 Total RNA Isolation from Patient Specimens

1. Prepare homogenization solution by adding 20 μL of 1-thioglycerol per 1 mL of homogenization solution. Store on ice or at 2–10 °C.

2. Prepare DNase I solution by adding 275 μL of nuclease-free water to lyophilized vial of DNase I. Invert to rinse residual DNase I off cap and swirl to mix. Add 5 μL of blue dye to resuspended DNase I as a visual cue for pipetting. Aliquot DNase I into 11 μL single-use aliquots and store at −20 °C.
3. Using a hematology analyzer, count the number of white blood cells (WBCs) from EDTA whole blood or bone marrow (*see* **Note 7**).
4. Transfer a specimen volume corresponding to 1×10^7 WBCs into a sterile 15 mL conical tube, and add 7.5 mL of cell lysis solution (*see* **Note 8**). Invert 5–6 times to mix.
5. Incubate at room temperature for 10 min. Invert to mix twice during incubation to facilitate lysis.
6. Centrifuge tube at 3000 × *g* for 10 min.
7. Remove and discard supernatant without disturbing WBC pellet. Briefly centrifuge tube, and remove and discard residual supernatant with a pipette without disturbing WBC pellet.
8. Add 200 μL chilled 1-thioglycerol/homogenization solution to WBC pellet and mix by vortexing or pipetting to resuspend.
9. Add 200 μL lysis buffer and 25 μL proteinase K to the resuspended pellet. Vortex for 20 s to thoroughly resuspend.
10. Incubate at room temperature for 10 min and prepare the simplyRNA Blood Cartridge during incubation. Remove one vial of DNase I solution per specimen from freezer and thaw on ice. Add 10 μL DNase I solution to well #4 of the simplyRNA Blood Cartridge.
11. Following incubation, add lysate to well #1 of the simplyRNA Blood Cartridge.
12. Place cartridge in Maxwell® 16 LEV Cartridge Rack with the label side facing away from the Elution Tubes. Press cartridge down to snap into position. Gently peel back seal and discard.
13. Place an LEV Plunger in well #8 of each cartridge.
14. Place a 0.5 mL Elution Tube in the front of the Maxwell® 16 LEV Cartridge Rack, and add 50 μL nuclease-free water to the bottom of the elution tube.
15. Place rack in Maxwell® instrument and close door.
16. Run the simplyRNA Blood protocol.
17. When run is complete, transfer RNA to an RNase-free 1.5 mL tube and store at −80 °C (*see* **Note 9**).

3.3 Reverse Transcription

1. Thaw RNA on ice and add 10 μL of total RNA to 0.2 mL PCR tube (*see* **Note 10**). Incubate at 65 °C for 5 min.
2. Place tube on ice for 5 min.

Table 2
Reverse transcription mastermix reagents

Reagent	Volume (μL)	Final concentration
Reverse transcriptase buffer	5.0	1×
dNTP mix (10 mM each)	2.0	0.8 μM
Random nonamers (100 μM)	5.25	21 μM
RNase inhibitor (40 U/μL)	0.5	0.8 U/μL
Reverse transcriptase (200 U/μL)	1.0	8 U/μL
DTT	1.25	
Final volume	15.0	

3. Pulse spin tube and replace on ice.
4. Prepare a reverse transcription mastermix by combining all reagents (*see* Table 2).
5. Add 15 μL reverse transcription mastermix to RNA and pipette to mix. Centrifuge briefly.
6. Run the following program in a thermocycler: 25 °C for 10 min followed by 50 °C for 60 min followed by 85 °C for 5 min and 4 °C for 5 min.
7. Store cDNA at −20 °C.

3.4 Preparation of Multiplex and Individual PCR Primer and Probe Mixes

1. Resuspend PCR primers (*see* Table 1) to 100 μM in 10 mM Tris–HCl, 0.5 mM EDTA, pH = 8.0 using a PCR primer, and probe resuspension calculator. Store at −20 °C long term.

3.5 Real-Time Quantitative PCR (RT-qPCR)

1. Thaw patient cDNA on ice and in dedicated amplicon laboratory; thaw working stock plasmid calibrators on ice.
2. Prepare a 96-well plate layout reflecting the analysis of each patient specimen and plasmid calibrator in duplicate and water control in singlet (*see* Fig. 4).
3. Prepare *PML-RARA* bcr1/2-*ABL1* and bcr1/ABL1 mastermixes following Table 3. Add 1–2 dead volumes.
4. Gently vortex *PML-RARA* bcr1/2-*ABL1* and bcr3-*ABL1* mastermixes and briefly centrifuge.
5. Pipette 20 μL of *PML-RARA* bcr1/2-*ABL1* mastermix into wells dedicated for bcr1/2 reactions and 20 μL of bcr3-*ABL1* mastermix into wells dedicated for bcr3 reactions (*see* Fig. 4).

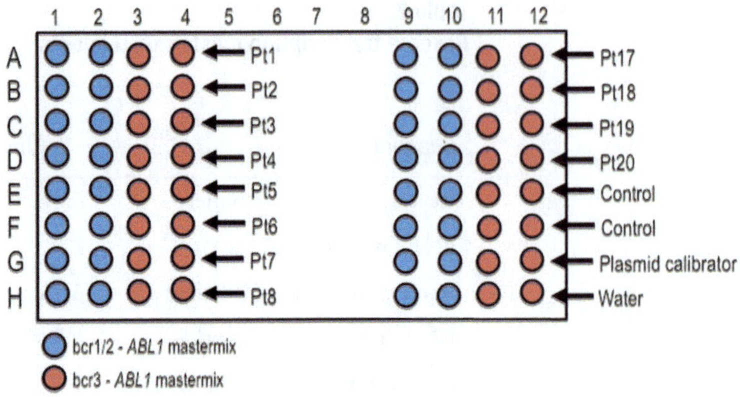

Fig. 4 Illustration of PCR plate setup for multiplex amplification of *PML-RARA* and *ABL1*. Patient specimens and controls are amplified in duplicate for both bcr1/2-*ABL1* and bcr3-*ABL1*

Table 3
25× primer-probe mastermix reagents

Component	Volume (μL)	Final concentration volume (μM)
PML bcr1/2 OR bcr3 F	12.5	5.0
RARA R	12.5	5.0
RARA P	2.5	1.0
ABL1 F	5.0	2.0
ABL1 R	5.0	2.0
ABL1 P	2.5	1.0
Water	160.0	
Final volume	200.0	

F forward, *R* reverse, and *P* probe

6. Pipette 5 μL of patient cDNA into the two wells corresponding to *PML-RARA* bcr1/2-*ABL1* and 2 wells corresponding to *PML-RARA* bcr3-*ABL1*.
7. Transition plate to dedicated amplicon laboratory and pipette 5 μL of plasmid calibrator into each designated well.
8. With a multichannel pipette set to 20 μL, mix each well 5×.
9. Cover plate with optical sealing film.
10. Centrifuge at 550 × *g* for 1 min.
11. Place plate in LightCycler® 480 real-time PCR instrument and program the following conditions:

- Under Setup:
  - Select Multi Color Hydrolysis Probe then Customize. Select Cyan 500 and FAM as active Filter Combinations and OK.
  - Change Reaction Volume to 25 μL.
- Under Program:
  - Add two Programs. The first, Hot Start, should consist of 1 cycle and None under Analysis Mode, and the second, Amplification, should consist of 45 cycles and Quantification under Analysis Mode.
- Under Temperature targets:
  - Select Hot Start from Program Name. Target temperature is 95 °C, Acquisition Mode of None, Hold for 2:00, and 0 for Set Target, Step Size, and Step Delay.
  - Select Amplification from Program Name. Target temperature is 95 °C, Acquisition Mode of None, Hold for 15 s, Ramp Rate of 4.4, and 0 for Set Target, Step Size, and Step Delay.
  - Add a second step with Target temperature of 60 °C, Acquisition Mode of Single, Hold for 60s, Ramp Rate of 4.4, and 0 for Set Target, Step Size, and Step Delay.

12. Start Run.
13. When the run is complete, open Subset Editor, and create 2 subsets: bcr1/2-*ABL1* and bcr3-*ABL1*. Select the specimens corresponding to each subset and Apply.
14. Open Sample Editor.
    - Under **Step 1**: Select Workflow, and select Rel Quant.
    - Under **Step 2**: Select Samples, and use the dropdown arrow to select the bcr1/2-*ABL1* subset.
    - In the right box, define replicate specimens and type specimen name. Identify patient specimen wells with the Filter Combination of FAM as bcr1/2 and designate as Target Unknown. Identify patient specimen wells with the Filter Combination of Cyan 500 as *ABL1* and designated as Reference Unknown. The bcr1/2 plasmid calibrator wells should be designated as Target PosCalibrator and Reference PosCalibrator, respectively. Water control should be designated as Target Negative and Reference Negative, respectively.
    - Under **Step 2**: Select Samples, and use the dropdown arrow to select the bcr3-*ABL1* subset.
    - In the right box, define replicate specimens and type specimen name. Identify patient specimen wells with the Filter Combination of FAM as bcr3 and designate as Target Unknown.

Identify patient specimen wells with the Filter Combination of Cyan 500 as *ABL1* and designated as Reference Unknown. The bcr3 plasmid calibrator wells should be designated as Target PosCalibrator and Reference PosCalibrator, respectively. Water control should be designated as Target Negative and Reference Negative, respectively.

15. Select Analysis using the Advanced Relative Quantification method for bcr1/2-*ABL1* subset and select Calculate. Under the Results tab, the NCN or ratio of bcr1/2 to *ABL1* will appear. Raw data may be viewed under the Sample View tab.
16. Select Add Item and under Analysis Type, select Advanced Relative Quantification method for bcr3-*ABL1* subset and select Calculate. Under the Results tab, the NCN or ratio of bcr3-*ABL1* will appear. Raw data may be viewed under the Sample View tab.
17. Specimens with amplification of *PML-RARA* bcr1/2 often exhibit amplification in the bcr3 reaction, whereas specimens with amplification in the bcr3 reaction should not exhibit amplification in the bcr1/2 reaction (*see* **Note 11**).
18. QC indicators should be validated per institution reflecting WBC input, RNA isolation and reverse transcription method, and real-time PCR instrumentation. No template (water) controls should not amplify, and patient specimens should amplify in duplicate with minimal validated C_p differences (ex: <1.0) between replicates.

4 Notes

1. Restriction sites were included in the event that individual fragments require cloning.
2. A hematology analyzer is used to enumerate WBCs for standardized cell input in RNA isolation.
3. Other validated RNA isolation methods may be used.
4. Other validated reverse transcription methods may be used.
5. Other validated real-time PCR instrumentation may be used but ensure that probe fluorescent dyes are compatible.
6. PCR primers probes may be ordered salt-free. HPLC purifies fluorescent probes to ensure highest purity.
7. RNA isolation must occur within 48 h of collection to ensure RNA integrity. Ethylenediaminetetraacetic acid (EDTA) is the recommended anticoagulant as heparin and citrate may contain PCR inhibitors.
8. A standard 1×10^7 WBCs generates lower *ABL1* C_ps and greater assay sensitivity. If 1×10^7 WBCs are not possible, use highest blood volume possible (up to 2.5 mL).

9. RNA is highly labile, and freeze-thaw cycles should be kept to a minimal to reduce degradation. Reverse transcription should be performed immediately upon completion of RNA isolation.
10. RNA solution may be discolored from bead carry-over during isolation, but beads should not impact assay performance.
11. Specimens expressing the bcr1 or 2 isoform retain *PML* exons 3–6. As a result, these cases will amplify in the bcr3 reaction, but because the *PML* region includes three exons, the product is longer and will yield higher C_p values due to relatively inefficient amplification. Specimens expressing the bcr3 isoform lack *PML* exon 6 and will not amplify in the bcr1/2 reaction.

References

1. Grossmann V, Schnittger S, Kohlmann A et al (2012) A novel hierarchical prognostic model of AML solely based on molecular mutations. Blood 120:2963–2972
2. Hahm C, Mun YC, Seong CM et al (2012) Additional genomic aberrations identified by single nucleotide polymorphism array-based karyotyping in an acute myeloid leukemia case with isolated del(20q) abnormality. Ann Lab Med 32:445–449
3. Messner HA (2006) How good is allogeneic transplantation for high-risk patients with AML? Best Pract Res Clin Haematol 19:329–332
4. Burnett AK, Russell NH, Hills RK et al (2015) Arsenic trioxide and all-trans retinoic acid treatment for acute promyelocytic leukaemia in all risk groups (AML17): results of a randomised, controlled, phase 3 trial. Lancet Oncol 16:1295–1305
5. Glassman AB (1995) Cytogenetics, gene fusions, and cancer. Ann Clin Lab Sci 25:389–393
6. Ravandi F, Estey E, Jones D et al (2009) Effective treatment of acute promyelocytic leukemia with all-trans-retinoic acid, arsenic trioxide, and gemtuzumab ozogamicin. J Clin Oncol 27:504–510
7. Imagawa J, Harada Y, Shimomura T et al (2010) Clinical and genetic features of therapy-related myeloid neoplasms after chemotherapy for acute promyelocytic leukemia. Blood 116:6018–6022
8. van Dongen JJ, Macintyre EA, Gabert JA et al (1999) Standardized RT-PCR analysis of fusion gene transcripts from chromosome aberrations in acute leukemia for detection of minimal residual disease. Report of the BIOMED-1 concerted action: investigation of minimal residual disease in acute leukemia. Leukemia 13:1901–1928
9. Jeziskova I, Razga F, Gazdova J et al (2010) A case of a novel PML/RARA short fusion transcript with truncated transcription variant 2 of the RARA gene. Mol Diag Ther 14:113–117
10. Zhang L, Cao Z, Zou Y et al (2012) Quantification of PML/RARa transcript after induction predicts outcome in children with acute promyelocytic leukemia. Int J Hematol 95:500–508
11. Nasilowska-Adamska B, Majewski M, Seferynska I et al (2007) Predictive value of RT-PCR PML-RARA transcript monitoring for extramedullary relapse of acute promyelocytic leukemia in the pleura, heart and pericardium after allogeneic SCT. Ann Transplant 12:33–38
12. Antonov J, Goldstein DR, Oberli A et al (2005) Reliable gene expression measurements from degraded RNA by quantitative real-time PCR depend on short amplicons and a proper normalization. Lab Investig 85:1040–1050
13. Schumacher JA, Scott Reading N, Szankasi P et al (2015) A novel approach to quantitating leukemia fusion transcripts by qRT-PCR without the need for standard curves. Exp Mol Pathol 99:104–108
14. Szankasi P, Reading NS, Vaughn CP et al (2013) A quantitative allele-specific PCR test for the BRAF V600E mutation using a single heterozygous control plasmid for quantitation: a model for qPCR testing without standard curves. J Mol Diagn 15:248–254

Chapter 11

Targeted Next-Generation Sequencing of Acute Leukemia

Eric Konnick, Christina M. Lockwood, and David Wu

Abstract

Mutation profiling of acute leukemias is a valuable tool for identifying genetic mutations with prognostic, predictive, therapeutic, and diagnostic utility. Technological advances, such as massively parallel sequencing, have allowed laboratories to assess for variation across dozens or hundreds of genes simultaneously with relatively low cost per target.

Here, we describe a procedure for designing and using a TruSeq Custom Amplicon assay targeting genes involved in acute leukemias. This method is a fully customizable, amplicon-based assay for targeted resequencing, allowing interrogation of selected genomic regions of interest. The most readily available form of the assay allows sequencing of up to 1536 amplicons in a single reaction using a straightforward workflow. The ability to multiplex up to 1536 amplicons per reaction allows coverage of up to 650 kb of cumulative sequence and supports up to 96 samples per batch, depending on library size and desired sequencing depth.

Key words Next-generation sequencing, TruSeq, Amplicon, Leukemia, Illumina

1 Introduction

Acute leukemias are generally defined as the presence of greater than 20% abnormal blasts in the peripheral blood or bone marrow and can often be classified based on the hematopoietic cell of origin. Approximately two-thirds of cases arise from myeloid lineage cells (acute myeloid leukemias [AML]), and one-third originate from lymphoid lineage cells (acute lymphoid leukemia [ALL]) [1]. There are numerous differences in the mutational spectrum of different types of acute leukemias that have been elucidated, many of which are recurrent in a given classification. Some genetic aberrations appear to be limited to a specific spectrum of entities, while other mutations are observed in a wider range of neoplasia.

In the context of AML, numerous mutations and structural alterations have been described, with some mutations, such as the *PML-RARA* translocation having diagnostic and therapeutic implications, while other mutations have a prognostic role in other AML subtypes. For example, internal tandem duplications of a

Paolo Fortina et al. (eds.), *Acute Myeloid Leukemia: Methods and Protocols*, Methods in Molecular Biology, vol. 1633, DOI 10.1007/978-1-4939-7142-8_11, © Springer Science+Business Media LLC 2017

Table 1
Examples of molecular or cytogenetic aberrations in tumors useful for pathologic classification, prognostication, or clinical targeting

	Molecular/cytogenetic aberrations
Acute myeloid leukemia	*CBFB-MYH11, DEK-NUP214, PML-RARA,* inv. [16], *RUNX1/RUNX1T1, FLT3, IDH1, IDH2, KIT, MLL-MLLT3, NPM1, CEBPA, KIT, DNMT3A, TP53, WT1, RPN1-EVI1, RBM15-MKL1, PTEN, PHF6, TP53, TET2, RAS, ASXL1, GATA2*
Acute lymphoid leukemia	*BCR-ABL, MLL, CRLF2, JAK2, JAK1, JAK3, IL7R, IKZF1, NOTCH1, FBXW7, IDH2, DNMT3A, ETV6, NF1*

Given the rapidity of change in this field, this represents at, best, an incomplete list of known and recently discovered molecular genetic aberrations present in the listed neoplasms

portion of the fms-related tyrosine kinase 3 (*FLT3*) gene (*FLT3*-ITD) have been associated with poor prognosis [2], while *CEBPA* and *NPM1* mutations have been associated with favorable prognosis [3, 4]. Other mutated genes that have been associated with poor prognosis include *KIT* [5], *DNMT3A* [6], *RUNX1* [7], and *TET2* [8]. Additional mutations have been identified that are associated with resistance to targeted therapies [9, 10], and other genes have been identified that offer prognostic information. A subset of the known clinically relevant genes and structural rearrangements known to be important in AML are presented in Table 1.

Similar to AML, genetic mutations have been discovered to have a meaningful impact on prognosis in ALL. Mutations in specific genes have been associated with poor prognosis in ALL, including *FBXW7* [11] and *IL7R* [12]. Other genes have also been observed to have mutations in a fraction of ALL cases, including in genes that may be amenable to therapeutic intervention, such as *JAK1* [13]. As scientific and medical knowledge expand, additional genes are likely to be identified that will have prognostic, diagnostic, and/or predictive utility [15]. A subset of the known clinically relevant genes and structural rearrangements known to be important in ALL are presented in Table 1.

Although many genes with mutations appear to be limited to distinct subsets of AML and ALL, the overall frequency of many of the meaningful variants may be low. With the advent of massively parallel sequencing (also known as next-generation sequencing [NGS]), large numbers of clinically relevant genes can be simultaneously evaluated in a single assay [14]. This technology allows for rapid, cost-efficient, and tissue-sparing identification of relevant mutations for a specific disease population that is especially useful when the spectrum of mutated genes and mutations is wide.

The TruSeq amplicon-based NGS method uses oligonucleotide probes to hybridize to targeted regions of interest on non-fragmented genomic sample DNA. In a subsequent extension-ligation step, a DNA polymerase extends from the upstream oligonucleotide through the targeted region followed by ligation to the 5′ end of the downstream oligonucleotide using a DNA ligase. The extension-ligation products are separated from genomic DNA in a wash step and subsequently amplified using primers that incorporate multiplexing index sequences as well as adapters required for cluster generation. Following the amplification and an indexing step, samples are purified and normalized with bead-based normalization. Pooled libraries are diluted and heat denatured prior to loading on the Illumina instrument for sequencing. Data analysis can be accomplished using onboard informatics, or raw data can be exported for analysis and annotation using a commercial or custom pipeline.

2 Materials

Prepare reagents as indicated in the methods. Freshly prepared solutions and reagents will result in optimal method performance.

1. Adjustable micropipettes with aerosol-resistant disposable pipette tips.
2. Microcentrifuge tubes—various sizes.
3. PCR eight-tube strips.
4. Microcentrifuges.
5. Thermal cycler.
6. 96-well skirted PCR plate, 0.2 mL, polypropylene.
7. Reagent and waste troughs.
8. 10 N NaOH.
9. Ethanol, 200 proof for molecular biology.
10. TruSeq Index Plate Fixture Kit (Illumina).
11. TruSeq Custom Amplicon Filter Plate (Illumina).
12. TruSeq Index Plate Fixture and Collar Kit (Illumina).
13. 96-well storage plates, 0.8 mL (MIDI plates) (Fisher Scientific).
14. Agencourt AMPureXP kit (Beckman Coulter).
15. Adhesive aluminum foil seal (Beckman Coulter).
16. Microseal "B" adhesive seals (Bio-Rad).
17. Agarose gel or Bioanalyzer system for quality assessment of PCR product.
18. Ice bucket.

19. 37° incubator.
20. Heat block for 1.5 mL centrifuge tubes (96 °C).
21. Hybex Microsample Incubator for PCR plate, 96-well (Scigene).
22. Tabletop centrifuge (plate centrifuge that can achieve 2400 × *g*).
23. Magnetic Stand-96 Side Skirted (Invitrogen).
24. BioShake iQ High-Speed Thermal Mixer (Q instruments).
25. Thermal cycler with heated lid.
26. Custom or manufacturer distributed TruSeq oligonucleotides targeting regions of interest (*see* **Notes 1** and **2**, Illumina).
27. TruSeq reagents (included with TruSeq oligonucleotides): OHS2, ACD1, ACP1, ELM4, SW1, UB1, ELM4, PMM2, i5 primers, i7 primers, TDP1, EBT, LNA1, LNB1, LNW1, LNS2, and HT1 (Illumina).
28. MiSeq reagent cartridge and kit (Illumina).
29. MiSeq instrument (Illumina).

3 Methods

3.1 DNA Isolation

DNA can be isolated using numerous methods. An important consideration is the source of the specimen (fresh, frozen, blood, plasma, formalin-fixed paraffin-embedded tissue, etc.) as specimens with more manipulation (i.e., FFPE) generally yield poorer-quality DNA. Numerous commercial kits are available for DNA extraction, or DNA can be extracted with a laboratory-developed procedure. We have had success using DNA extraction kits from Qiagen for FFPE, blood, plasma, and bone marrow applications.

3.2 Hybridization of Oligonucleotide Pool

During this step, a custom pool containing upstream and downstream oligonucleotide probes specific to the targeted regions of interest is hybridized to genomic DNA extracted from the samples (Table 2).

1. Remove the reagents (CAT, ACD1, ACP1, OHS2) and genomic DNA from −15 to −25 °C storage and thaw at room temperature. The OHS2 reagent may require more time to thaw than the other reagents.
2. Set the Hybex 96-well heat block to 95 °C (*see* **Note 3**).
3. Preheat an incubator to 37 °C to prepare for the extension-ligation step.
4. Mix all reagents well by vortexing and quick spin using a tabletop centrifuge prior to use.
5. Label a new 96-well hybridization plate with the date, run identifier, and wells in use.

Table 2
Reagents and consumables required for hybridization of oligonucleotide pool

Item	Quantity	Storage (°C)	Supplied
Custom amplicon oligonucleotide tube (CAT)	1 tube	−15 to −25	Illumina
OHS2 (Oligo Hybridization for Sequencing 2)	1 tube	−15 to −25	Illumina
Amplicon Control DNA (ACD1)	1 tube	−15 to −25	Illumina
Amplicon Control Oligo Pool 1 (ACP1)	1 tube	−15 to −25	Illumina
Genomic DNA	As needed	−15 to −25	User
96-well skirted PCR plate	1 plate	Room temperature	User
Adhesive aluminum foil seal	2 seals	Room temperature	User
Troughs	As needed	Room temperature	User

6. Pipette 5 μL of custom amplicon oligonucleotide tube (CAT) to the sample wells and 5 μL of Amplicon Control Oligo Pool 1 (ACP1) to the ACD1 control well (if used).
7. Add 250 ng (up to 10 μL) of genomic or FFPE DNA to each sample well of the hybridization plate to be used in the assay. For more dilute samples (<25 ng/μL), up to 15 μL of DNA can be used.
8. If used, add 5 μL of Amplicon Control DNA (ACD1) and 5 μL of water the ACD1 control well in the hybridization plate for the assay control. ACD1 is a pool of known amplicons that will be amplified by ACP1 primers and can be included to assess the assay performance. The generated data are primarily used by Illumina technical support for troubleshooting. Note that the targets and primers used for these reagents do not overlap with the genomes that can be used in the online assay design software.
9. If samples are not positioned at the bottom of the well, seal the hybridization plate with adhesive aluminum foil and centrifuge to 1000 × *g* at 20 °C for 1 min.
10. After ensuring that any crystals or precipitate in the OHS2 reagent have dissolved, use a single channel pipette to pipette 35 μL of OHS2 to each sample in the hybridization plate. Change tips after each sample to avoid cross-contamination. When finished, gently pipette up and down 3–5 times to mix with a multichannel pipette.
11. Seal the hybridization plate securely with plastic optical Polyolefin Sealing Film and centrifuge to 1000 × *g* at 20 °C for 1 min.

12. Place the hybridization plate in the preheated Hybex block at 95 °C and incubate for 1 min (*see* **Note 3**).
13. While the plate remains on the preheated block, set the temperature to 40 °C and continue incubating for 80 min.
14. It is helpful to return 20–30 min before the end of the incubation to prepare for the next steps of the procedure.

3.3 Removal of Unbound Oligonucleotide Probes

Unbound oligonucleotide probes are removed from template DNA using a size selection filter and two washes with a stringent wash solution (SW1). A final wash using a buffered solution (UB1) removes the residual wash solution and prepares samples for the extension-ligation reaction (Table 3).

1. Remove ELM4 from −15 to −25 °C storage and thaw at room temperature. This reagent will be used for the subsequent extension-ligation reaction.
2. Remove stringent wash solution (SW1) and Universal Buffer 1 solution (UB1) from 2 to 8 °C storage and set aside at room temperature.
3. Assemble the filter plate assembly unit (FPAU) in the order from top to bottom: lid, filter plate, adapter collar, and 96-well storage plates (0.8 mL).
4. Mix all reagents well by vortexing and quick spin prior to use.
5. Prewash the FPAU plate membrane as follows: Using a multichannel pipette, add 45 μL of SW1 to each well; cover the FPAU plate with the filter plate lid and keep it covered during each centrifugation step; and centrifuge the FPAU at 2400 × *g* at 20 °C for 10 min.

Table 3
Reagents and consumables required for removal of unbound oligonucleotide probes

Item	Quantity	Storage (°C)	Supplied
ELM4 (thawed in preparation for extension-ligation)	1 tube	−15 to −25	Illumina
SW1 (Stringent Wash 1) contains formamide	1 tube	2–8	Illumina
UB1 (Universal Buffer 1)	1 tube	2–8	Illumina
Filter plate with lid	1 plate	Room temperature	Illumina
Adapter collar (reusable)	1 plate	Room temperature	Illumina
96-well storage plates, 0.8 mL (MIDI plates)	1 plate	Room temperature	User
Troughs	As needed	Room temperature	User

6. Inspect the filter plate: if there is >15 μL/well of residual buffer in ≥10 wells/plate, discard the current plate and repeat the above process with a fresh filter plate.
7. After the 80-min incubation of the sample DNA and probe oligonucleotides, confirm that the heat block has cooled to 40 °C. Do not proceed until the heat block has cooled to 40 °C.
8. While the HYB plate is still in the heat block, reinforce the seal using a rubber roller or sealing wedge (*see* **Note 4**).
9. Remove the HYB plate from the heat block and centrifuge to 1000 × *g* at 20 °C for 1 min to collect condensation.
10. Using a multichannel pipette set to 65 μL, using aerosol barrier pipette tips, transfer the entire volume (50 μL) of each sample onto the center of the corresponding prewashed wells of the FPAU plate. Change tips after each column to avoid cross-contamination.
11. Cover the FPAU plate with the filter plate lid and centrifuge the FPAU at 2400 × *g* at 20 °C for 2 min.
12. Wash the FPAU plate as follows: Using a multichannel pipette, add 45 μL of SW1 to each sample well (*see* **Note 5**); cover the FPAU plate with the filter plate lid and centrifuge the FPAU at 2400 × *g* for 2 min; and inspect the FPAU. If there is residual SW1 reagent present in the filter plate, centrifuge the plate at 2400 × *g* for 2 min for up to 10 min (*see* **Note 6**); repeat the wash procedure one more time.
13. Using a pipette, discard all the flow-through (containing formamide waste and unbound oligonucleotides) collected up to this point in a biohazard waste container, and then reassemble the FPAU. The same MIDI plate can be reused for the remaining pre-amplification steps.
14. Using a multichannel pipette, add 45 μL of Universal Buffer 1 (UB1) to each sample well.
15. Cover the FPAU plate with the filter plate lid and centrifuge the FPAU at 2400 × *g* for 2 min.

3.4 Extension-Ligation of Bound Oligonucleotides

At the end of the previous wash step, sample DNA and bound oligonucleotide probes specific for the targets of interest are present in the membrane of the filter plate, with unbound oligonucleotides washed away. This step will ligate the hybridized upstream and downstream oligonucleotide probes (oligos) via an enzymatic reaction. A DNA polymerase is used to extend from the upstream oligo through the targeted region, followed by ligation to the 5′ end of the downstream oligo using a DNA ligase. The extension-ligation results in the formation of products containing the targeted regions

Table 4
Reagents and consumables required for extension-ligation of bound oligonucleotides step

Item	Quantity	Storage (°C)	Supplied
ELM4 (Extension-Ligation Mix 4)	1 tube	−15 to −25	Illumina
Adhesive aluminum foil seal	1 seal	Room temperature	User
Troughs	As needed	Room temperature	User

of interest flanked by sequences on both the 5′ and 3′ ends that facilitate amplification using indexed PCR primers in the next step (Table 4).

1. Using a multichannel pipette, add 45 μL of Extension-Ligation Mix 4 (ELM4) to each sample well of the FPAU plate (*see* **Note 7**).
2. Seal the FPAU plate with adhesive aluminum foil, and then cover with the lid to secure the foil during incubation.
3. Incubate the entire FPAU assembly in the preheated 37 °C incubator for 45 min.
4. While the FPAU plate is incubating, prepare the Indexed Amplification Plate (IAP) as described in the following Subheading.

3.5 Polymerase Chain Reaction Amplification

Once the oligonucleotide probes flanking the targeted regions of DNA have been extended and ligated, each oligonucleotide probe contains nontarget genome primer binding sites that will allow the extension-ligation products to be amplified using primers that add sample multiplexing index sequences (i5 and i7) as well as common adapters required for sequencing cluster generation (P5 and P7). Common adapters allow the amplified products to hybridize to the sequencing instrument flow cell, and the incorporation of unique index sequences allows multiple samples to be multiplexed on the same flow cell (Table 5).

1. Determine the index primers to be used in the assay and record index primer positions for downstream use in the bioinformatics pipeline.
2. Remove PCR Master Mix 2 (PMM2) and the index primers (i5 and i7) from −15 to −25 °C storage and thaw on a bench at room temperature. Vortex each tube to mix and briefly centrifuge the tubes in a microcentrifuge.
3. Arrange i5 primer tubes (white-green caps, clear solution) vertically in a rack, aligned with rows A through H.

Table 5
Reagents and consumables required for polymerase chain reaction amplification

Item	Quantity	Storage (°C)	Supplied
PMM2 (PCR Master Mix 2)	1 tube	−15 to −25	Illumina
i5 primers (A5XX)	1 tube per primer	−15 to −25	Illumina
i7 primers (A7XX)	1 tube per primer	−15 to −25	Illumina
TDP1 (TruSeq DNA Polymerase 1)	1 tube	−15 to −25	Illumina
Microseal "B" adhesive film	1	Room temperature	User
50 mM NaOH (fresh; prepared from 10 N NaOH)	3.5 mL for 96 samples, 25 μL/sample 10 N to 50 mM 1:200 dilution	Room temperature	User
96-well skirted PCR plate	1 plate	Room temperature	User
Troughs	As needed	Room temperature	User

4. Arrange i7 primer tubes (orange caps, yellow solution) horizontally in a rack, aligned with columns 1 through 12.
5. Prepare fresh 50 mM NaOH (1:200 dilution of 10 N NaOH). For example, for 16 samples, use 7 μL 10 N NaOH diluted into 1393 μL Molecular Grade water (*see* **Note 8**).
6. Combine TruSeq DNA Polymerase 1 (TDP1) and PCR Master Mix 2 (PMM2) for the number of samples in your run, plus two additional samples to account for volume loss, as follows:

   # of samples × 22 μL = Volume of PMM2 needed.

   Volume of PMM2 ÷ 50 = Volume of TDP1 needed.
7. Mix all reagents well to create the PMM2/TDP1 PCR master mix and quick spin prior to use.
8. When the 45-min extension-ligation reaction is complete, remove the FPAU from the incubator. Remove the aluminum foil seal and replace with the filter plate lid.
9. Centrifuge the FPAU at 2400 × *g* for 2 min.
10. Using a multichannel pipette, add 25 μL of 50 mM NaOH to each sample well on the FPAU plate to denature the double-stranded DNA product. Ensuring that pipette tips come in contact with the membrane, pipette the NaOH up and down 5–6 times. Tips must be changed after each column (*see* **Note 9**).
11. Incubate the FPAU plate at room temperature for 5 min.
12. While the FPAU plate is incubating, use a multichannel pipette to transfer 22 μL of the PMM2/TDP1 PCR master mix to each well of the Indexed Amplification Plate (IAP) (*see* **Note 10**).

13. Using a multichannel pipette, add 4 μL of i5 primers (clear solution) to each column of the IAP plate.
14. To avoid index cross-contamination, discard the original white caps and apply new white-green caps provided in the TruSeq Custom Amplicon Index Kit (*see* **Note 11**).
15. Using a multichannel pipette, add 4 μL of i7 primers (yellow solution) to each row of the IAP plate. Tips must be changed after each row to avoid index cross-contamination (*see* **Note 9**).
16. To avoid index cross-contamination, discard the original orange caps and apply new orange caps provided in the TruSeq Custom Amplicon Index Kit (*see* **Note 9**).
17. Transfer samples eluted from the FPAU plate to the IAP plate. Set a multichannel P20 pipette to 20 μL. Using fine tips, pipette the NaOH in the first column of the FPAU plate up and down 5–6 times. Then transfer 20 μL from the FPAU plate to the corresponding column of the IAP plate. Gently pipette up and down 5–6 times to combine the DNA with the PCR master mix (*see* **Note 12**). Transfer the samples from the remaining columns from the FPAU plate to the IAP plate in a similar manner. Tips must be changed after each column to avoid index and sample cross-contamination.
18. After all the samples have been transferred, the waste collection MIDI plate of the FPAU can be discarded. Put the metal adapter collar away for future use. If only a partial FPAU plate is used, clearly mark which wells have been used. Store the FPAU plate and lid in a sealed plastic bag to avoid contamination of the filter membrane.
19. Cover the IAP plate with Microseal "B" film and seal with a rubber roller.
20. Centrifuge to 1000 × *g* at 20 °C for 1 min.
21. Transfer the IAP plate to the post-amplification area.
22. Perform PCR on a thermal cycler using the following program:

    95 °C for 3 min.

    24 cycles of:

        95 °C for 30 s.

        66 °C for 30 s.

        72 °C for 60 s.

    72 °C for 5 min.

    Hold at 10 °C.

23. Immediately proceed to PCR cleanup or store PCR product (*see* **Note 13**).

3.6 PCR Cleanup

Unbound primers and unused PCR reagents are removed from dual indexed, double-stranded PCR product using AMPure XP beads (Table 6).

1. Turn on a heat block suitable for 1.5 mL centrifuge tubes to 96 °C and allow to preheat for **step 8**.
2. Bring the AMPure XP beads to room temperature and mix prior to use (*see* **Note 14**).
3. Prepare fresh 80% ethanol from absolute ethanol. 400 μL will be required for each sample (*see* **Note 15**).
4. Label a new 0.8 mL 96-well storage plate (MIDI plate) for use during the PCR cleanup and normalization procedures.
5. Centrifuge the IAP plate at 1000 × *g* at 20 °C for 1 min to collect condensation.
6. To confirm that the library successfully amplified, run an aliquot of the control and selected test samples on a 4% agarose (5 μL) or on a Bioanalyzer (1 μL). The expected PCR product size depends on the design parameters (e.g., 175 bp design should have a ~310 bp band).
7. Using a multichannel pipette, add 60 μL of AMPure XP beads to each well of the cleanup plate.
8. Using a multichannel pipette set to 60 μL, transfer the entire PCR product from the IAP plate to the 96-well skirted PCR plate, 0.2 mL (CLP) plate. Change tips between samples.
9. Seal the CLP plate with a foil adhesive seal.
10. Shake the CLP plate on a microplate shaker at 1800 rpm for 2 min.
11. Incubate at room temperature without shaking for 10 min.
12. Place the plate on an appropriate magnetic stand for 2 min or until the supernatant has cleared.

Table 6
Reagents and consumables required for PCR cleanup

Item	Quantity	Storage (°C)	Supplied
EBT (Elution Buffer with Tris)	1 tube	Room temperature	Illumina
AMPure XP beads	As needed	2–8	User
Freshly prepared 80% ethanol	400 μL per sample	Room temperature	User
96-well storage plates, 0.8 mL (MIDI plates)	2	Room temperature	User
Foil adhesive seal	As needed	Room temperature	User
Troughs	As needed	Room temperature	User

13. Using a multichannel pipette set to 100 μL and with the CLP plate on the magnetic stand, carefully remove and discard the supernatant. Change tips between samples.
14. With the CLP plate on the magnetic stand, wash the beads with freshly prepared 80% ethanol. Using a multichannel pipette, add 200 μL of freshly prepared 80% ethanol to each sample well (*see* **Note 16**). Incubate the plate on the magnetic stand for 30 s or until the supernatant appears clear. Carefully remove and discard the supernatant. Repeat the 80% ethanol wash described in the previous step. After repeating the ethanol wash, use a P20 multichannel pipette set to 20 μL to remove any remaining excess ethanol.
15. Remove the CLP plate from the magnetic stand and allow the beads to air-dry for 10 min or until cracks form (*see* **Note 17**).
16. Using a multichannel pipette, add 30 μL of EBT to each well of the CLP plate (*see* **Note 15**).
17. Seal the CLP plate with foil seal and shake on a microplate shaker at 1800 rpm for 2 min. After shaking, if any samples are not resuspended, gently pipette up and down or lightly tap the plate on the bench to mix, and then repeat this step.
18. Incubate at room temperature without shaking for 2 min.
19. Place the plate on the magnetic stand for 2 min or until the supernatant has cleared.
20. Carefully transfer 20 μL of the supernatant from the CLP plate to the bottom of the wells of a new MIDI plate (Library Normalization Plate [LNP]). Alternatively, an unused set of wells on the CLP plate can be used. Change tips between samples.

3.7 Library Normalization

In order to multiplex samples on a single flow cell, the relative amounts of sequencing library for each sample must be similar to ensure approximately equal library representation in the final pooled sample. This step uses a bead-based procedure to normalize the libraries of the samples prior to combining and sequencing (Table 7).

1. Prepare fresh 0.1 N NaOH (*see* **Note 18**).
2. Set a heat block suitable for 1.5 mL centrifuge tubes to 96 °C and allow to preheat for **step 3.8**.
3. Remove Library Normalization Additives 1 (LNA1) and Library Normalization Storage Buffer 2 (LNS2) from −15 to −25 °C storage and bring to room temperature. When at room temperature, vortex vigorously and make sure that all precipitates have dissolved.
4. Remove Library Normalization Beads 1(LNB1) and Library Normalization Wash 1 (LNW1) from 2 to 8 °C storage and bring to room temperature.

Table 7
Reagents and consumables required for library normalization

Item	Quantity	Storage (°C)	Supplied
LNA1 (Library Normalization Additives 1)	1 tube	−15 to −25	Illumina
LNB1 (Library Normalization Beads 1)	1 tube	2–8	Illumina
LNW1 (Library Normalization Wash 1)	2 tubes	2–8	Illumina
LNS2 (Library Normalization Storage Buffer 2)	1 tube	Room temperature	Illumina
0.1 N NaOH (fresh)	30 μL per sample	Room temperature	User
96-well skirted PCR plate	1 plate	Room temperature	User
15 mL conical tube	1 tube	Room temperature	User
Foil adhesive film	As needed	Room temperature	User

5. Vigorously vortex LNB1 for at least 1 min with intermittent inversion until the beads are well resuspended, and no pellet is found at the bottom of the tube when the tube is inverted.
6. Use a P1000 pipette set to 1000 μL to resuspend LNB1 thoroughly by pipetting up and down 15–20 times, until the bead pellet at the bottom is resuspended (*see* **Note 19**).
7. Calculate the volume of LNA1 and LNB1 needed to prepare enough of the LNA1/LNB1 solution for the number of samples being processed as follows, being sure to prepare extra for volume loss during pipetting:

   Volume LNA1 per sample = 45 μL.

   Volume LNB1 per sample = 8.2 μL.
8. Immediately after LNB1 is thoroughly resuspended, use a P1000 pipette transfer LNB1 to the tube containing LNA1. Mix well by inverting the tube 15–20 times.
9. Add 45 μL of the combined LNA1/LNB1 mixture to each well of the LNP plate containing the individual sequencing libraries (*see* **Note 20**).
10. Seal the LNP plate with a foil adhesive seal and shake on a microplate shaker at 1800 rpm for 30 min (*see* **Note 21**).
11. Place the plate on a magnetic stand for 2 min or until the supernatant has cleared.

12. With the LNP plate on the magnetic stand, use a multichannel pipette set to 80 μL to remove the supernatant and then discard in the normalization biohazard waste container.
13. Remove the LNP plate from the magnetic stand and wash the beads with LNW1. Using a multichannel pipette, add 45 μL of LNW1 to each sample well. Seal the LNP plate with a foil adhesive seal. Shake the LNP plate on a microplate shaker at 1800 rpm for 5 min. Place the plate on the magnetic stand for 2 min or until the supernatant has cleared. Carefully remove and discard the supernatant in normalization biohazard waste container. Use a P20 multichannel pipette to remove excess LNW1 (*see* **Note 22**). Repeat the LNW1 wash.
14. Remove the LNP plate from the magnetic stand and add 30 μL of fresh 0.1 N NaOH to each well to elute the sample.
15. Seal the LNP plate with a foil adhesive seal and shake on a microplate shaker at 1800 rpm for 5 min (*see* **Note 8**).
16. During the 5-min elution, designate clean wells of the 96-well plate as storage plate (SGP) or prepare a separate storage plate.
17. Add 30 μL LNS2 to each well to be used in the SGP plate.
18. After the 5-min elution, make sure that all samples in the LNP plate are resuspended completely. If the samples are not resuspended, gently pipette up and down or lightly tap the plate on the bench to resuspend the beads. Then shake for another 5 min.
19. Place the LNP plate on the magnetic stand for 2 min or until the liquid is clear.
20. Using a multichannel pipette set to 30 μL, transfer the supernatant containing the released sequencing libraries from the LNP plate to the SGP plate wells containing LNS2. Change tips between samples to avoid cross-contamination.
21. If stopping is not avoidable, seal the SGP plate with foil seal and then centrifuge to 1000 × *g* for 1 min. Store at −20 °C for a maximum of 2 h (*see* **Note 23**).

3.8 Library Pooling and MiSeq Sample Loading

Equal volumes of normalized library are combined, diluted in hybridization buffer, and heat denatured in preparation for cluster generation and sequencing (Table 8).

1. Set a heat block suitable for 1.5 mL centrifuge tubes to 96 °C, as indicated in **steps 3.6** and **3.7**.
2. Remove a MiSeq reagent cartridge from −15 to −25 °C storage and thaw at room temperature.
3. In an ice bucket, prepare an ice-water bath by combining three parts ice and one part water.

Table 8
Reagents and consumables required for library pooling and MiSeq sample loading

Item	Quantity	Storage (°C)	Supplied
HT1 (hybridization buffer)	1 tube	−15 to −25	Illumina
1.5 mL Eppendorf tubes (screw-cap recommended)	2 tubes	Room temperature	User
PCR eight-tube strip	1	Room temperature	User
2.5 L ice bucket	1	Room temperature	User
Ice	As needed	Room temperature	User
Water	As needed	Room temperature	User

4. If stored, centrifuge the SGP plate at 1000 × *g* at 20 °C for 1 min to collect condensation.
5. Label a clean 1.5 mL low retention Eppendorf tube with the name and date of your run and Pooled Amplicon Library (PAL).
6. Determine the samples to be pooled for sequencing.
7. Using a P20 multichannel pipette, transfer 5 μL of each library to be sequenced from the SGP plate, column by column, to a single unused column. Change tips after each column to avoid cross-contamination.
8. Combine and transfer the contents of the combined sample column into the PAL tube. Mix PAL well. Seal the SGP plate and store the sealed plate at −15 to −25 °C.
9. Label two new 1.5 mL low retention Eppendorf tubes with the date, name of run, and "DAL-1" and "DAL-2" (Dilute Amplicon Library).
10. Create DAL-1 by combining 590 μL of HT1 and 10 μL PAL. Upon transferring PAL, using the same tip, pipette up and down 3–5 times to rinse the tip and ensure complete transfer. Close cap tightly (*see* **Note 24**).
11. Do the same for DAL-2 using 15 μL of PAL and 585 μL HT1. This will be stored in case of low cluster density of DAL-1 (*see* **Note 24**).
12. Mix DALs by vortexing the tube at top speed. Continue to the next step with DAL-1 (*see* **Note 25**) and place the PAL and DAL-2 at −15 to −25 °C after sealing the containers.
13. Using a heat block, incubate the DAL-1 tube at 96 °C for 2 min.
14. After the incubation, invert DAL 1–2 times to mix and immediately place in the ice-water bath.
15. Keep the DAL-1 tube in the ice-water bath for a minimum of 5 min.

3.9 Loading the MiSeq

1. Remove one MiSeq reagent cartridge (MiSeq Reagent Kit v2, 300 cycles box 1 of 2) from the freezer and thaw in room temperature water. Remove one MiSeq Reagent Kit v2 (box 2 of 2) from the refrigerator immediately prior to loading.
2. After the reagent cartridge has thawed, invert the cartridge gently 5–10 times to mix the reagents. Visually confirm that the reagents are completely thawed in all reagent trays and that reagents are well mixed.
3. After a minimum of 5-min ice-water incubation, transfer the 600 μL contents of the DAL to the designated sample position on the Illumina cartridge.
4. Follow the manufacturer's instructions for MiSeq and run setup. Components of setting up the system are as follows: Load the PR2 fluid and waste bottle, remove the wash cartridge, load the prepared sample cartridge, and identify the samples being tested.
5. Prepare flow cell. Remove flow cell from the vial with clean forceps. Only touch the plastic casing. Hold it over a beaker and rinse thoroughly with Molecular Grade water. Make sure all traces of buffer are washed off. Using a Kimwipe, carefully dry all surfaces. Make sure the flow cell glass surface is free of smudges, lint, moisture, or other foreign material. Hold it up against the light to visually double check. Following the prompt on MiSeq, remove the used flow cell from the instrument and insert the new flow cell (*see* **Note 26**). Close the outer door of the MiSeq.
6. After the MiSeq has passed the internal self-check routine, start the sequencing run.

3.10 Data Analysis

After completion of sequencing, the data must be manipulated, aligned to a reference genome, and variants called before analysis by qualified professionals. Numerous options exist for this process that include software packaged with the instrumentation, separate third-party packages, cloud-computing platforms, or custom in-house developed bioinformatics pipelines. All approaches have the following common processes:

1. Demultiplexing (DEMUX), base calling, and quality assessment of raw sequence data of the individual sequencing data to generate FASTQ files.
2. Mapping sequencing reads from a given sample to a reference genome sequence to generate BAM and/or Sequence Alignment/Map format (SAM) file.
3. Variant calling and annotation programs to generate a Variant Call File (VCF).

Additional software packages can be used to identify structural changes that are larger than can be reliably identified using many of the common variant calling programs (e.g., VarScan, GATK). These programs often have unique output files.

The analysis methods chosen by the laboratory to perform the above tasks are highly dependent on the specific experimental application, the expertise of the laboratory, the availability of bioinformatics and computational resources, and the time available to assemble vs. purchase bioinformatics pipelines. Our laboratory uses a modification of the custom pipeline previously described pipeline [16] that includes the PINDEL [17] package, but excludes Breakdancer [18], CREST [19], and CONTRA [20].

Basic quality metric information for a given MiSeq run can be obtained as follows:

1. Open the Sequence Analysis Viewer program from the computer desktop of the MiSeq personal computer (PC).
2. Click the "Browse" icon and locate the data file in the MiSeq Data folder in the pop-up window. Select ok.
3. Click the "Refresh" icon on Sequence Analysis Viewer.
   (a) Select the summary tab and record the following run metrics on the run worksheet: cluster density (k/mm^2), clusters passing filter %, final yield (GB), and final Q score %.

4 Notes

1. The design of the custom TruSeq Custom Amplicon assay can be accomplished using the design studio application available from Illumina (http://designstudio.illumina.com). This design method allows the user to customize amplicon-based assays for a total target size up to 650 kilobases (kb) and sequence up to 1536 amplicons in a single reaction using the Illumina MiSeq or NextSeq instruments. The software allows the user to select several parameters that are used to create the oligonucleotides for the design. The software allows the user to use either DBSNP 138 or 1000 genomes project data to avoid probes being placed over variable sites, which would potentially alter annealing and ligation in a subset of subjects. The software also allows the user to select amplicons of varying sizes. In general, shorter amplicon sizes should be used in applications where use of DNA from formalin-fixed paraffin-embedded tissues (FFPE) is anticipated. Since the design restrictions are greater with designs using 150 base pair (bp) amplicons, it is suggested to use 175 bp amplicons as the minimum design size, if possible. Larger design sizes offer the ability to interrogate regions with small stretches of repetitive

or complex sequence but require higher-quality DNA input, such as fresh tissue, frozen tissue, blood, or bone marrow, and longer sequencing protocols. Two versions of assay are available, the TruSeq Custom Amplicon (TSCA) 1.5 and the TSCA low input. The TSCA 1.5 requires 50 ng or more of input DNA, can accommodate amplicon designs ranging from 150–425 bp, and can use read lengths up to 2 × 300 bp. The TSCA low input is designed for lower-quality DNA and can accept down to 10 ng of input DNA but is limited to 150–250 bp designs and only 2 × 150 bp reads. The assay used as the basis of the described method uses a 175-bp amplicon design incorporating all or part of the following genes: *ABL1, ASXL1, CALR, CBL, CEBPA, CSFR3, DNMT3A, EZH2, FLT3-ITD/FLT3-TKD, IDH1, IDH2, JAK2, KIT, MLL, MPL, NPM1, PHF6, RB1, SF3B1, SRSF2, STAG2, TET2, TP53, U2AF1, WT1,* and *ZRSR2.*

2. Gene targets can be added by HG19 coordinates or by specifying the gene of interest and either the coding region (CDS), exons, or entire gene. Selecting CDS restricts the design specifically to coding regions and will not include probes for exon sequence that does not result in protein as well as the 3′ and 5′ untranslated regions (UTR). Selecting exons includes all coding and noncoding exons as well as the 3′ and 5′ untranslated regions. Selecting the whole region will target all coding and noncoding regions, including introns. There is an option to include additional bases upstream and downstream of the selected region, which could allow detection of splice site changes. While these options are convenient, the algorithm used to design oligonucleotide probes may design probes to off-target regions with homology to the region of interest when these choices are employed. These off-target oligonucleotides will consume reagents, flow cell space, and sequencing capacity; so to reduce the possibility of such interferences, we recommend that the user select specific target regions, including additional bases up- and downstream of the desired region. The manufacturer also offers services to aid laboratories in the design process for a fee. Once the design is created and ordered, synthesis can take up to 8–10 weeks. The end product of the synthesis is a pool of oligonucleotides, so individual targets cannot be excluded after synthesis but will require a repeat synthesis.

3. The 96-well heat block used for annealing the oligonucleotide probes to the target DNA sequence is critically important. The specified Hybex block has a heated lid that does not contact the sealed 96-well plate and has a heat ramp feature that decreases the lid temperature as the block cools. Heat blocks without a heated lid will allow condensation on the sealing

material, which results in decreased annealing and ligation efficiency. The use of a thermocycler with a heated lid is not recommended because the heated lid for most thermocyclers will be in contact with the sealant and typically is maintained at a high temperature. This situation results in heat transfer to the plate and reagents, which decreases the annealing and ligation efficiency of the oligonucleotide probes, which will result in suboptimal sequencing coverage. Gradual cooling is critical for proper hybridization; therefore, PCR thermal cyclers with active cooling must not be used for this process. A standard heat block is not recommended because they typically lack heated lids. The heated lid on the specified Hybex incubator prevents large amounts of condensation from collecting on the underside of the 96-well plate seal. Large amounts of condensation will cause uneven heating and negatively affect uniform hybridization.

4. Reinforcing the plate seal before removing the 0.8 mL MIDI block from the Hybex heat block is important to help decrease cross-contamination between samples. Any cross-contamination or splash-over at this stage may result in false-positive results because sample indices have not been uniquely added to the sample DNA.
5. When adding wash solutions, changing pipette tips between columns is not necessarily required if care is used to avoid contact with the surfaces of the destination plate, and do not observe splashing or splattering of reagents as they are dispensed from the pipette. However, having a low threshold to change pipette tips will help avoid cross-contamination.
6. The presence of residual SW1 after the centrifugation steps will compromise target enrichment specificity.
7. The Extension-Ligation Mix 4 (ELM4) reagent generally has a short shelf life, and optimum performance is critical to achieve optimum target amplification. Do not use this reagent after the expiration date and pay careful attention to assay performance as the expiration date approaches.
8. Always prepare fresh 0.1 N NaOH. After the addition of NaOH, the DNA is single-stranded (ssDNA). As such, it is more fragile and will shear if vortexed too vigorously.
9. Adequate rinsing of the filter plate with 50 mM NaOH during the elution following the ELM4 incubation is important for ensuring good yield from the PCR step.
10. Tilting the filter plate when aspirating and transferring the extension-ligation product aids in transferring the product volume.

11. Contamination of index reagents will cause incorrect sequence data to be assigned to incorrect specimens.
12. Slightly tilting the FPAU plate will ensure complete aspiration of the targeted DNA and will help avoid air bubbles.
13. If you do not plan to proceed to PCR cleanup immediately, the plate can remain on the thermal cycler overnight or can be stored at 2–8 °C up to 2 days.
14. Always allow the AMPure XP beads to come to room temperature (30 min is recommended) and mix well so that the beads are completely resuspended and form a homogenous solution.
15. Always prepare fresh 80% ethanol from absolute ethanol. Eighty percent ethanol is hygroscopic and will become dilute over time. Using the improper alcohol dilution will decrease DNA yield.
16. Do not touch the side of the reaction tube or the beads that are attracted to the side of the tube. Changing tips is not required at this stage if you use care to avoid cross-contamination. The beads do not need to be resuspended at the time of pipetting.
17. After the second 80% ethanol wash, allow the beads to air-dry only until visible cracks form in the bead pellet. Waiting the full 10 min may result in overdrying and will make resuspension of sequencing libraries more difficult. If overdrying occurs, after addition of EBT (elution buffer), pipette up and down and mix on the microplate shaker until all beads are resuspended regardless of the time it takes (potentially up to 30 min).
18. Always prepare fresh 0.1 N NaOH and have a low tolerance for using a fresh stock reagent since the concentration of NaOH can dramatically impact the quality of sequence data generated. In cases where a high concentration of NaOH is used, troubleshooting will reveal that increasing the amount of DNA presented to the flow cell will result in a similar low cluster density and low-quality sequencing data.
19. It is critical to completely resuspend the LNB1 bead pellet at the bottom of the tube. The use of a P1000 ensures that the beads are homogeneously resuspended and that there is no bead mass at the bottom of the tube. Resuspension is essential for achieving consistent cluster density on the flow cell. If you do not plan to use full tubes for 96 samples, a P1000 set to 1000 μL is required to resuspend the beads completely. Mix only the required amounts of LNA1 and LNB1 for the current experiment. Do not use a P200 pipette to handle LNB1. Store the remaining LNA1 and LNB1 separately at their respective recommended temperatures. To preserve stability, never freeze LNB1 beads or mix with LNA1 if not used immediately.

20. Do not use a reagent trough for this step; the total volume of reagent needed for samples and dead volume is insufficient.
21. The foil seal can be reused during the cleanup procedure if care is taken not to cross-contaminate sample wells. If the foil is reused, a low tolerance for using a fresh seal is imperative. If there is any possibility of contamination, a fresh seal should be used.
22. Using a P20 multichannel to remove residual LNW1 is important to avoid reagent carryover into the storage buffer and to reduce volume variability, which would affect library normalization.
23. Post normalization and resuspension in NaOH, proceed directly to pooling and sequencing on the MiSeq or NextSeq instrument. Post-library normalization is NOT A SAFE STOPPING POINT because ssDNA will adhere to the sides of plastic tubes/wells if stored more than a few hours. This will negatively affect uniform sample pooling and result in lower cluster densities. If stopping is unavoidable, proceed to creation of Pooled Amplicon Library (PAL) and sequence as soon as possible (preferably next day, within 1 week max). In addition, on the day of sequencing, before diluting PAL to Diluted Amplicon Library (DAL), heat the 1.5 mL PAL tube at 96 °C for 2 min, and then invert PAL tube to mix well and immediately cool in ice bath (this helps releases ssDNA from the sides of the PAL tube). Dilute PAL to DAL immediately and heat DAL at 96 °C for 2 min.
24. Volumes for diluting PAL with HT1 were established using recommended equipment (e.g., plate shaker calibrated for shaking speed) and typical laboratory conditions (e.g., 20–25 °C) during the normalization procedure. If cluster density is too high or too low, adjustment of the dilution ratio may be necessary to accommodate the equipment and conditions in the testing laboratory.
25. Make sure that the diluted library DAL is freshly prepared and used immediately for MiSeq loading. Storage of the DAL results in a significant reduction of cluster density.
26. After removal of the spent flow cell, make sure the platform is free of debris. Gently wipe the flow cell platform with a moist Kimwipe followed with ethanol-moistened Kimwipe (do not squirt water or ethanol directly onto the platform). Gently place the new flow cell on the platform. The flow cell will only fit in one direction (use the arrow on the flow cell as a guide). Make sure the position of the flow cell is correctly aligned and flat on the platform. Gently close the lid. Do not force the lid. It should close easily with a "click."

Acknowledgments

Special thanks to the members of the University of Washington Genetics and Solid Tumor Laboratory and the Molecular Hematopathology Laboratory who offered their help and insight, especially Jennifer Hempelmann, Eric Hoyle, and Lena Mulillo.

References

1. Jemal A, Siegel R, Ward E et al (2009) Cancer statistics, 2009. CA Cancer J Clin 59:225–249
2. Whitman SP, Archer KJ, Feng L et al (2001) Absence of the wild-type allele predicts poor prognosis in adult de novo acute myeloid leukemia with normal cytogenetics and the internal tandem duplication of FLT3: a cancer and leukemia group B study. Cancer Res 61:7233–7239
3. Döhner K, Schlenk RF, Habdank M et al (2005) Mutant nucleophosmin (NPM1) predicts favorable prognosis in younger adults with acute myeloid leukemia and normal cytogenetics: interaction with other gene mutations. Blood 106:3740–3746
4. Preudhomme C, Sagot C, Boissel N et al (2002) Favorable prognostic significance of CEBPA mutations in patients with de novo acute myeloid leukemia: a study from the acute leukemia French association (ALFA). Blood 100:2717–2723
5. Paschka P, Marcucci G, Rupper AS et al (2006) Adverse prognostic significance of KIT mutations in adult acute myeloid leukemia with inv(16) and t(8;21): a cancer and leukemia group B study. J Clin Oncol 24:3904–3911
6. Shivarov V, Gueorguieva R, Stoimenov A et al (2013) DNMT3A mutation is a poor prognosis biomarker in AML: results of a meta-analysis of 4500 AML patients. Leuk Res 37:1445–1450
7. Mendler JH, Maharry K, Radmacher MD et al (2012) RUNX1 mutations are associated with poor outcome in younger and older patients with cytogenetically normal acute myeloid leukemia and with distinct gene and MicroRNA expression signatures. J Clin Oncol 30:3109–3118
8. Gaidzik VI, Paschka P, Späth D et al (2012) TET2 mutations in acute myeloid leukemia (AML): results from a comprehensive genetic and clinical analysis of the AML study group. J Clin Oncol 30:1350–1357
9. Alvarado Y, Kantarjian HM, Luthra R et al (2014) Treatment with FLT3 inhibitor in patients with FLT3-mutated acute myeloid leukemia is associated with development of secondary FLT3-tyrosine kinase domain mutations. Cancer 120:2142–2149
10. Lee HK, Kim HW, Lee IY et al (2014) G-749, a novel FLT3 kinase inhibitor can overcome drug resistance for the treatment of acute myeloid leukemia. Blood 123:2209–2210
11. Yuan L, Lu L, Yang Y et al (2015) Genetic mutational profiling analysis of T cell acute lymphoblastic leukemia reveal mutant FBXW7 as a prognostic indicator for inferior survival. Ann Hematol 94:1817–1828
12. Zenatti PP, Ribeiro D, Li W et al (2011) Oncogenic IL7R gain-of-function mutations in childhood T-cell acute lymphoblastic leukemia. Nat Genet 43:932–939
13. Flex E, Petrangeli V, Stella L et al (2008) Somatically acquired JAK1 mutations in adult acute lymphoblastic leukemia. J Exp Med 205:751–758
14. Voelkerding KV, Dames S, Durtschi JD (2009) Next-generation sequencing: from basic research to diagnostics. Clin Chem 55:641–658
15. Mullighan CG, Downing JR (2009) Genome-wide profiling of genetic alterations in acute lymphoblastic leukemia: recent insights and future directions. Leukemia 23:1209–1218
16. Pritchard CC, Salipante SJ, Koehler K et al (2013) Validation and implementation of targeted capture and sequencing for the detection of actionable mutation, copy number variation, and Gene rearrangement in clinical cancer specimens. J Mol Diagn 16:56–67
17. Ye K, Schulz MH, Long Q et al (2009) Pindel: a pattern growth approach to detect break points of large deletions and medium sized insertions from paired-end short reads. Bioinformatics 25:2865–2871
18. Chen K, Wallis JW, McLellan MD et al (2009) BreakDancer: an algorithm for high-resolution mapping of genomic structural variation. Nat Methods 6:677–681
19. Wang J, Mullighan CG, Easton J et al (2011) CREST maps somatic structural variation in cancer genomes with base-pair resolution. Nat Methods 8:652–654
20. Li J, Lupat R, Amarasinghe KC et al (2012) CONTRA: copy number analysis for targeted resequencing. Bioinformatics 28:1307–1313

Chapter 12

Bioinformatics Data Analysis of Next-Generation Sequencing Data from Heterogeneous Tumor Samples

Sean R. Landman and Tae Hyun Hwang

Abstract

Tumor heterogeneity is a major challenge when it comes to treating cancer and also complicates research aimed at determining genetic sources for tumorigenesis. Leveraging high-throughput sequencing technology has been an effective approach for advancing our understanding of genetic diseases, and this type of data can also be used to better understand and make inferences about tumor heterogeneity. Here we describe the basics of genomics data analysis, as well as analysis pipelines for investigating tumor heterogeneity with next-generation sequencing data.

Key words Tumor heterogeneity, Subclone, Subpopulation, Structural variation, Bioinformatics, Genomics, Next-generation sequencing

1 Introduction

The aggressive cell growth characteristic in tumor tissue often leads to an accumulation of many new mutations in genomes of the rapidly dividing cells. Some of these mutations will establish a selective advantage for certain tumor cells over neighboring cells, resulting in an evolutionary battle between different genetic subpopulations within a tumor, also known as tumor subclones. This phenomenon is known as intra-tumor heterogeneity, and it is a complicating factor in the study of cancer genetics for a number of reasons. When treating a tumor, such as via drug therapy or chemotherapy, a treatment may be affective against some, but not all, subclones within the tumor. As a result, treatment may appear to be successful in abolishing the tumor, though this could be due to effectivity against only the primary subclones. Smaller subclones harboring resistive traits may yet rise up to take their place, resulting in the reemergence of the tumor. Additionally, the heterogeneous mix of genetic material present in a tumor tissue sample makes it difficult to adequately predict the most relevant causal mutations that drove

Paolo Fortina et al. (eds.), *Acute Myeloid Leukemia: Methods and Protocols*, Methods in Molecular Biology, vol. 1633,
DOI 10.1007/978-1-4939-7142-8_12, © Springer Science+Business Media LLC 2017

the initial tumor growth. Thus, it is important to account for tumor heterogeneity when studying DNA from tumor tissue.

Next-generation sequencing has become the prevailing approach for collecting DNA data due to its rising throughput and efficiency coupled with its increasingly affordable cost. Sequencing data consists of many short DNA sequences (called reads) fragmented from amplified copies of the original genetic sequence(s) of interest. The first step in any sequencing data analysis is often to align these reads against a reference genome in order to determine which section of the genome they each originated from. Inferences can be made from this data by detecting clusters of abnormally aligned reads. For example, regions of the genome that have far fewer reads aligned to it than expected might be indicative of a deletion that is present in that sample.

Recently there have been a number of algorithms and software developed that utilize this discordant alignment information to make inferences related to tumor heterogeneity. One such program is sample heterogeneity estimation and assembly by reference (SHEAR) [1], which predicts structural variations (SVs) while also estimating the portion of the sequencing sample that each SV occurs in. SHEAR works by predicting SVs via a split-read approach in which single reads are partially mapped to two different regions of the genome, indicating a novel fusion event. The heterogeneity estimation for each SV is then calculated using information about the number of spanning and soft-clipped reads at each SV breakpoint. Another complementary program for helping to understand tumor heterogeneity in a tumor tissue sample is tumor heterogeneity analysis (THetA) [2, 3]. Rather than estimating heterogeneity frequencies variant by variant, THetA estimates the number of subclones present as well as the integer copy numbers for different regions of the genome for each subclone. Unlike SHEAR, THetA does not deal with copy-neutral SVs, such as inversions or translocations, but does group variants together into their respective subclones. Thus, the two can be complementary to one another in a tumor heterogeneity analysis pipeline.

Here we describe a simple workflow for analyzing next-generation sequencing data and making inferences about intratumor heterogeneity from tumor tissue samples. This description is far from comprehensive, but is instead designed to get a beginner user comfortable working with next-generation sequencing data and to help familiarize the user with some of the capabilities available through next-generation sequencing data analysis.

2 Materials

Next-generation sequencing data analysis typically begins with FASTQ files, which contain the read sequences along with their quality strings (i.e., the quality score of each base in each read). We will not describe the process of sequencing itself, nor the low-level analysis that results in the generation of FASTQ files, but we will instead focus on the downstream bioinformatics analysis of next-generation sequencing data. In the methods described, we will assume that we are working with Illumina data, as that is typically most common.

All steps of the Subheading 3 describe commands to be entered at the command line of a UNIX/Linux operating system. We assume that users are familiar with this style of operating system, as well as comfortable working with command line programs.

2.1 Software Applications (Publically Available for Download)

1. Trimmomatic (http://www.usadellab.org/cms/?page=trimmomatic).
2. Burrows-Wheeler Aligner (BWA: https://sourceforge.net/projects/bio-bwa/).
3. Picard Tools (https://github.com/broadinstitute/picard/releases/tag/2.6.0).
4. SAMtools (http://www.htslib.org/download/).
5. Genome Analysis ToolKit (GATK: https://software.broadinstitute.org/gatk/download/).
6. DELLY (https://github.com/tobiasrausch/delly).
7. SHEAR (http://vk.cs.umn.edu/SHEAR/).
8. THetA (http://compbio.cs.brown.edu/projects/theta/).

3 Methods

Each step explains one component of the data analysis pipeline by describing what is being done, giving the command to perform the step, and then explaining aspects of the command itself and/or the meaning behind different output files from the command. This assumes all required programs are already installed on the user's system. Generic file paths (e.g., `<path to trimmomatic.jar>`) should be replaced with the proper paths on the user's specific system.

3.1 Data Preparation

1. Trim and filter read sequences for quality control using Trimmomatic [4]. This will trim low-quality ends of reads (quality often drops off toward the end of a read) and remove reads that fall below a certain threshold length as a result of trimming.

```
java -jar <path to trimmomatic.jar> PE reads-1.fq
    reads-2.fq \
filtered-reads-1.fq filtered-reads-unpaired-1.fq \
filtered-reads-2.fq filtered-reads-unpaired-2.fq \
LEADING:3 TRAILING:3 SLIDINGWINDOW:4:15 MINLEN:36
```

This command applies filters to remove leading and trailing bases marked as "low quality" by Illumina (LEADING:3 and TRAILING:3), examines the average quality across the read using a 4 bp sliding window and trims the read at the point where that average quality drops below 15 (SLIDINGWINDOW:4:15), and removes reads that are smaller than 36 bp after trimming (MINLEN:36) (*see* **Note 1**). The relevant output files are filtered-reads-1.fq and filtered-reads-2.fq, which contain the trimmed reads that are still paired after filtering.

2. Align reads against the reference genome using BWA [5]. This creates an alignment file in SAM/BAM format [6] (*see* **Note 2**), which contains the read sequences along with additional information about where and how each read aligns to the reference genome.

```
bwa mem -R '@RG\tID:sample\tSM:sample' <path to reference.fa> \ filtered-reads-1.fq filtered-reads-2.fq > alignment.sam
```

You can replace 'sample' with relevant read group information, if desired (*see* **Note 3**). This assumes that a BWA index is available for the hg19.fa reference genome (*see* **Note 4**).

3. Correct potential formatting errors in the alignment file and sort the alignment using Picard Tools [7]. This will ensure that downstream analyses work correctly (*see* **Note 5**).

```
java -jar <path to picard.jar> CleanSam
   I=alignment.sam \ O=alignment.cleaned.bam
java -jar <path to picard.jar> FixMateInformation \
    I=alignment.cleaned.bam O=alignment.final.bam
   SO=coordinate
```

The CleanSam command will fix various common SAM format problems, as well as automatically convert from SAM to BAM (*see* **Note 6**). The FixMateInformation command will ensure that read pair information is consistent while also sorting the alignment, which is required for indexing (next step).

4. Index the Alignment Using SAMtools [6].

```
samtools index alignment.final.bam
```

This creates a new file, alignment.final.bam.bai, which contains the index and will be used by any programs that process the alignment file.

3.2 Variant Prediction

1. Predict SNPs and small Indels using GATK HaplotypeCaller [8] (*see* **Note 7**). SNPs and small Indels are predicted by determining areas in the alignment where aligned reads consistently contain the same sequence differences relative to the reference sequence.

```
java -jar <path to GenomeAnalysisTK.jar> -T
HaplotypeCaller \            -R <path to reference.
fa> -I alignment.final.bam -o snps_indels.vcf
```

This will produce a VCF file [9] (snps_indels.vcf) that contains the predicted SNPs and small Indels for your sample (*see* **Note 8**).

2. Predict structural variations (SVs) using DELLY [10] (*see* **Note 9**). This program predicts SVs by locating regions in the alignment where read pairs align in a consistent but discordant way (i.e., many read pairs align in an unexpected way, but all do so in the same way, thus supporting evidence of a large-scale SV) and other read pairs align partially to two different regions of the reference sequence (to identify the SV breakpoints).

```
delly -t DEL -o sv-predictions.del.vcf -f <path to
reference.fa> \ alignment.final.bam
delly -t DUP -o sv-predictions.dup.vcf -f <path to
reference.fa> \ alignment.final.bam
delly -t INV -o sv-predictions.inv.vcf -f <path to
reference.fa> \ alignment.final.bam
delly -t TRA -o sv-predictions.tra.vcf -f <path to
reference.fa> \ alignment.final.bam
```

This set of commands produces several VCF files (`sv-predictions.*.vcf`), one for each SV type, that contain the predicted SVs of that type.

3.3 Tumor Heterogeneity Estimation

1. Predict variants, along with their estimated heterogeneity percentage, using SHEAR [1]. SHEAR works by estimating variants using external programs (usually DELLY [10] and GATK's HaplotypeCaller [8]), refining the variant predictions using an iterative local realignment at SV breakpoint regions, and finally estimating the heterogeneity percentage of each variant separately using the counts of clipped and spanning reads at each SV breakpoint.

```
java -jar <path to SHEAR.jar> sv -p shear-results \
-b alignment.final.bam -f <path to reference.fa>
```

The shear-results.report file contains the main SHEAR results, which includes final variant calls and their associated heterogeneity percentage estimations (*see* **Note 10**).

2. Predict tumor subclones and their respective integer copy number intervals using THetA [2, 3]. THetA works by taking a DNA segmentation and predicting the most likely collection of subclones to support the data using a maximum likelihood estimation for a multinomial distribution. The input to THetA is an interval count file, which contains information about the numbers of reads from tumor and normal tissue samples aligning in different segments of the genome (*see* **Note 11**).

```
RunTHetA -OUTPUT_PREFIX theta-results interval_
count_file
```

The theta-results.BEST.results output file contains the optimal solution to the heterogeneity estimation for the sample. This file contains information about the copy number of each interval segment in each normal and tumor subclone for the optimal solution. A more detailed description of this output file is provided in the official documentation that comes bundled with THetA.

3.4 Discussion

At the end of this process, there will be results from several analyses (HaplotypeCaller, DELLY, SHEAR, and THetA) that can then be examined in detail in order to better understand the underlying genetic background of the tumor sample. The results from HaplotypeCaller and DELLY will contain SNPs/Indels and SVs, respectively, that are predicted to be present without taking tumor heterogeneity into account. SHEAR's results will contain variant predictions (which may or may not overlap with those predictions from HaplotypeCaller and DELLY) along with the estimated percentage of the sample that each is present in. Finally, THetA's results will contain the estimated copy number for different regions of the genome for different tumor subclones.

All of these programs and algorithms have their respective strengths and weaknesses. Thus, running different analyses concurrently allows for complementary approaches and can strengthen supporting evidence for findings. This is just a small sampling of the types of analyses that are available, but it should hopefully begin to demonstrate the many possibilities of next-generation sequencing data analysis.

4 Notes

1. The necessary level of quality control will differ for every data set. For additional available options, please refer to the Trimmomatic manual (http://www.usadellab.org/cms/uploads/supplementary/Trimmomatic/TrimmomaticManual_V0.32.pdf). It may also be informative to examine the overall quality trends of your sequencing data using a tool such as FastQC [11].
2. Detailed information about the SAM/BAM file format specification can be found at http://samtools.github.io/hts-specs/SAMv1.pdf.
3. Whether or not accurate read group is specified, the read group headers are required to be present for many downstream analyses (such as GATK), so specifying read groups via the "-R" flag should be done regardless.

4. See the BWA manual (http://bio-bwa.sourceforge.net/bwa.shtml) for information about creating a BWA index, as well as information about additional BWA options.
5. Most modern alignment programs sufficiently conform to proper file format standards. However, it is still generally good practice to use programs such as Picard Tools' CleanSam and FixMateInformation to ensure valid formatting, especially for alignment files that were processed or prepared by other parties.
6. BAM is a more condensed version of the SAM file format. BAM files should be used for all downstream analyses, as well as for storage space considerations.
7. For more information about running HaplotypeCaller, see the GATK Best Practices guide on the subject (http://www.broadinstitute.org/gatk/guide/article?id=2803).
8. VCF is a file format used for storing information about variants. Detailed information about the VCF file format can be found at http://www.broadinstitute.org/gatk/guide/article?id=1268, and it may also be informative to refer to the GATK Best Practices guide on the subject (http://www.broadinstitute.org/gatk/guide/article?id=1268).
9. DELLY is used here as just one example, but there are numerous other programs and algorithms available that can be used for predicting SVs. It is generally good practice to predict SVs using a variety of programs and then select consistently predicted variants for downstream analyses.
10. The heterogeneity estimations produced by SHEAR reflect the total portion of the DNA mass that contains the particular variant. Thus, a 50% heterogeneity estimation could be due to a heterozygous variant present in 100% of the tumor subclones in a diploid case, a homozygous variant present in 50% of the tumor subclones, or other possibilities in situations involving aneuploidy in tumor subclone(s).
11. The expected format for the interval count file is provided in the official documentation that comes bundled with THetA. There are many ways to prepare this file, though it is recommended to use a DNA segmentation program called BIC-Seq [12] and to then post-process the BIC-Seq results using the runBICSeqToTHetA.jar utility program that comes bundled with THetA. This is beyond the scope of this chapter, but instructions for how to do this can be found in the official THetA documentation.

References

1. Landman SR, Hwang TH, Silverstein KAT, Li Y, Dehm SM, Steinbach M, Kumar V (2014) SHEAR: sample heterogeneity estimation and assembly by reference. BMC Genomics 15(1):84
2. Oesper L, Mahmoody A, Raphael BJ (2013) THetA: inferring intra-tumor heterogeneity from high-throughput DNA sequencing data. Genome Biol 14(7):R80
3. Oesper L, Satas G, Raphael BJ (2014) Quantifying tumor heterogeneity in whole-genome and whole-exome sequencing data. Bioinformatics 30(24):3532–3540
4. Bolger AM, Lohse M, Usadel B (2014) Trimmomatic: a flexible trimmer for Illumina sequence data. Bioinformatics 30(15): 2114–2120
5. Li H, Durbin R (2009) Fast and accurate short read alignment with burrows-Wheeler transform. Bioinformatics 25(14):1754–1760
6. Li H, Handsaker B, Wysoker A, Fennell T, Ruan J, Homer N, Marth G, Abecasis G, Durbin R (2009) The sequence alignment/map format and SAMtools. Bioinformatics 25(16):2078–2079
7. "Picard" [Online]. http://picard.sourceforge.net
8. McKenna A, Hanna M, Banks E, Sivachenko A, Cibulskis K, Kernytsky A, Garimella K, Altshuler D, Gabriel S, Daly M, DePristo MA (2010) The genome analysis Toolkit: a MapReduce framework for analyzing next-generation DNA sequencing data. Genome Res 20(9):1297–1303
9. Danecek P, Auton A, Abecasis G, Albers CA, Banks E, DePristo MA, Handsaker RE, Lunter G, Marth GT, Sherry ST, McVean G, Durbin R (2011) The variant call format and VCFtools. Bioinformatics 27(15):2156–2158
10. Rausch T, Zichner T, Schlattl A, Stutz AM, Benes V, Korbel JO (2012) DELLY: structural variant discovery by integrated paired-end and split-read analysis. Bioinformatics 28(18): i333–i339
11. "FastqQC" [Online]. http://www.bioinformatics.babraham.ac.uk/projects/fastqc
12. Xi R, Hadjipanayis AG, Luquette LJ, Kim T-M, Lee E, Zhang J, Johnson MD, Muzny DM, Wheeler DA, Gibbs RA, Kucherlapati R, Park PJ (2011) Copy number variation detection in whole-genome sequencing data using the Bayesian information criterion. PNAS 108(46):E1128–E1136

Chapter 13

A Zebrafish Model for Evaluating the Function of Human Leukemic Gene *IDH1* and Its Mutation

Alvin C.H. Ma, Xiangguo Shi, Bai-Liang He, Yuhan Guo, and Anskar Y.H. Leung

Abstract

The recent advent of next-generation sequencing (NGS) has greatly accelerated identification of gene mutations in myeloid malignancies at unprecedented speed that will soon outpace their functional validation by conventional laboratory techniques and animal models. A high-throughput whole-organism model is useful for the functional validation of new mutations. We recently reported the use of zebrafish to evaluate the hematopoietic function of isocitrate dehydrogenase 1 (*IDH1*) and the effects of expressing human IDH1-R132H that is frequently identified in human acute myeloid leukemia (AML), in myelopoiesis, with a view to develop zebrafish as a model of AML. Here, we use *IDH1* as an example to describe a comprehensive approach to evaluate hematopoietic gene function and the effects of mutations using zebrafish as a model.

Key words Zebrafish, Hematopoiesis, Myelopoiesis, Myeloid malignancy, Mutation, Transient expression

1 Introduction

The recent advent of next-generation sequencing (NGS) has led to the identification of novel gene mutations with hitherto unknown pathogenetic role in myeloid malignancies [1–4]. This new information has resolved mechanisms of pathogenesis as well as potential therapeutic strategies for myeloid malignancies. However, with the expected decrease in cost and increased availability of NGS technologies, the emergence of new genetic information has outpaced our ability to perform functional validation by conventional laboratory techniques and animal models. Therefore, a novel and clinically relevant animal model with high-throughput capacity is needed. Zebrafish (*Danio rerio*) exhibits unique features and has emerged as an ideal model for the study of life processes and human diseases. In particular, the cellular and molecular features of

Paolo Fortina et al. (eds.), *Acute Myeloid Leukemia: Methods and Protocols*, Methods in Molecular Biology, vol. 1633, DOI 10.1007/978-1-4939-7142-8_13, © Springer Science+Business Media LLC 2017

embryonic hematopoiesis are remarkably similar to those in human. Technically, the embryos are externally fertilized and optically transparent and are highly amendable to pharmacological and genetic manipulations [5–8]. The small size of adult animals and their high fecundity have also made it an affordable and cost-effective model organism that can be exploited for the functional validation of gene mutations discovered by NGS.

Isocitrate dehydrogenase 1 and 2 (IDH1/IDH2) are key metabolic enzymes that convert isocitrate to α-ketoglutarate (α-KG) in the citric acid cycle (TCA cycle). In particular, arginine substitution at IDH1 R132 or IDH2 R140/R172 confers novel substrate specificity to the mutant enzymes by which α-KG is converted to the oncogenic metabolite 2-hydroxyglutarate (2-HG). Increase in 2-HG results in an aberrant epigenetic landscape and contributes to leukemic transformation [9–12]. In mice, IDH1 R132H knock-in has been shown to expand the hematopoietic progenitor population [13]. However, the role of IDH1 in hematopoiesis and its pathogenetic link with human leukemia remain unclear. We previously reported the use of zebrafish model in the study of IDH1 and its mutations in hematopoiesis [14] and herein describe the protocols of the study.

2 Materials

2.1 Molecular Cloning

1. TRIzol reagent (Life Technologies, Grand Island, NY).
2. SuperScript First-Strand Synthesis System (Life Technologies).
3. 293T cell line (ATCC, Manassas, VA).
4. Wild-type (WT) zebrafish embryos at 24-h post-fertilization (hpf).
5. Primers for cloning human *IDH1* into pCS2+ expression vector (pCS2-IDH1): pCS2-IDH1-BamHI-F (CGG GAT CCT CAG AAG CGG AGG CA) and pCS2-IDH1-XbaI-R (GCG CGC TCT AGA CAA AGG TGG CAA TAA CT).
6. Primers for cloning zebrafish *idh1-egfp* fusion construct (pidh1-egfp): zidh1-HindIII-F (GGG CCC AAG CTT CTC CTC CTT ACT GCT AAA ATA G) and zidh1-BamHI-R (GTC GCG GAT CCA AGT TTG GGT TGG CTT GAT AG).
7. Primers for subcloning zebrafish *idh1-egfp* fusion into pCS2+ expression vector (pCS2-idh1-egfp): pCS2-zidh1-egfp-ClaI-F (CCA TCG ATC TCC TCC TTA CTG CTA AAA TAG) and pCS2-zidh1-egfp-EcoRI-R (CGG AAT TCT CTA CAA AAT GTG GTA TGG C).
8. Primers for TA cloning of zebrafish *idh1* with mutated (*see* **Note 1**) MO targeting sequence (pGEMT-idh1): zidh1-rescue-F (CGT GAT TTG AGA ACA TGG ATT CCT CAC

GAA AC) and zidh1-rescue-R (CAT TTG TGG TAA AGT GAC AGA CCG TAA TGA GTG TG).

9. Primers for TA cloning of zebrafish *idh1* partial sequence (412 b.p.) for antisense probe synthesis (pGEMT-idh1P): zidh1-probe-F (AAC AGT TGA GGC AGC AGA A) and zidh1-probe-R (AGC AAA GTC CCG GAT TGA C).
10. Standard agarose gel electrophoresis setup.
11. Restriction enzymes: BamHI, ClaI, EcoRI, HindIII, XbaI (New England Biolabs, Ipswich, MA).
12. T4 DNA ligase (400,000 units/mL, New England Biolabs).
13. pGEM-T Easy Vector Systems (Promega, Fitchburg, WI).
14. Heat-shock competent DH5α *E. coli* cell.
15. QIAprep Spin Miniprep Kit (Qiagen, Valencia, CA).
16. QIAquick Gel Extraction Kit (Qiagen).
17. Sequencing Primers: CMV (CGC AAA TGG GCG GTA GGC GTG), SP6 (ATT TAG GTG ACA CTA TAG), T3 (GCA ATT AAC CCT CAC TAA AGG), and T7 (TAA TAC GAC TCA CTA TAG GG).

2.2 Site-Directed Mutagenesis

1. Primers for human *IDH1* R132H site-directed mutagenesis: IDH1-R132H-F (GTA AAA CCT ATC ATC ATA GGT CAT CAT GCT TAT GGG GAT CAA TAC) and IDH1-R132H-R (GTA TTG ATC CCC ATA AGC ATG ATG ACC TAT GAT GAT AGG TTT TAC).
2. Primers for zebrafish *idh1* R146H site-directed mutagenesis: zidh1-R146H-F (GTA CTG GTC CCC ATG TGC ATG ATG GCC GAT AAT TAT AGG CTT GAT) and zidh1-R146H-R (ATC AAG CCT ATA ATT ATC GGC CAT CAT GCA CAT GGG GAC CAG TAC).
3. Platinum *Pfx* DNA polymerase (Life Technologies).
4. DpnI (New England Biolabs).
5. QIAquick PCR Purification Kit (Qiagen).
6. T4 DNA ligase (400,000 units/mL, New England Biolabs).

2.3 Zebrafish Embryo Husbandry

1. E3 medium (5 mM NaCl, 0.17 mM KCl, 0.33 mM $CaCl_2$, 0.33 mM $MgSO_4$).
2. 0.003% PTU (1-phenyl-2-thiourea) (Sigma-Aldrich, St. Louis, MO).
3. 4% paraformaldehyde (PFA).
4. 25% (in PBS), 50% (in PBS), 75% (in deionized water), and 100% ethanol.
5. 0.016% tricaine methanesulfonate (MS-222, Sigma-Aldrich) in E3 medium.
6. 3% methylcellulose (Sigma-Aldrich).

2.4 Morpholino (MO) Knockdown of Zebrafish idh1

1. MO targeting start codon of *idh1* (TCT GTT TCT TGA AGA GTC CAT ATG C) (Gene Tools, LLC, Philomath, OR).
2. Standard control MO (CCT CTT ACC TCA GTT ACA ATT TAT A) (Gene Tools, LLC).
3. Danieau's solution (17.4 mM NaCl, 0.21 mM KCl, 0.12 mM $MgSO_4$, 0.18 mM $Ca(NO_3)_2$, 1.5 mM HEPES, pH 7.2).
4. pidh1-egfp (MO efficiency testing).
5. pGEMT-idh1 (in vitro transcription of WT *idh1* mRNA for rescue experiment).
6. Ambion mMESSAGE mMACHINE Transcription Kit (Life Technologies).
7. Ambion Poly(A) Tailing Kit (Life Technologies).
8. SalI (20,000 units/mL, New England Biolabs).

2.5 Denaturing Formaldehyde RNA Gel Electrophoresis

1. 10× MOPS buffer (0.2 M MOPS, 10 mM sodium acetate, pH 5.0, 10 mM EDTA, pH 8.0).
2. Formaldehyde gel-loading buffer (For 100 μL: 62.5 μL formamide, 9.3 μL 37% formaldehyde, 12.5 μL 10× MOPS, 1 μL 1% bromophenol blue, 5 μL 1 mg/mL ethidium bromide, 9.7 μL deionized water).
3. 0.5–10 Kb RNA Ladder (Life Technologies).

2.6 Transcription Activator-like Effector Nuclease (TALEN) Synthesis

1. Golden Gate TALEN and TAL Effector Kit 2.0 (Addgene Kit #1000000024, Cambridge, MA).
2. RCIscript-GoldyTALEN backbone (Addgene #38142).
3. T4 DNA ligase (2,000,000 units/mL, New England Biolabs).
4. BsaI (New England Biolabs).
5. Plasmid-Safe ATP-Dependent DNase (Epicentre Biotechnologies, Madison, WI).
6. 10 mM ATP.
7. Esp3I (Thermo Fisher Scientific, Waltham, MA).
8. SacI (New England Biolabs).
9. Heat-shock competent *E. coli* cell.
10. LB medium and agar plate with spectinomycin (100 μg/mL).
11. LB medium and agar plate with ampicillin (100 μg/mL).
12. X-Gal (5-bromo-4-chloro-3-indolyl-β-D-galactoside) (20 mg/mL).
13. IPTG (isopropylthio-β-galactoside) (0.1 M).
14. Primers (colony PCR and sequencing): pCR8_F1 (TTG ATG CCT GGC AGT TCC CT), pCR8_R1 (CGA ACC GAA CAG GCT TAT GT), TAL_F1 (TTG GCG TCG GCA AAC AGT GG), and TAL_R2 (GGC GAC GAG GTG GTC GTT GG) [15].

15. QIAquick PCR Purification Kit (Qiagen).
16. Ambion T3 mMESSAGE mMACHINE Transcription Kit (Life Technologies).
17. Lithium chloride precipitate solution (7.5 M LiCl, 50 mM EDTA, pH 8.0).
18. 70% ethanol.

2.7 Zebrafish Embryo/Adult Genotyping and RFLP Assay for TALEN Mutagenic Activity

1. Genomic DNA (gDNA) extraction buffer (10 mM Tris-HCl, pH 8.3, 50 mM KCl).
2. 10% Tween 20.
3. 10% NP-40.
4. Proteinase K solution (recombinant, PCR grade, 14–22 mg/mL in 10 mM Tris–HCl, pH 7.5, Roche Life Science, Indianapolis, IN).
5. Primers for genotyping *idh1* Exon-1: zidh1-E1-gF (CAA ACT GCT CGT TTT CAT G) and zidh1-E1-gR (TTT CCA CTC ACC TTT ATC G).
6. BsmI (New England Biolabs).
7. pGEM-T Easy Vector Systems (Promega).

2.8 Overexpression of Human IDH1 R132H and Zebrafish idh1 R146H

1. pCS2-IDH1 and pCS2-IDH1R132H.
2. pCS2-idh1-egpf and pCS2-idh1R146H-egfp.
3. NotI-HF (20,000 units/mL, New England Biolabs).
4. QIAquick PCR Purification Kit (Qiagen).
5. Ambion mMESSAGE mMACHINE SP6 Transcription Kit (Life Technologies).
6. Ambion Poly(A) Tailing Kit (Life Technologies).
7. Lithium chloride precipitate solution (7.5 M LiCl, 50 mM EDTA, pH 8.0).
8. 70% ethanol.

2.9 Pharmacological Treatment of Zebrafish Embryos

1. DMSO
2. IDH1 R132H-specific inhibitor, AGI-5198 (10 mM in DMSO, Xcess Biosciences, San Diego, CA).

2.10 Generation of Antisense RNA Probe

1. pGEMT-idh1P.
2. SacII (20,000 units/mL, New England Biolabs).
3. QIAquick PCR Purification Kit (Qiagen).
4. SP6 DIG RNA Labeling Kit (Roche Life Science).
5. Lithium chloride precipitate solution (7.5 M LiCl, 50 mM EDTA, pH 8.0).
6. 70% ethanol.

2.11 Whole-Mount In Situ Hybridization (WISH)

1. Phosphate-buffered saline (PBS) (137 mM NaCl, 2.7 mM KCl, 4.3 mM Na_2HPO_4, 1.4 mM KH_2PO_4, pH 7.3).
2. PBST (PBS with 0.2% Tween 20).
3. 25% (in PBS), 50% (in PBS), 75% (in deionized water), and 100% ethanol.
4. Proteinase K solution (1:1000 diluted in PBST, Roche Life Science).
5. 4% PFA.
6. 20× SSC buffer (3 M NaCl, 0.3 M sodium citrate, pH 7.0).
7. Pre-hybridization buffer (PHB) (50% formamide, 5× SSC, 50 μg/mL heparin, 500 μg/mL yeast rRNA, 5 mM EDTA, 0.1% Tween 20, 9.2 μL/mL 1 M citric acid).
8. DIG-labeled RNA probes for zebrafish *idh1*, *scl*, *lmo2*, *pu.1*, *l-plastin*, *mpo*, *mpeg1*, *gata1*, *gata2*, *ahe1*, *cebpa*, *c-myb*, *rag1*, *runx1*, *efnb2a*, and *flt4* [14, 16–22].
9. Anti-digoxigenin-AP, Fab fragments (Roche Life Science).
10. Alkaline phosphatase (AP) buffer (100 mM NaCl, 50 mM $MgCl_2$, 100 mM Tris–HCl, pH 9.5, 0.1% Tween 20).
11. Lamb serum (Life Technologies).
12. NBT/BCIP stock solution (Roche Life Science).

2.12 Whole-Mount Fluorescent Immunostaining

1. Acetone (ice cold).
2. PBS with 1% Triton X-100 (PBSTX).
3. 25% (in PBS), 50% (in PBS), 75% (in deionized water), and 100% ethanol.
4. Blocking solution (10% FBS in PBSTX).
5. Primary antibody (1:500 dilution): rabbit anti-spi1 antibody [23] and rabbit anti-phospho-histone H3 (Ser10) (Upstate, Lake Placid, NY).
6. Secondary antibody (1:1000 dilution): goat anti-rabbit IgG Alexa Fluor 488 (Life Technologies) and goat anti-rabbit IgG Alexa Fluor 594 (Life Technologies).

2.13 Quantitative PCR

1. TRIzol reagent (Life Technologies).
2. SuperScript First-Strand Synthesis System (Life Technologies).
3. Power SYBR Green PCR master mix (Life Technologies).
4. StepOnePlus Real-Time PCR System (Life Technologies).
5. MicroAmp Optical 96-Well Reaction Plate (0.1 mL, Life Technologies).
6. MicroAmp Optical Adhesive Film (Life Technologies).
7. Primer sequences:

β-actin-F	TTC CTT CCT GGG TAT GGA ATC
β-actin-R	GCA CTG TGT TGG CAT ACA GG
scl-F	CTA TTA ACC GTG GTT TTG CTG G
scl-R	CCA TCG TTG ATT TCA ACC TCA T
lmo2-F	GGA CGC AGG CTT TAC TAC AAA C
lmo2-R	CCG GAT CCT CTT TTC ACA GGA A
gata1-F	AAG ATG GGA CAG GCC ACT AC
gata1-R	TGC TGA CAA TCA GCC TCT TTT
αhe1-F	TGC TCT CTC CAG GAT GTT GA
αhe1-R	TCA CAG TCT TGC CGT GTT TC
βhe1-F	AGG CTC TGG CAA GGT GTC TCA
βhe1-R	CAT TGG GTT TCC CAG GAT
pu.1-F	GGG CAG TTT TAA CCA AAG ATC A
pu.1-R	CCC AAG AGT GAT CGT TCT GAC
l-plastin-F	GAA GCT CTG ATC GCT CTG CT
l-plastin-R	GTT GTT GAT TTT GGG GCA TC
mpeg1-F	CCC ACC AAG TGA AAG AGG
mpeg1-R	GTG TTT GAT TGT TTT CAA TGG
mpo-F	GGG GCA GAA GAA GAA AGT CC
mpo-R	CCC TTG CTA AAC TCT CAT CTC G

2.14 Whole-Mount BrdU Incorporation Assay

1. 10 mM BrdU.
2. E3 medium.
3. 4% PFA.
4. PBST.
5. 25% (in PBS), 50% (in PBS), 75% (in deionized water), and 100% ethanol.
6. Proteinase K solution (1:1000 diluted in PBST, Roche Life Science).
7. 2 N HCl.
8. Blocking solution (1% BSA in PBST).
9. PE-conjugated anti-mouse BrdU antibody (1:500 dilution) (BD Biosciences, San Jose, CA).

2.15 Whole-Mount TUNEL Assay

1. ApopTag Fluorescein Direct In Situ Apoptosis Detection Kit (equilibration buffer, reaction buffer, TdT enzyme, and stop/wash buffer included; Millipore, Billerica, MA).

2. 4% PFA.
3. Proteinase K solution (1:1000 diluted in PBST, Roche Life Science).
4. PBST.

2.16 Flow Cytometry Quantification and Cell Sorting from Fluorescent Transgenic Embryo

1. Transgenic zebrafish line Tg(*mpo:gfp*) [24] (ZIRC).
2. Trypsin-EDTA (0.05%), phenol red (Life Technologies).
3. 100 mM $CaCl_2$.
4. 40 μm cell strainer (BD Biosciences).
5. 0.9× PBS with 2% FBS.
6. Cytocentrifuge.
7. Wright-Giemsa stain (Sigma-Aldrich).

2.17 Western Blot

1. CelLytic MT Cell Lysis Reagent (Sigma-Aldrich).
2. Protease and phosphatase inhibitor cocktail (100×, Thermo Fisher Scientific).
3. 5× loading buffer (0.25% bromophenol blue, 0.5 M dithiothreitol (DTT), 50% glycerol, 10% sodium dodecyl sulfate (SDS)).
4. Standard SDS-PAGE (polyacrylamide gel electrophoresis) system.
5. 12% resolving Tris-glycine polyacrylamide gel.
6. Protran Nitrocellulose Transfer Membranes (PerkinElmer, Waltham, MA).
7. TBST (20 mM Tris, pH 7.5, 500 mM NaCl, 0.1% Tween 20).
8. Blocking buffer: 5% (Wt/Vol) milk in TBST.
9. Primary antibody: mouse anti-β-actin (1:5000 dilution) (Sigma-Aldrich) and rabbit anti-idh1 (1:3000) (GeneTex, Irvine, CA).
10. Secondary antibody (1:5000 dilution): sheep anti-mouse IgG-HRP antibody (GE Healthcare Life Sciences, Pittsburgh, PA) and goat anti-rabbit IgG-HRP antibody (Thermo Fisher Scientific).
11. Luminata Forte Western HRP substrate (Millipore).

2.18 Adult Zebrafish Kidney Marrow Analysis

1. Adult *idh1* mutants and WT siblings.
2. 5 mL syringe with 18G needle.
3. 40 μm cell strainer (BD Biosciences).
4. 0.9× PBS with 5% FBS.
5. Cytocentrifuge.
6. Wright-Giemsa stain (Sigma-Aldrich).

2.19 GC-Mass Spectrometry of 2-HG

1. 80% methanol (in deionized water).
2. Ultrasonic Processor (Cole-Parmer, Vernon Hills, IL).
3. *N*-methyl-*N*-tertbutyldimethylsilyltrifluoroacetamide (MTBSTFA) (Regis Technologies, Morton Grove, IL).
4. 450-GC system (Bruker).
5. VF-5 ms inert capillary column (30 m length × 0.25 mm inner diameter with 0.25 μM film thickness) (Varian, Palo Alto, CA).
6. 320-MS triple quadrupole mass spectrometer (Bruker, Billerica, MA).
7. 2-HG standard (Sigma-Aldrich).

2.20 ELISA Assay for 5-Hydroxy methylcytosine

1. QIAamp DNA Mini Kit (Qiagen).
2. Quest 5-hmC DNA ELISA Kit (Zymo Research, Irvine, CA).
3. Standard microplate reader.

3 Methods

3.1 Molecular Cloning of Human and Zebrafish Idh1

1. To clone human and zebrafish *Idh1*, total RNA is prepared using TRIzol reagent from 293FT cell line and WT zebrafish embryos at 24 hpf (hours post-fertilization).
2. Synthesize first-strand complementary DNA (cDNA) from total RNA using SuperScript First-Strand Synthesis System following manufacturer's recommendations.
3. To subclone human IDH1 into pCS2+ expression vector (pCS2-IDH1), full coding sequence is PCR amplified with primer pair pCS2-IDH1-BamHI-F and pCS2-IDH1-XbaI-R with the following PCR program (*see* **Note 2**):
   (a) 95 °C, 5 min.
   (b) 95 °C, 30 s; 58 °C, 30 s; and 72 °C, 2 min → 35 cycles.
   (c) 72 °C, 7 min.
   (d) 4 °C and hold.
4. Check PCR product size and purity by agarose gel electrophoresis.
5. Digest PCR product and pCS2+ vector with BamHI and XbaI at 37 °C for 2 h.
6. Resolve digested products with agarose gel electrophoresis and purify them by QIAquick Gel Extraction Kit following manufacturer's recommendations.
7. Set up ligation reaction and incubate the reaction product at room temperature (RT) for 2 h or at 16 °C overnight:

Reagents	Standard reaction	Background control
10× T4 DNA ligase reaction buffer	1 μL	1 μL
T4 DNA ligase	0.5 μL	0.5 μL
Digested vector	25 ng	25 ng
Digested PCR product	75 ng	–
Deionized water to a total volume of	10 μL	10 μL

8. Transform 5 μL of the ligation reaction into DH5α competent cells by heat shock.
9. Pick and grow 3–5 colonies at 37 °C overnight and purify plasmid DNA from bacterial culture using QIAprep Spin Miniprep Kit.
10. To clone the zebrafish *idh1-egfp* fusion gene (pidh1-egfp), PCR amplify the full coding sequence without stop codon with primer pair zidh1-HindIII-F and zidh1-BamHI-R following **steps 3–9**. Digest PCR products with HindIII/BamHI followed by ligation into pEGFP-N3 vector in frame between the HindIII and BamHI sites.
11. To subclone*idh1-egfp* fusion gene into pCS2+ expression vector (pCS2-idh1-egfp), PCR amplify the fusion construct idh1-egfp with primer pair pCS2-zidh1-egfp-ClaI-F and pCS2-zidh1-egfp-EcoRI-R from pidh1-egfp following **steps 3–9**. PCR product was then restriction digested with ClaI/EcoRI and ligated into pCS2+ vector between the ClaI and EcoRI sites.
12. To clone WT zebrafish *idh1* (pGEMT-idh1) for in vitro mRNA transcription, PCR amplify full coding sequence with primer pair zidh1-rescue-F and zidh1-rescue-R (*see* **Note 1**) with the following PCR program:

    (a) 95 °C, 5 min.

    (b) 95 °C, 30 s; 55 °C, 30 s; and 72 °C, 2 min → 35 cycles.

    (c) 72 °C, 7 min.

    (d) 4 °C hold

    And the PCR product is TA-cloned into pGEM-T Easy Vector following manufacturer's recommendations.
13. To clone zebrafish *idh1* partial sequence (pGEMT-idh1P) for antisense RNA probe synthesis, PCR amplify full coding sequence with primer pair zidh1-probe-F and zidh1-probe-R with the following PCR program:

(a) 95 °C, 5 min.

(b) 95 °C, 30 s; 64 °C, 30 s and 72 °C, 2 min → 35 cycles.

(c) 72 °C, 7 min.

(d) 4 °C hold.

And the PCR product is TA-cloned into pGEM-T Easy Vector following manufacturer's recommendations.

14. All the subcloned constructs are confirmed by bidirectional sequencing using appropriate sequencing primers:

pCS2+: CMV, T3.

pEGFP-N3: CMV, EGFP-N.

pGEM-T Easy: T7, SP6.

3.2 Site-Directed Mutagenesis of Human and Zebrafish Idh1

1. Design primer pair for site-directed mutagenesis with Agilent QuikChange Primer Design software (http://www.genomics.agilent.com/primerDesignProgram.jsp), as shown in Subheading 2.2, Primers for site-directed mutagenesis.
2. For generating human IDH1 R132H mutation (pCS2-IDH1R132H), set up the following PCR reaction with primer pair IDH1-R132H-F and IDH1-R132H-R:

Reagents	Volume (μL)
10× *Pfx* amplification buffer	5
10 mM dNTP mixture	1.5
50 mM $MgSO_4$	1
Forward primer (10 μM)	1
Reverse primer (10 μM)	1
Platinum *Pfx* DNA polymerase	0.5
pCS2-IDH1 DNA template (60 ng)	
Deionized water to a total volume of	50

3. PCR with the following program:

(a) 95 °C, 1 min.

(b) 95 °C, 50 s; 60 °C, 50 s; and 68 °C, 6 min → 17 cycles.

(c) 68 °C, 7 min.

(d) 4 °C hold.

4. Check PCR product size and purity by agarose gel electrophoresis (*see* **Note 3**).
5. Eliminate plasmid DNA template by DpnI digestion at 37 °C for 2 h:

Reagents	Volume (μL)
10× NEB CutSmart buffer	5
PCR product	40
DpnI (20,000 units/mL)	1
Deionized water to a total volume of	50

6. Purify the reaction with QIAquick Gel Extraction Kit and ligate the purified PCR product with T4 DNA ligase by overnight at 16 °C.

Reagents	Standard reaction (μL)
10× T4 DNA ligase reaction buffer	5
T4 DNA ligase	1
Purified PCR product	44

7. Transform 5 μL of the ligation reaction with DH5α competent cells by heat shock.
8. Pick and grow 3–5 colonies at 37 °C overnight and purify plasmid DNA from bacterial culture using QIAprep Spin Miniprep Kit.
9. Confirm sequence by bidirectional sequencing using primers CMV and T3.
10. To generate zebrafish idh1 R146H mutation (pCS2-idh1R146H-egfp), repeat **steps 2–9** with primer pair zidh1-R146H-F and zidh1-R146H-R using pCS2-idh1-egfp construct as PCR template.

3.3 Zebrafish Embryo Handling

1. All embryos are raised in E3 medium at 28.5 °C.
2. For whole-mount in situ hybridization, whole-mount immunostaining, or whole-embryo fluorescence microscopy, embryos are treated from 6 hpf onward with 0.003% PTU in E3 medium to suppress pigmentation.
3. Embryos at appropriate stages are dechorionated, fixed with 4% PFA at RT for 4 h (or at 4 °C overnight), and dehydrated stepwise from 25%, 50%, and 75% to 100% ethanol. Dehydrated embryos are stored at −20 °C in 100% ethanol until subsequent analysis.
4. For whole-mount imaging, live or fixed zebrafish embryos are mounted in 3% methylcellulose. Live embryos are anesthetized with 0.016% MS-222 prior to mounting.

3.4 Morpholino Knockdown of Zebrafish idh1

1. Dilute MOs to appropriate working concentration with Danieau's solution.
2. Determine optimal MO dosage by microinjecting MO into 1- to 4-cell stage zebrafish embryos at different doses ranging from 1 to 9 ng. Approximately 90% of the embryos should tolerate up to 6 ng of *idh1* MO without obvious toxicity and lethality, and the maximum tolerable dose should be chosen for subsequent experiments.
3. The same amount of standard control MO is injected to sibling embryos as control.
4. To test the efficiency of *idh1* MO, pidh1-egfp construct is injected into 1-cell stage embryos with or without *idh1* MO. A quenching of mosaic egfp expression in co-injected embryos demonstrated the molecular targeting of *idh1* MO (Fig. 1a).

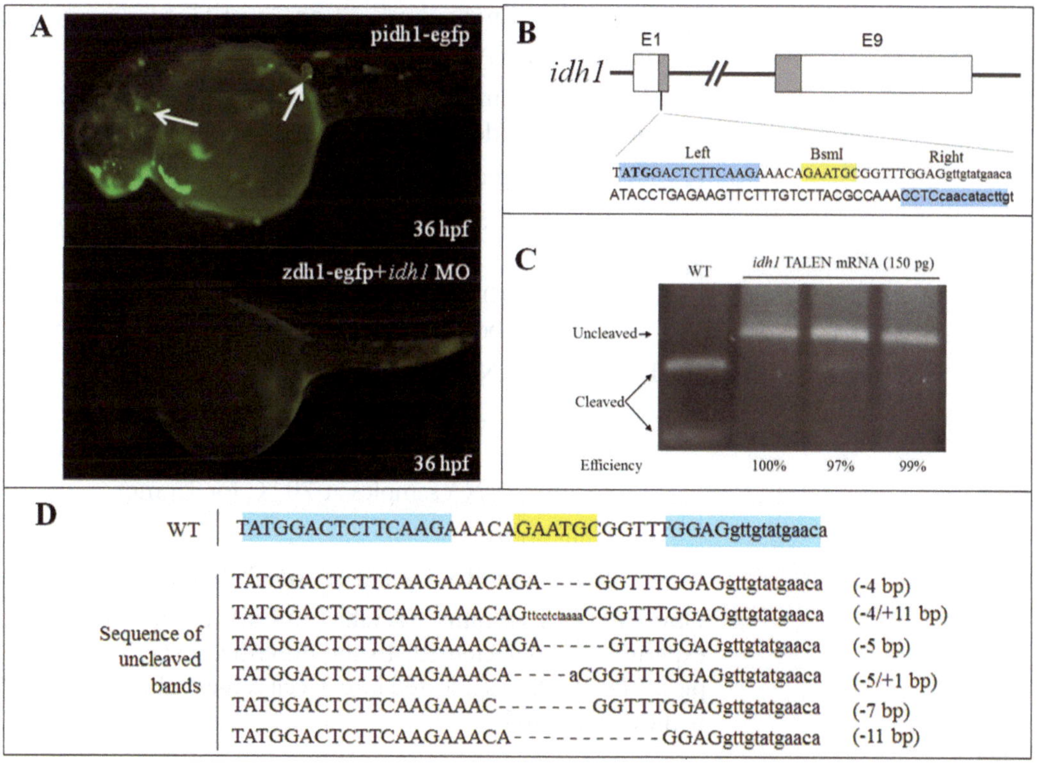

Fig. 1 Morpholino-mediated knockdown and TALEN-mediated knockout of *idh1*. (**a**) Mosaic fluorescent pattern (*white arrows*) in embryos injected with pidh1-egfp was almost completely abolished (*lower panel*) by *idh1* MO co-injection. (**b**) Target site of *idh1* TALEN. *Cyan*: binding sequence for the TALEN pair (indicated by "*left*" and "*right*"); *yellow*: BsmI site; *bold*: The start codon of *idh1*; *E*: exon. (**c**) RFLP assay with BsmI digestion from pooled gDNA of five embryos injected with *idh1* TALEN in three separate experiments. Cleaved and uncleaved PCR products are indicated by *arrows*. (**d**) Representative sequences of mutated *idh1* locus. These figures were originally published in Blood. Shi X, He BL, Ma AC, Guo Y, Chi Y et al. Functions of idh1 and its mutation in the regulation of developmental hematopoiesis in zebrafish. Blood. 2015; 125(19): 2974-2984. © the American Society of Hematology

5. For rescue experiment, capped WT *idh1* mRNA not targetable by *idh1* MO (*see* **Note 1**) is in vitro transcribed from pGEMT-idh1 linearized with SalI using Ambion mMESSAGE mMACHINE T7 Transcription Kit (*see* **Note 4**).
6. Polyadenylate freshly synthesized mRNA using Ambion Poly(A) Tailing Kit.
7. Purify and quantify in vitro-transcribed mRNA:
   (a) Add 100 μL LiCl precipitation solution to each transcription reaction.
   (b) Precipitate at −20 °C ≥ 1 h.
   (c) Centrifuge at 4 °C, 12,000 × *g* for 15 min.
   (d) Remove supernatant and wash with 70% ethanol.
   (e) Centrifuge at 4 °C, 12,000 × *g* for 5 min.
   (f) Remove supernatant and air-dry pellet.
   (g) Resuspend mRNA pellet in 50 μL deionized water and quantify mRNA.
8. Check size and integrity of in vitro-transcribed mRNA by denaturing formaldehyde RNA gel electrophoresis, briefly:
   (a) 1% denaturing agarose RNA gel.
      - Dissolve 1.5 g agarose in 72 mL water and cool down to 55 °C.
      - Mix with 10 mL 10× MOPS buffer and 18 mL 37% formaldehyde (both pre-warmed to 55 °C) and cast the gel.
   (b) Denaturing RNA sample.
      - Mix RNA sample (up to ~200 ng) with formaldehyde gel-loading buffer-loading dye at 1:8 (Vol/Vol) ratio.
      - Incubate RNA samples at 70 °C for 15 min.
      - Chill on ice.
      - Resolve on RNA gel in 1× MOPS buffer at 4–5 V/cm.
9. Optimal or maximum tolerable mRNA dosage for rescue experiment is determined. In the published experiments, 100 pg *idh1* mRNA was injected into 1-cell stage embryos with and without *idh1* MO.

3.5 TALEN-Mediated Mutagenesis of Zebrafish idh1

1. To induce loss-of-function *idh1* mutation, TALEN targeting *idh1* is designed based on the following parameters described previously [25] (Fig. 1b) (*see* **Note 5**):
   (a) Length of TAL-binding domain with 15 RVDs.
   (b) Spacer length between 14 and 18 b.p.
   (c) Unique restriction site within the spacer for RFLP assay of NHEJ-mediated mutagenesis.

(d) T nucleotide upstream of both TAL-binding domains.

2. TALEN pair in GoldyTALEN scaffold [25] is assembled through Golden Gate method with the Golden Gate TALEN and TAL Effector Kit 2.0 as described [15] (*see* **Note 6**).
3. Linearize the TALEN constructs with SacI and purify the digested plasmids with QIAquick PCR Purification Kit.
4. Synthesize capped mRNA encoding the TALEN pairs with Ambion T3 mMESSAGE mMACHINE Transcription Kit (*see* **Note 7**).
5. Purify and quantify in vitro-transcribed mRNA as in Subheading 3.4, **step 7**.
6. Check mRNA size and integrity as in Subheading 3.4, **step 8**.
7. Mix and dilute mRNA pair to working concentration for microinjection (final concentration 50 ng/μL of each TALEN mRNA).
8. Microinject 3 nl of working mRNA solution (150 pg of each TALEN arm; *see* **Note 8**) into the yolk of 1-cell stage embryos.

3.6 Genotyping Targeted Genomic Locus

1. Extract gDNA from zebrafish embryos or adult fin tissue:
   (a) Prepare working extraction buffer (freshly add 30 μL 10% Tween 20, 30 μL 10% NP-40, and 10 μL proteinase K solution to 930 μL gDNA extraction buffer 1 mL working buffer).
   (b) Transfer embryo or fin tissue to PCR tube and remove excess water carryover.
   (c) Add working extraction buffer (50 μL per embryo, 100 μL per fin tissue).
   (d) Incubate at 55 °C with shaking ≥4 h until complete digestion of embryo or fin tissue followed by 10 min at 98 °C to inactivate proteinase K.
   (e) gDNA can be stored at −20 °C until PCR (5 μL of extracted gDNA are typically used in 25 μL PCR reaction).
2. PCR amplify *idh1* Exon-1 locus with primers zidh1-E1-gF and zidh1-E1-gR (*see* **Note 9**) with the following program:
   (a) 95 °C, 5 min.
   (b) 95 °C, 30 s; 58 °C, 30 s and 72 °C, 2 min → 35 cycles.
   (c) 72 °C, 7 min.
   (d) 4 °C hold.
3. Digest 10 μL PCR product directly with BsmI at 37 °C for 2 h (Fig. 1c).
4. Resolve digested PCR product on 1.5% agarose gel and quantify mutagenic activity by Image Analysis software (e.g., Image J, http://imagej.nih.gov/ij/).

5. To confirm small indels introduced in target locus, TA-clone the remaining undigested PCR product with pGEM-T Easy Vector Systems and sequence ~10 colonies per sample bidirectionally with sequencing primer T7 and SP6 (Fig. 1d).

3.7 Overexpression of Human IDH1 R132H and Zebrafish idh1 R146H

1. Linearize expression construct with NotI-HF and purify the digested plasmids with QIAquick PCR Purification Kit.
2. Synthesize capped mRNA encoding WT or mutant IDH1 (idh1) with Ambion SP6 mMESSAGE mMACHINE Transcription Kit.
3. Polyadenylate freshly synthesized mRNA using Ambion Poly(A) Tailing Kit.
4. Purify and quantify in vitro-transcribed mRNA as in Subheading 3.4, **step 7**.
5. Check mRNA size and integrity as in Subheading 3.4, **step 8**.
6. Dilute mRNA working concentration and microinjecting 100 pg of either WT or mutant IDH1 (idh1) encoded mRNA (*see* **Note 8**) into the yolk of 1-cell stage sibling embryos.

3.8 Pharmacological Inhibition of IDH R132H

1. Plate 30–50 embryos overexpressing human WT or IDH1 R132H as in Subheading 3.7 into 6-well plate.
2. Treat the embryos with AGI-5198 at 10 μM from 6 hpf onward. Treat the vehicle control embryos with equivolume amount of DMSO.
3. Collect the embryos at appropriate time points for further analysis.

3.9 Generation of Antisense RNA Probe Against Zebrafish idh1

1. Linearize 2 μg of pGEMT-idh1P with SacII at 37 °C for 2 h.
2. Purify the linearized plasmid with QIAquick PCR Purification Kit.
3. Setup the following SP6 in vitro transcription reaction and incubate at 37 °C for 2 h:

Reagents	Volume
Linearized pGEMT-idh1P	0.6–1 μg
10× transcription buffer	2 μL
10× DIG-UTP labeling mix	2 μL
RNAse inhibitor (20 units/μL)	1 μL
SP6 RNA polymerase (20 units/μL)	2 μL
Deionized water to a total volume of	20 μL

4. Remove plasmid template by adding 1 μL DNase I (10 units/μL) and incubate at 37 °C for 15 min.

5. Purify RNA probe by LiCl solution as in Subheading 3.4, **step 7**.
6. Check size and integrity of RNA probe as in Subheading 3.4, **step 8**.

3.10 Whole-Mount in Situ Hybridization

1. Rehydrate the fixed and dehydrated embryos stepwise (5 min each) from 100, 75, 50, and 25% ethanol to PBST.
2. Embryos beyond 24 hpf are further permeabilized with working proteinase K solution at RT (*see* **Note 10**), refixed with 4% PFA for 30 min (RT), and then washed with PBST four times (5 min).
3. Wash in PHB for 5 min and then pre-hybridize in PHB at 65 °C for 4–6 h.
4. Hybridize embryos in DIG-labeled RNA probe diluted in PHB (0.5 ng/μL) at 65 °C overnight.
5. Wash sequentially with the 100% PHB; 75% PHB, 0.5× SSC; 50% PHB, 1× SSC; and 25% PHB, 1.5× SSC and 2× SSC at 65 °C, 15 min each.
6. Wash twice with 0.2× SSC for 30 min at RT.
7. Wash sequentially with the 0.15× SSC, 25% PBST; 0.1× SSC, 50% PBST; and 0.05× SSC, 75% PBST at RT, 5 min each.
8. Wash twice with PBST at RT, 5 min each.
9. Incubate with alkaline phosphatase-conjugated anti-DIG antibody (diluted 1:5000 in PBST) with 5% lamb serum at 4 °C overnight with constant shaking.
10. Wash four times with PBST at RT, 30 min each.
11. Wash three times with AP buffer at RT, 5 min each.
12. Develop staining with 0.01× NBT/BCIP stock solution (diluted in AP buffer) with inspections at regular interval to avoid overstaining (*see* **Note 11**).
13. Stop staining by washing in PBST and dehydrate embryos stepwise from 25, 50, and 75 to 100% ethanol to remove background staining. Embryos can be stored in 100% ethanol until imaging.
14. Rehydrate embryos stepwise from 100% ethanol to PBST before imaging (Fig. 2).

3.11 Whole-Mount Fluorescent Immunostaining

1. Rehydrate fixed and dehydrated embryos stepwise (5 min each) from 100, 75, 50, and 25% ethanol to PBST.
2. Permeabilize embryos with ice-cold acetone for 5 min.
3. Wash four times in PBST at RT, 5 min each.
4. Incubate with blocking solution for 1 h at RT with constant shaking.

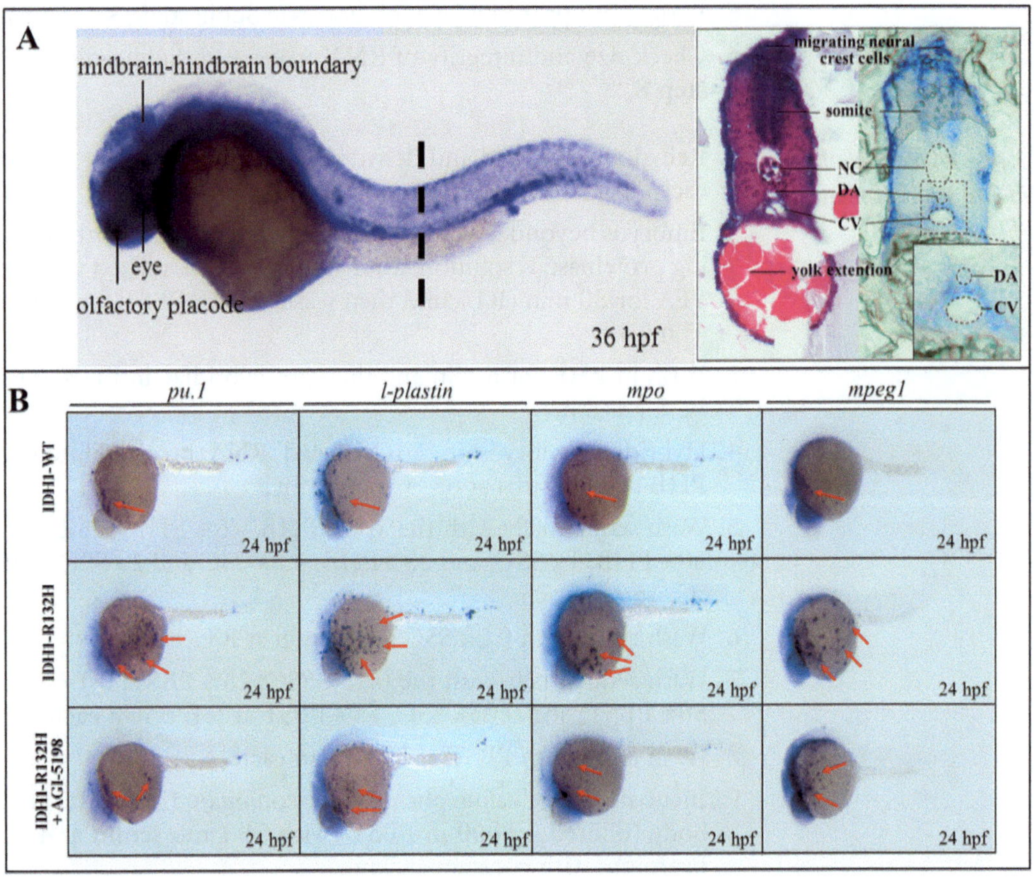

Fig. 2 WISH showing expression pattern of *idh1* and genes associated with myeloid lineages in zebrafish embryos. (**a**) *Left panel*: spatial expression pattern of *idh1* at 36 hpf. *Dashed line* indicates the level of the histological paraffin section in *right panel* showing *idh1* expression around the ventral wall of the dorsal aorta (DA). (**b**) WISH showing the expression of early myeloid progenitor marker *pu.1* and late myelomonocytic differentiation markers *l-plastin, mpo,* and *mpeg1* at 24 hpf in embryos injected with pCS2-IDH1 (IDH1-WT) or pCS2-IDH1R132H (IDH1-R123H), with or without AGI-5198 (10 mM) treatment starting from bud stage. *Red arrows* indicate myeloid cells on the yolk sac. These figures were originally published in Blood. Shi X, He BL, Ma AC, Guo Y, Chi Y et al. Functions of idh1 and its mutation in the regulation of developmental hematopoiesis in zebrafish. Blood. 2015; 125(19): 2974-2984. © the American Society of Hematology

5. Incubate with primary antibody at 4 °C overnight with constant shaking.
6. Wash four times in blocking solution at RT, 30 min each.
7. Incubate with secondary antibody at 4 °C overnight in the dark with constant shaking.
8. Wash four times in PBSTX at 4 °C in the dark, 30 min each.
9. Mount embryos in 3% methylcellulose for fluorescent microscopy (Fig. 3a). Stained embryos should be kept in 4 °C in the dark.

3.12 Quantitative PCR

1. Extract total RNA from control or treated embryos at 18 hpf (at least 30 embryos were pooled for each sample) using TRIzol reagent according to the manufacturer's recommendations.
2. Synthesize cDNA from total RNA using SuperScript First-Strand Synthesis System following manufacturer's recommendations.
3. Setup the following reaction in 96-well plate with triplicates:

Reagents	Volume (μL)
2× SYBR Green PCR master mix	6.5
Forward primer	0.26
Reverse primer	0.26
cDNA (0.01×, *see* **Note 12**)	1
Deionized water to a total volume of	13

4. Run the following program with StepOnePlus Real-Time PCR System:
   (a) 95 °C, 10 min.
   (b) 95 °C, 15 s; 60 °C, 1 min → 40 cycles.
5. Analyze gene expression using comparative C^T method with *β-actin* as the housekeeping gene.

3.13 Whole-Mount BrdU Incorporation Assay

1. Incubate the dechorionated embryos at 24 hpf with BrdU (10 mM) in 1× E3 for 1 h at 28 °C.
2. Fix and dehydrate embryo as in Subheading 3.3, **step 3**.
3. Rehydrate embryos stepwise (5 min each) from 100, 75, 50, and 25% ethanol to PBST.
4. Digest with proteinase K for 20 min at RT.
5. Refix with 4% PFA at RT for 20 min.
6. Incubate with 2 N HCl for 1 h at RT.
7. Incubate with blocking solution for 2 h at RT.
8. Incubate with PE-conjugated anti-BrdU antibody at 4 °C overnight.
9. Wash three times with PBST at RT, 5 min each.
10. Mount embryos in 3% methylcellulose for fluorescent microscopy (Fig. 3b).

3.14 Whole-Mount TUNEL Assay

1. Rehydrate fixed and dehydrated embryos stepwise (5 min each) from 100, 75, 50, and 25% ethanol to PBST.
2. Digest with proteinase K for 5 min at RT.

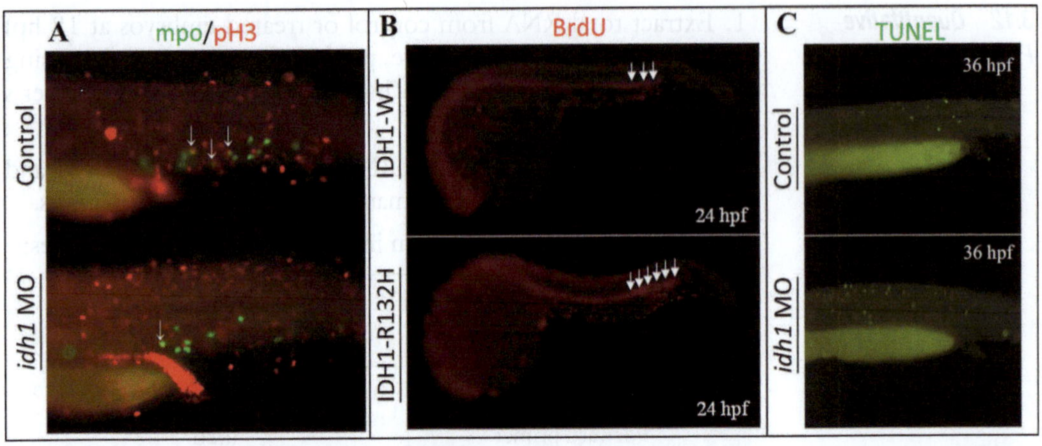

Fig. 3 Fluorescent immuno- and biochemical staining to examine proliferation and apoptosis in zebrafish embryos. (**a**) Tg(*mpo:gfp*) embryo at the caudal hematopoietic tissue (CHT) region stained for phospho-histone H3 (pH 3) at 28 hpf injected with control or *idh1* MO. *Arrows* indicate pH 3 and mpo double-positive proliferating myeloid cells. (**b**) BrdU incorporation assay showing cellular proliferation (*white arrows*) embryos injected with pCS2-IDH1 (IDH1-WT) or pCS2-IDH1R132H (IDH1-R132H) at 24 hpf. (**c**) Whole-mount TUNEL assay showing apoptosis cells along the CHT in embryo at 48 hpf injected with control or *idh1* MO. These figures were originally published in Blood. Shi X, He BL, Ma AC, Guo Y, Chi Y et al. Functions of idh1 and its mutation in the regulation of developmental hematopoiesis in zebrafish. Blood. 2015; 125(19): 2974-2984. © the American Society of Hematology

3. Wash three times with PBST at RT, 5 min each.
4. Incubate in 50 μL equilibration buffer for 1 h at RT.
5. Incubate with 50 μL of working strength TdT solution (35 μL reaction buffer and 15 μL TdT enzyme) at 37 °C for 1 h.
6. Wash four times with working strength stop/wash buffer (1:34 Vol/Vol diluted in deionized water) at RT, 5 min each.
7. Mount embryos in 3% methylcellulose for fluorescent microscopy (Fig. 3c).

3.15 Flow Cytometry Quantification and Sorting of Neutrophils in Transgenic Embryos

1. Dechorionate Tg(*mpo:gfp*) transgenic embryos (and wild-type as negative control) at 36 hpf.
2. Rinse embryos in E3 medium and digest with 0.05% trypsin-EDTA solution for 15 min at 28.5 °C.
3. Completely dissociate embryos into single-cell suspension by pipetting up and down.
4. Add $CaCl_2$ (final concentration 2 mM) to inactivate trypsin digestion.
5. Filter cell suspension through 40 μm cell strainer to remove debris and cell clumps.
6. Centrifuge cell suspension at 1200 rpm for 5 min at RT and resuspend cell pellet in 0.9× PBS (with 2% FBS) and keep it on ice.

7. Enumerate percentage of GFP^+ cell population with flow cytometer (acquired >10,000 total cells) or isolate GFP^+ cell population by fluorescence-activated cell sorting (FACS) (Fig. 4a)
8. To examine morphology of sorted neutrophils, centrifuge cells at 300 rpm using standard cytocentrifuge, then stain cytospin with Wright-Giemsa stain, and observe under microscope (Fig. 4b).

3.16 Western Blot

1. Homogenize 30 dechorionated zebrafish embryos in 100 μL CelLytic MT Cell Lysis Reagent with 1× protease and phosphatase inhibitor cocktail (~2–5 μL lysis buffer per embryo).
2. Centrifuge lysate at top speed for 15 min at 4 °C and collect supernatant.
3. Add 25 μL 5× loading buffer.
4. Boil the protein lysate for 10 min.
5. Resolve protein sample with SDS-PAGE on 12% resolving polyacrylamide gel.
6. Electro-transfer resolved protein onto nitrocellulose membranes.
7. Incubate membrane in blocking buffer at RT for 1 h with constant shaking.
8. Incubate with primary antibody at 4 °C overnight with constant shaking.
9. Wash four times with TBST at RT, 15 min each with constant shaking.
10. Incubate with secondary antibody for 2 h at RT.
11. Wash four times with TBST at RT, 15 min each with constant shaking.
12. Detect target protein by chemiluminescence with Luminata Forte Western HRP substrate according to manufacturer's recommendations.

3.17 Adult Zebrafish Kidney Marrow Analysis

1. Euthanize 3 months old *idh1* mutants and their WT siblings on ice.
2. Dissect kidney marrow from euthanized fish and rinse it in ice cold 0.9× PBS with 5% FBS.
3. Dissociate kidney marrow by trituration using pipette and then syringe with 18G needle.
4. Filter cell suspension through 40 μm cell strainer to remove debris and cell clumps.
5. Centrifuge cell suspension at 1200 rpm for 5 min at RT and resuspend cell pellet in 0.9× PBS (with 5% FBS) and keep it on ice.

6. Analyze and enumerate different hematopoietic populations in the kidney marrow by flow cytometry as described [26, 27] (Fig. 4c).
7. Particular population can be isolated through cell sorting to examine cell morphology through cytospin as in Subheading 3.15, **step 8** (Fig. 4d).

3.18 GC-Mass Spectrometry of 2-HG

1. Sonicate embryos at 24 hpf in 1 mL 80% methanol (ice cold) on ice at 3 s on and 3 s off cycle for 5 min.
2. Incubate methanol extract at −80 °C for 30 min.
3. Centrifuge extract at top speed for 30 min at 4 °C to remove precipitated protein and cellular debris.

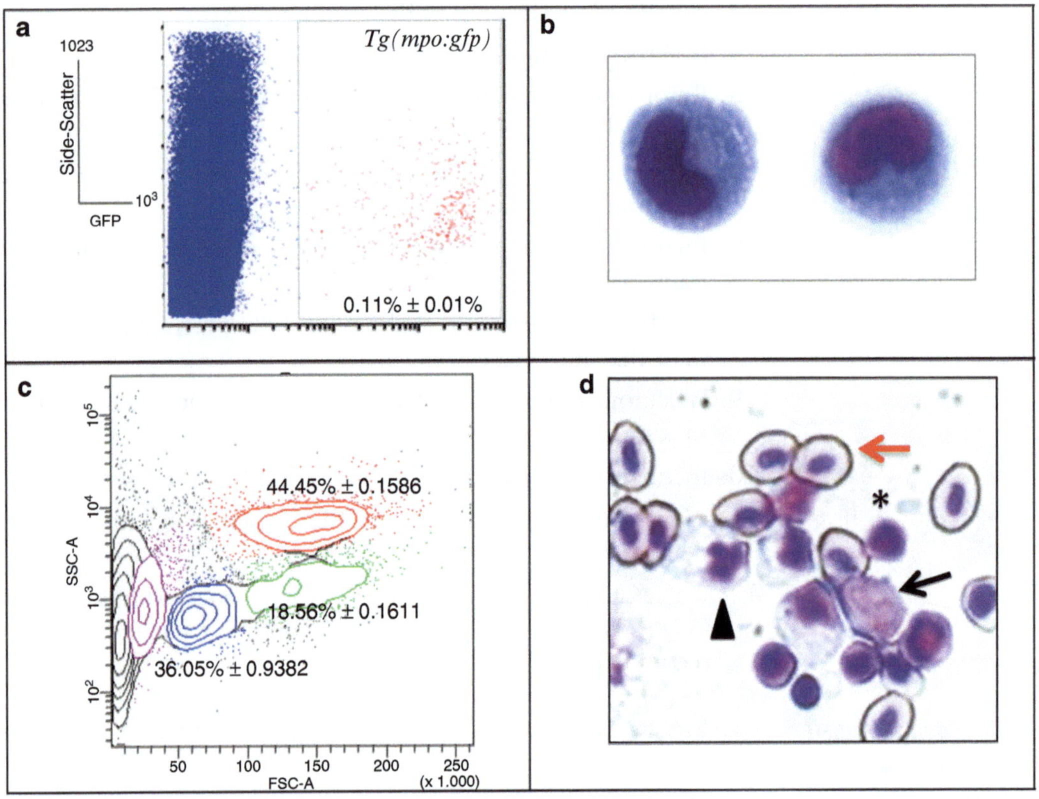

Fig. 4 Examination of hematopoietic lineages at cellular level in embryonic and adult zebrafish with flow cytometry and cytospins. (**a**) Flow cytometry result quantifying percentage of gfp-positive cells in Tg(*mpo:gfp*) embryos at 36 hpf. (**b**) Morphology of FACS-sorted gfp-positive cells in dissociated Tg(*mpo:gfp*) embryos. (**c**) Contour plot of flow cytometry showing myelomonocytic (*red*), precursor (*green*), lymphocytic (*blue*), and erythroid lineages (*purple*) from dissociated adult kidney marrow. (**d**) Morphology of hematopoietic cells from kidney marrow of *idh1* TALEN-injected adult zebrafish. *Red arrows*, erythrocytes; *black arrows*, precursor cells; *arrowheads*, myelomonocytes; *asterisks*, lymphocytes. These figures were originally published in Blood. Shi X, He BL, Ma AC, Guo Y, Chi Y et al. Functions of idh1 and its mutation in the regulation of developmental hematopoiesis in zebrafish. Blood. 2015; 125(19): 2974-2984. © the American Society of Hematology

4. Evaporate the aqueous metabolites in the supernatant layer to dryness under nitrogen gas (stored at −80 °C until GC/MS analysis).
5. Resuspend dried extract with 1:1 (Vol/Vol) acetonitrile and MTBSTFA mixture.
6. Heat the mixture at 70 °C for 75 min.
7. Inject 1 μL of derivatized materials into 450-GC system equipped with a VF-5 ms capillary column and connected to a 320-MS triple quadruple mass spectrometer in a splitless model with the following setting:
   (a) Injection, interface, and ion source temperatures at 310 °C, 250 °C, and 200 °C, respectively.
   (b) Initial GC oven temperature at 100 °C for 3 min, then raise to 230 °C at 4 °C/min (hold for 4 min) and maintain at 300 °C for 5 min.

   Measure with electronic ionization (70 eV) in the full-scan mode (m/z: 50–550 amu) and detector voltage at 1200 V

8. Confirm 2-HG peak with standard.
9. Quantify 2-HG and glutamate signal intensity by integration of peak areas and determine relative 2-HG level with the ratio of 2-HG to glutamate normalized by number of embryos.

3.19 ELISA Assay for5-Hydroxy methylcytosine in Zebrafish Genome

1. Extract gDNA from embryos with QIAamp DNA Mini Kit.
2. Quantify 5-hmC DNA by using Quest 5-hmC DNA ELISA Kit briefly:
   (a) Coat reaction wells with anti-5-hmC polyclonal antibody (1 ng/μL in coating buffer, 100 μL/well) with 1 h incubation at 37 °C.
   (b) Wash three times with 1× ELISA buffer at RT, 5 min each.
   (c) Incubate with 200 μL 1× ELISA buffer at 37 °C for 30 min.
   (d) Denature sample and control DNA at 98 °C for 5 min, and then cool on ice for 10 min.
   (e) Remove all liquid from wells, add 100 μL denatured sample or control DNA (1 ng/μL in 1× ELISA buffer) to each well, and incubate at 37 °C for 1 h.
   (f) Wash three times with 200 μL 1× ELISA buffer at RT, 5 min each.
   (g) Incubate with 100 μL anti-DNA HRP antibody (1:100 diluted in 1× ELISA buffer) at 37 °C for 1 h.
   (h) Wash three times with 200 μL 1× ELISA buffer at RT, 5 min each.

(i) Incubate with 100 μL 1× Developer at RT for 30 min.

(j) Measure absorbance at 405 nm by microplate reader.

3. Generate standard curve using absorbance from control DNAs and quantify percentage of 5-hmC in each sample with the standard curve.

4 Notes

1. To generate *idh1* mRNA that is not targetable by *idh1* MO during rescue experiment, silent mutations (5 b.p. mismatch) should be introduced into the MO-binding sequence through primer zidh1-rescue-F.
2. PCR program can be modified to suit different PCR systems or DNA polymerases. All the PCR reactions described in the protocol are based on AmpliTaq Gold 360 (Life Technologies) unless otherwise stated.
3. Although a band with a size corresponding to the plasmid is usually seen in electrophoresis, procedures can be carried on and correct mutant clone may be obtained even if initial PCR fail to produce any visible band. However, PCR conditions should be optimized if multiple bands are observed.
4. For pGEMT-idh1 and pGEMT-idh1P, orientation during TA cloning is random and should be confirmed by sequencing. The construct should be linearized with appropriate enzyme and in vitro transcribed with correct RNA polymerase. Briefly, to synthesize mRNA, construct should be linearized at 3′ end and RNA polymerase at 5′ end should be chosen, while for antisense RNA probe, construct should be linearized at 5′ end and RNA polymerase at 3′ end should be chosen.
5. To generate loss-of-function mutation, TALEN should be designed to target early exons after the start codon (or alternate start codon) or particular functional domain. TALEN will potentially introduce frame-shifting small indels at target site through nonhomologous end joining (NHEJ). Recent development in microhomology-mediated end joining (MMEJ) prediction algorithm [28] greatly enhanced the possibility of out-of-frame mutation and should be taken into consideration during TALEN design. Zebrafish line or colonies in use should be genotyped to avoid polymorphism that will otherwise affect TALEN activity. Online software Mojo Hand (www.talendesign.org) is available to facilitate TALEN design [29].
6. A new version of Golden Gate TALEN assembling system (FusX) has been developed recently. It has streamlined the original Golden Gate system to a single reaction with higher efficiency. Corresponding plasmid libraries may soon be available through Addgene.

7. A half (10 μL) in vitro transcription reaction will produce sufficient mRNA for TALEN applications.
8. Optimum dose of mRNA should be determined by dose-response trials. Typically, the highest dose compatible with normal development in more than 50% embryos is chosen.
9. Although any PCR reagent can be use, ready-to-use PCR master mix will facilitate large-scale genotyping.
10. Proteinase K digestion time depends on the developmental stage of embryos as well as the specific batch of proteinase K solution. Typically, embryos at 36, 48, 72, and 96 hpf are digested for 5, 10, 15, and 20 min, respectively.
11. If embryo is subjected to paraffin sectioning after whole-mount in situ hybridization (Fig. 2a), significant overstaining is needed to ensure adequate staining on individual section.
12. cDNA sample synthesized from a standard 20 μL reaction with the SuperScript First-Strand Synthesis System is usually diluted 100-fold to use as template for quantitative PCR.

Acknowledgments

Zebrafish research was supported by Faculty Core Zebrafish Facility, LKS Faculty of Medicine, HKU. This work was supported by HKU771613M, HKUST5/CRF/12R, CityU9/CRF/13G, HMRF02132326, HMRF03143756 and HKU Seed Funding for Basic Research (201401159004, 201411159098). AYHL is the Li Shu Fan Medical Foundation Professor in Haematology and received funding from its endowment.

References

1. Mardis ER, Ding L, Dooling DJ et al (2009) Recurring mutations found by sequencing an acute myeloid leukemia genome. N Engl J Med 361(11):1058–1066
2. Ley TJ, Ding L, Walter MJ et al (2010) DNMT3A mutations in acute myeloid leukemia. N Engl J Med 363(25):2424–2433
3. Patel JP, Gonen M, Figueroa ME et al (2012) Prognostic relevance of integrated genetic profiling in acute myeloid leukemia. N Engl J Med 366(12):1079–1089
4. Cancer Genome Atlas Research Network (2013) Genomic and epigenomic landscapes of adult de novo acute myeloid leukemia. N Engl J Med 368(22):2059–2074
5. Martin CS, Moriyama A, Zon LI (2011) Hematopoietic stem cells, hematopoiesis and disease: lessons from the zebrafish model. Genome Med 3(12):83
6. de Jong JL, Zon LI (2005) Use of the zebrafish system to study primitive and definitive hematopoiesis. Annu Rev Genet 39:481–501
7. Davidson AJ, Zon LI (2004) The 'definitive' (and 'primitive') guide to zebrafish hematopoiesis. Oncogene 23(43):7233–7246
8. Paw BH, Zon LI (2000) Zebrafish: a genetic approach in studying hematopoiesis. Curr Opin Hematol 7(2):79–84
9. Im AP, Sehgal AR, Carroll MP et al (2014) DNMT3A and IDH mutations in acute myeloid leukemia and other myeloid malignancies: associations with prognosis and potential treatment strategies. Leukemia 28(9):1774–1783
10. Lasho TL, Jimma T, Finke CM et al (2012) SRSF2 mutations in primary myelofibrosis: significant clustering with IDH mutations and independent association with inferior overall and leukemia-free survival. Blood 120(20):4168–4171

11. Pardanani A, Patnaik MM, Lasho TL et al (2010) Recurrent IDH mutations in high-risk myelodysplastic syndrome or acute myeloid leukemia with isolated del(5q). Leukemia 24(7):1370–1372
12. Caramazza D, Lasho TL, Finke CM et al (2010) IDH mutations and trisomy 8 in myelodysplastic syndromes and acute myeloid leukemia. Leukemia 24(12):2120–2122
13. Sasaki M, Knobbe CB, Munger JC et al (2012) IDH1(R132H) mutation increases murine haematopoietic progenitors and alters epigenetics. Nature 488(7413):656–659
14. Shi X, He BL, Ma AC et al (2015) Functions of idh1 and its mutation in the regulation of developmental hematopoiesis in zebrafish. Blood 125(19):2974–2984
15. Cermak T, Doyle EL, Christian M et al (2011) Efficient design and assembly of custom TALEN and other TAL effector-based constructs for DNA targeting. Nucleic Acids Res 39(12):e82
16. He BL, Shi X, Man CH, Ma AC et al (2014) Functions of flt3 in zebrafish hematopoiesis and its relevance to human acute myeloid leukemia. Blood 123(16):2518–2529
17. Ma AC, Chung MI, Liang R et al (2010) A DEAB-sensitive aldehyde dehydrogenase regulates hematopoietic stem and progenitor cells development during primitive hematopoiesis in zebrafish embryos. Leukemia 24(12):2090–2099
18. Ma AC, Fan A, Ward AC et al (2009) A novel zebrafish jak2a(V581F) model shared features of human JAK2(V617F) polycythemia vera. Exp Hematol 37(12):1379.e4–1386.e4
19. Ma AC, Chung MI, Liang R et al (2009) The role of survivin2 in primitive hematopoiesis during zebrafish development. Leukemia 23(4):712–720
20. Ma AC, Ward AC, Liang R et al (2007) The role of jak2a in zebrafish hematopoiesis. Blood 110(6):1824–1830
21. Ma A, Lin R, Chan PK et al (2007) The role of survivin in angiogenesis during zebrafish embryonic development. BMC Dev Biol 7:50
22. Ma AC, Liang R, Leung AY (2007) The role of phospholipase C gamma 1 in primitive hematopoiesis during zebrafish development. Exp Hematol 35(3):368–373
23. Jin H, Li L, Xu J et al (2012) Runx1 regulates embryonic myeloid fate choice in zebrafish through a negative feedback loop inhibiting Pu.1 expression. Blood 119(22):5239–5249
24. Renshaw SA, Loynes CA, Trushell DM et al (2006) A transgenic zebrafish model of neutrophilic inflammation. Blood 108(13):3976–3978
25. Ma AC, Lee HB, Clark KJ et al (2013) High efficiency in vivo genome engineering with a simplified 15-RVD GoldyTALEN design. PLoS One 8(5):e65259
26. Kobayashi I, Kobayashi-Sun J, Kim AD et al (2014) Jam1a-Jam2a interactions regulate haematopoietic stem cell fate through Notch signalling. Nature 512(7514):319–323
27. Stachura DL, Reyes JR, Bartunek P et al (2009) Zebrafish kidney stromal cell lines support multilineage hematopoiesis. Blood 114(2):279–289
28. Nakade S, Tsubota T, Sakane Y et al (2014) Microhomology-mediated end-joining-dependent integration of donor DNA in cells and animals using TALENs and CRISPR/Cas9. Nat Commun 5:5560
29. Neff KL, Argue DP, Ma AC et al (2013) Mojo hand, a TALEN design tool for genome editing applications. BMC Bioinformatics 14:1

Chapter 14

Measurement of Oncometabolites D-2-Hydroxyglutaric Acid and L-2-Hydroxyglutaric Acid

Patricia M. Jones, Richard Boriack, Eduard A. Struys, and Dinesh Rakheja

Abstract

We describe a liquid chromatography-tandem mass spectrometry assay for measurement of D-2-hydroxyglutaric acid and L-2-hydroxyglutaric acid. These metabolites are increased in specific inborn errors of metabolism and are now recognized as oncometabolites. The measurement of D-2-hydroxyglutarate in peripheral blood may be used as a biomarker for screening and follow-up of patients with *IDH*-mutated acute myeloid leukemia.

Key words 2-Hydroxyglutaric acid, 2HG, Biomarker, D-2-Hydroxyglutaric acid, D-2HG, L-2-Hydroxyglutaric acid, L-2HG, Liquid chromatography-tandem mass spectrometry, LC-MS/MS, Oncometabolite

1 Introduction

2-Hydroxyglutaric acid (2HG) is a 5-carbon dicarboxylic acid with a hydroxyl group at the second or alpha carbon (2-hydroxypentanedioic acid). The second carbon is thus a chiral or asymmetric carbon, resulting in two stereoisomers: D-2HG (or R-2HG or [+]-2HG) and L-2HG (or S-2HG or [−]-2HG). The stereoisomers have identical physical properties. However, they have different three-dimensional spatial configurations and are therefore recognized by different enzymes (Fig. 1), whose deficiencies lead to distinct inborn errors of metabolism. L-2HG is thought to be formed by the oxidation of alpha-ketoglutarate (2KG) by L-malate dehydrogenase (and by lactate dehydrogenase A under hypoxic conditions) and is converted back to 2KG by L-2-hydroxyglutarate dehydrogenase (L2HGDH) [1–5]. An inherited, autosomal recessive, deficiency of L2HGDH, caused by mutations in *L2HGDH*, results in the metabolic disorder L-2-hydroxyglutaric aciduria (OMIM #236792) [6–8]. D-2HG is

Paolo Fortina et al. (eds.), *Acute Myeloid Leukemia: Methods and Protocols*, Methods in Molecular Biology, vol. 1633, DOI 10.1007/978-1-4939-7142-8_14, © Springer Science+Business Media LLC 2017

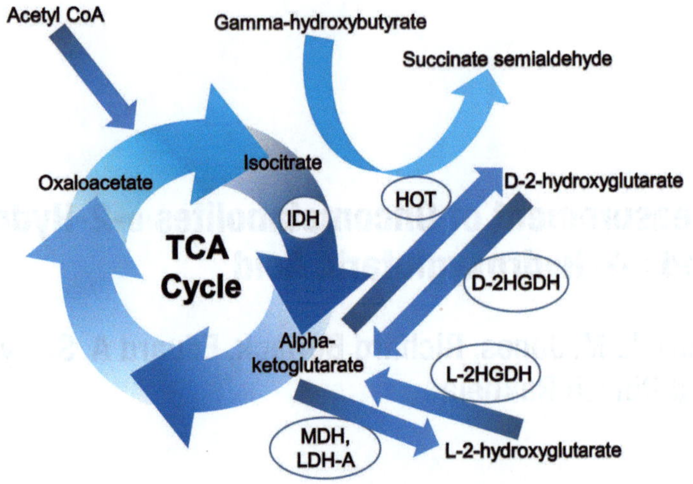

Fig. 1 Metabolic pathway. *TCA* tricarboxylic acid, *IDH* isocitrate dehydrogenase, *HOT* hydroxyacid-oxoacid transhydrogenase, *D2HGDH* D-2-hydroxyglutarate dehydrogenase, *L2HGDH* L-2-hydroxyglutarate dehydrogenase, *MDH* malate dehydrogenase, *LDH-A* lactate dehydrogenase A

formed by the oxidation of 2KG by hydroxyacid-oxoacid transhydrogenase (which simultaneously catalyzes the conversion of γ-hydroxybutyrate to succinate semialdehyde) and converted back to 2KG by D-2-hydroxyglutarate dehydrogenase (D-2HGDH) [9]. An inherited, autosomal recessive, deficiency of D2HGDH, caused by mutations in *D2HGDH*, produces the metabolic disorder D-2-hydroxyglutaric aciduria-1 (OMIM #600721) [9–12]. An inherited, autosomal recessive, deficiency of mitochondrial citrate carrier, caused by mutations in *SLC25A1*, produces the metabolic disorder combined D- and L-2-hydroxyglutaric aciduria (OMIM #615182) [13]. Interestingly, R140 mutations in *IDH2* (that encodes mitochondrial isocitrate dehydrogenase 2 [IDH2]) give rise to the autosomal dominant D-2-hydroxyglutaric aciduria-2 (OMIM #613657) [14]. Somatic R140 or R172 mutations in *IDH2* and R132 mutations in *IDH1* (that encodes cytoplasmic isocitrate dehydrogenase 1 [IDH1]) have been reported in multiple cancers including glioma [15, 16], acute myeloid leukemia [17–20], intrahepatic cholangiocarcinoma [21, 22], and central chondrosarcoma [23]. The mutant IDH1 and IDH2 acquire a new enzymatic activity of reduction of 2KG to D-2HG (in preference to oxidation of isocitrate to 2KG) resulting in high levels of D-2HG in tumors with *IDH* mutations [24–27]. Even before the discovery of somatic *IDH1* and *IDH2* mutations in cancer, there was a known association of L-2-hydroxyglutaric aciduria with brain tumors [28–30]. Recently, increased levels of L-2-hydroxyglutaric acid have been described in renal cell carcinoma [31]. Thus, both

D-2HG and L-2HG are oncometabolites predicted to effect epigenetic changes resulting in hypermethylation phenotype in affected cancer cells [31–36]. In addition, they can serve as sensitive and specific biomarkers for *IDH*-mutated cancers [27, 37–45].

Here, we describe a liquid chromatography-tandem mass spectrometry (LC-MS/MS) assay for measurement of D-2HG and L-2HG [20, 31, 46, 47]. The method is an adaptation of the method by Struys [48, 49]. This method utilizes (+)-Di-*O*-acetyl-L-tartaric anhydride (DATAN), a chiral derivatizing agent, to modify the D- and L-stereoisomers of 2HG, allowing separation and quantification by LC-MS/MS. Deuterated stable-isotope internal standard, D,L-[3,3,4,4-$^{2}H_{4}$)-2-hydroxyglutaric acid, is made from 2-ketopentanedioic acid-[$^{2}H_{6}$] and used in the quantification of the D- and L-2HG. The internal standard is added to the samples which are then vortexed. Plasma and homogenized tissue and cell pellets are extracted (urine requires no extraction), and the extract is dried under a gentle stream of nitrogen. The dried residue is then derivatized with DATAN, dried under nitrogen again, dissolved in water, and injected onto the LC-MS/MS system. The samples are injected onto a C18 column to separate the D- and L-stereoisomers and then introduced into the tandem mass spectrometer where the compounds are identified, and their abundances reported and quantified using a standard curve.

2 Materials

2.1 Samples

1. Serum, anti-coagulated plasma (heparin or EDTA) from peripheral blood or bone marrow, and urine are acceptable.
2. Samples of cell culture media, cultured cells, and tissues are also acceptable.
3. Serum and plasma samples should be centrifuged, separated from the cells, and frozen as soon after collection as possible. All other sample types should be frozen as soon as possible. Samples are stable for 1 year if frozen at <−10 °C. Samples are shipped frozen.

2.2 Native and Stable-Isotope D- and L-2-Hydroxyglutaric Acids

Native D-2HG (Sigma-Aldrich, St. Louis, MO, ≥95.0%) stock solution is made to 10 mmol/L in Optima® LC/MS grade water (Fisher Scientific, Pittsburgh, PA). 1 mmol/L native D-2HG is then made by diluting the 10 mmol/L stock solution in Optima® LC/MS grade water. Both stock solutions are stable for 1 year below −10 °C.

Native L-2HG (Sigma-Aldrich, St. Louis, MO, ≥98.0%) stock solution is made to 10 mmol/L in Optima® LC/MS grade water. 1 mmol/L native L-2HG is made by diluting the 10 mmol/L stock solution in Optima® LC/MS grade water. Both stock solutions are stable for 1 year below −10 °C.

Deuterated stable-isotope mixed D,L-[3,3,4,4-$^2H_4$] internal standard (D,L-IS) is made as follows:

1. 0.12 g of zinc powder (Riedel-de-Haën, Seelze, Germany (Sigma-Aldrich now owns)) is added to 1 mL of ice-cold, Optima® LC/MS grade water in a 16 × 100 mm glass screw cap tube and stirred using a flea (tiny magnetic stirrer) and a magnetic stir plate. The tube is kept on ice with stirring throughout.
2. Completely dissolve 0.15 g of 2-ketopentanedioic acid-[$^2H_6$] (Isotec, now also Sigma-Aldrich) in 0.5 mL of ice-cold, Optima® LC/MS grade water in a second glass screw cap tube. Vortex to ensure completely dissolved.
3. Slowly add the 0.5 mL of dissolved 2-ketopentanedioic acid-[$^2H_6$] to the stirring zinc solution and continue stirring for 30 min after addition is complete.
4. Centrifuge the sample at 750 × *g* for 2 min at room temperature to precipitate the excess zinc.
5. Remove the supernatant with a Pasteur pipette and save in a third glass tube held on ice.
6. Wash the zinc pellet two times with 1 mL ice-cold Optima® LC/MS grade water each time, centrifuging after each wash and combining the supernatants with the original supernatant. The total volume of saved supernatants should be approximately 3.5 mL.
7. Add three volumes (approximately 10.5 mL) of acetone to the saved supernatant mixture to precipitate the D,L-2-hydroxyglutaric acid-[$^2H_4$]-Zn salt. Note: The terminal deuterium ions are lost during this process of converting the keto-groups to OH-groups, resulting in a $^2H_4$ product from the $^2H_6$ starting compound (Fig. 2).

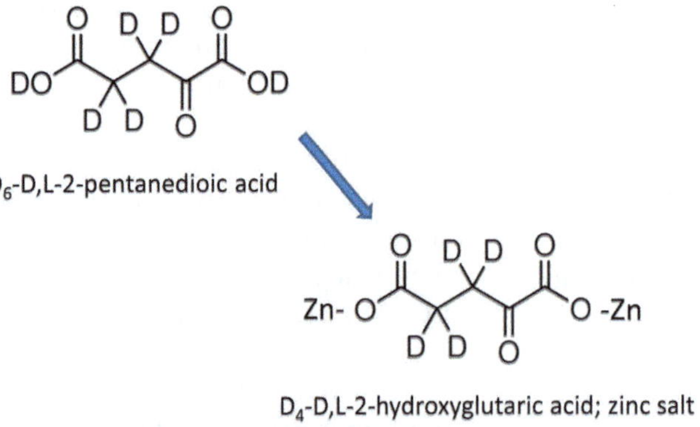

Fig. 2 2-Ketopentandioc acid conversion to 2-hydroxyglutaric acid

8. Centrifuge for 5 min at 2200 × *g*.
9. Remove the supernatant by Pasteur pipette and discard it.
10. Wash the pellet two times with 10 mL acetone each time, resuspending the pellet and then recentrifuging at 2200 × *g* for 5 min each time (*see* **Notes 1** and **2**).
11. Dry the resulting pellet under a very gentle stream of nitrogen, under the chemical hood at room temperature to avoid loss of product, and store below −10 °C until use. The D,L-IS is stable for 1 year below −10 °C (*see* **Note 3**).
12. Reaction yield is approximately 150 mg. Determine reaction success by dissolving 1.5 mg of product into 10 mL reagent grade water (making 1 mmol/L). Transfer 20 μL to a screw cap tube, dry down, and derivatize with DATAN as described in Subheading 3.2. After derivatization, dry down and dissolve in 1 mL Optima® LC/MS grade water. Infuse on the LC-MS/MS along with a previous batch of D,L-IS, monitoring the base ions. First infuse the previous batch of D,L-IS, monitoring the 367.2 and 151.14 base ions in negative mode. Repeat the process with the new batch of D,L-IS and compare the abundances. The 151.14 abundance represents the unreacted 2-ketopentanedioic acid, and the 367.2 abundance represents the DATAN-derivatized D,L-[3,3,4,4,-$^{2}H_{6}$]-2HG (*see* **Note 4**).
13. 10 mM deuterated D,L-IS stock solution is made by weighing 10.9 mg and diluting to 5 mL in Optima® LC/MS grade water. This solution is frozen at ≤−10 °C and is stable for 1 year at this temperature.
14. D,L-IS is used at a concentration of 40 μM. This is made by diluting 40 μL of the 10 mM D,L-IS stock solution into 10 mL of methanol. This solution is stable for 1 year at ≤−10 °C.

2.3 Calibrators and Quality Controls

A five-point calibration curve is run with every assay. The calibrators are made as follows:

1. Label 16 × 100 mm glass screw cap tubes as 1 mM, 100 μM, 10 μM, 1 μM, and 100 nM.
2. For 1 mM add 100 μL of 10 mM L-2HG stock solution and 100 μL of 10 mM D-2HG stock solution to 800 μL of Optima® LC/MS grade water. Vortex and dilute for the other calibrators as follows:
3. For 100 μM, add 100 μL of the 1 mM mixture in Subheading 2.3, **step 2** to 900 μL Optima® LC/MS grade water. Vortex.
4. For 10 μM, add 100 μL of the 100 μM mixture in Subheading 2.3, **step 3** to 900 μL Optima® LC/MS grade water. Vortex.
5. For 1 μM, add 100 μL of the 10 μM mixture in Subheading 2.3, **step 4** to 900 μL Optima® LC/MS grade water. Vortex.

6. For 100 nM, add 100 μL of the 1 μM mixture in Subheading 2.3, **step 5** to 900 μL Optima® LC/MS grade water. Vortex.
7. These calibrators are stable for 2 years if frozen at ≤−10 °C (*see* **Note 5**).
8. Transfer 10 μL of each calibrator into a separate, labeled screw cap tube. Add 25 μL of 40 μM D,L-IS to each tube, mix, and dry down at 37 °C under a gentle stream of nitrogen. The calibrator concentrations correspond to 1481 ng (10 nmol), 148 ng (1 nmol), 14.8 ng (100 pmol), 1.48 ng (10 pmol), and 0.15 ng (1 pmol) L- and D-2HG.
9. Once dried, the calibrators are ready to be derivatized with the rest of the samples as described below.

Two concentrations of controls that are assayed along with clinical patient samples are made from the D-2HG and L-2HG stock solutions as follows:

1. For serum/plasma controls, obtain expired fresh frozen plasma (FFP) from transfusion services.
2. Serum/plasma quality control (QC) level 1 (~19,000 ng/mL L-2HG and ~100 ng/mL D-2HG) (*see* **Notes 6** and 7). To 20 mL of FFP, add 200 μL of 10 mmol/L L-2HG stock solution and 10 μL of 1 mmol/L D-2HG stock solution. Vortex well to mix, aliquot into labeled tubes, and store frozen at ≤−70 °C. Stable for 5 years at ≤−70 °C.
3. Serum/plasma quality control (QC) level 2 (~100 ng/mL L-2HG and ~19,000 ng/mL D-2HG): To 20 mL of FFP, add 10 μL of 1 mmol/L L-2HG stock solution and 200 μL of 10 mmol/L D-2HG stock solution. Vortex well to mix, aliquot into labeled tubes, and store frozen at ≤−70 °C. Stable for 5 years at ≤−70 °C.
4. For each level of control to be analyzed in the run, transfer 100 μL into a separate, labeled 1.5 mL microfuge tube. Treat these QC samples as serum/plasma samples and extract and derivatize with them as described below.

2.4 Extraction and Derivatization Reagents

1. 6.0 M hydrochloric acid (HCl) (Ricca Chemical, Arlington, TX).
2. 0.1 M hydrochloric acid (HCl): Add 0.5 mL of 6.0 M HCl to 29.5 mL Optima® LC/MS grade water. Stable for 1 year at room temperature.
3. Optima® LC/MS grade methanol (Fisher Scientific, Pittsburgh, PA).
4. Methanol/water (80:20): Mix 200 mL of Optima® LC/MS grade methanol with 50 mL of Optima® LC/MS grade water. Stable for 1 year at room temperature.

5. Methylene chloride (Optima® grade, Fisher Scientific).
6. Acetic acid, J. T. Baker (VWR International, Radnor, PA).
7. Formic acid, Fluka (Sigma-Aldrich, St. Louis, MO).
8. 10 M ammonium formate (Sigma-Aldrich, St. Louis, MO).
9. Oasis HLB solid phase extraction (SPE) reverse phase columns (Waters Corp. Milford, MA).
10. Derivatizing agent: DATAN ((+)-Di-*O*-acetyl-L-tartaric anhydride) (Sigma-Aldrich, St. Louis, MO) 20 mg/mL in methylene chloride/acetic acid (80:20). This is made under a hood immediately before use. Only as much as is needed to derivatize the current set of samples in the run is made. DATAN is weighed on an analytical balance and placed into a 16 × 100 mm glass screw cap tube, into which methylene chloride and acetic acid is added as shown below:

Number of samples	Methylene chloride (μL)	Acetic acid (μL)	DATAN (mg)
1–15	800	200	20
16–35	1600	400	40
36–55	2400	600	60

If exactly 20, 40, or 60 mg of DATAN is not weighed, the amount of methylene chloride and acetic acid to be used can be calculated using the following formulas:

mg of DATAN weighed ÷ 20 × 800 = μL of methylene chloride to add.

mg of DATAN weighed ÷ 20 × 200 = μL of acetic acid to add.

2.5 Liquid Chromatography Buffers

1. Buffer A: 125 mg/L ammonium formate, pH 3.6. Dilute 400 μL of 10 M ammonium formate in 2 L Optima® LC/MS grade water. Adjust pH to 3.6 using concentrated formic acid and a pH meter. Stable for 2 weeks at room temperature.
2. Buffer B: Acetonitrile (Optima® LC/MS grade, Fisher Scientific). Stable for 3 months at room temperature.

2.6 Cell Culture Media

1. Dulbecco's Modified Eagle Medium (DMEM) (Gibco/BRL, Bethesda, MD) is used for all cell culture with 10% fetal bovine serum (FBS) (Gibco/BRL, Bethesda, MD) added.

3 Methods

The method is calibrated, and the linearity, precision, and lower limit of detection are established using the prepared native stock solutions. The assay is linear from 1.5 to 15,000 ng/mL and has a lower limit of detection of 1.5 ng/mL. Precision ranged from 1 to 31% across the range of concentrations (*see* **Notes 8** and **9**). Once validated, the assay can be used for testing various sample types including serum, plasma, urine, tissue, cultured cells, and culture media from cell culture.

Clinical patient samples of serum or plasma are pipetted into test tubes, into which is added internal standard and methanol/water (80:20) for extraction of the D,L-2HG. After extraction, the samples are centrifuged and dried down under nitrogen and then derivatized with DATAN. The derivatized samples are dried down under nitrogen again and then diluted in water, centrifuged, and transferred to autosampler vials to be run on the LC-MS/MS.

The LC-MS/MS method separates the D- and L-2HG isomers on a C18 column in a 30-min run using a slight gradient of 125 mg/L ammonium formate and acetonitrile. After separation on the column, the sample is introduced into the tandem MS using electrospray ionization, and transitions are monitored at m/z – 363.2 → m/z – 147.1 and m/z – 367.2 → m/z – 151.1 for the native 2HGs and the stable-isotope standard, respectively. Quantification is done using the abundances of the product ions of the transitions. The amount of native D- or L-2HG is calculated using a standard curve which is assayed with each run. The ratio of native to isotope abundances are calculated and then plotted against the standard to isotope concentration to create the standard curve. In the patient samples, the ratio of native abundance to isotope abundance is calculated and the 2HG concentration is derived from the standard curve equation.

3.1 Sample Extraction

3.1.1 Serum/Plasma Extraction

1. Pipette 100 μL of each serum, plasma, or QC sample into an appropriately labeled, 1.5 mL polypropylene microfuge tube.
2. Add 25 μL of 40 μmol/L D,L-IS to each tube.
3. Add 1 mL methanol/water (80:20) which has been precooled in the −80 °C freezer to each tube.
4. Cap tightly and vortex vigorously for 30 s.
5. Incubate the tubes in the −80 °C freezer for 30 min.
6. Remove tubes from freezer and centrifuge on high (16,100 × *g*) for 5 min in the microfuge at room temperature.
7. Transfer 500 μL of the supernatant from each tube to its respective, properly labeled 16 × 100 mm glass screw cap tube.
8. Dry samples down at 37 °C under a gentle stream of nitrogen.
9. Derivatize samples with DATAN as described in Subheading 3.2.

3.1.2 Urine Extraction

1. Pipette 20 μL of each duplicate urine sample into an appropriately labeled, 16 × 100 mm glass screw cap tube.
2. Add 25 μL of 40 μmol/L D,L-IS to each tube.
3. Vortex vigorously for 30 s.
4. Dry samples down at 37 °C under a gentle stream of nitrogen.
5. Derivatize samples with DATAN as described in Subheading 3.2.

3.1.3 Tissue or Cell Culture Pellet Extraction

1. Prepare a cell culture pellet by centrifuging 2×10^6 to 10×10^6 cultured cells at 500 × *g* for 7 min at room temperature. Carefully aspirate off the medium or buffer.
2. The cell pellet or 50 mg of frozen tissue is placed into an appropriately labeled, 50 mL polypropylene conical centrifuge tube.
3. Add 25 μL of 40 μmol/L D,L-IS to each tube.
4. Add 1 mL methanol/water (80:20) which has been precooled on ice.
5. Homogenize the sample on ice for 30 s using the appropriate plastic omni tip (Omni International, Kennesaw, GA). Alternatively, the tissue may be sonicated on ice.
6. Incubate samples in the −80 °C freezer for 30 min.
7. Two 5 μL aliquots of each homogenate are transferred to labeled 1.5 mL microfuge tubes and dried by placing open under the hood for 30–60 min until dry. These are used to determine protein concentration as previously described [50].
8. The remaining homogenates are each transferred to labeled 1.5 mL microfuge tubes and centrifuged at 16,100 × *g* for 5 min in a microfuge at room temperature.
9. Transfer 500 μL of the supernatant from each tube to its respective, properly labeled 16 × 100 mm glass screw cap tube.
10. Dry samples down at 37 °C under a gentle stream of nitrogen.
11. Derivatize samples with DATAN as described in Subheading 3.2.

3.1.4 Cell Culture/Cell Culture Medium Extraction

1. Oasis HLB columns are conditioned by placing a column for each sample in a labeled 16 × 125 mm glass tube. A 750 μL of Optima® LC/MS grade methanol is added to each column and let drain through. A 750 μL of 0.1 M HCl is then added and let drain through.
2. Pipette 1 mL of each media sample into a labeled 1.5 mL microfuge tube and acidify to a pH of <1 by adding 30 μL of 6 M HCl.

3. Add 25 μL of 40 μM D,L-IS to each sample and vortex for 30 s.
4. Using a transfer pipette, transfer each sample onto its appropriately labeled, conditioned column.
5. After the samples drain through the columns, wash the columns with 750 μL of 0.1 M HCl.
6. Let drain and then make sure all wash fluid is through the column by applying pressure to the column with a pipette bulb or by applying a vacuum using a manifold.
7. Transfer the columns to a second, clean, labeled 16 × 100 mm glass tube.
8. Elute the samples from the columns by adding 850 μL of Optima® LC/MS grade methanol to each column.
9. Dry samples down at 37 °C under a gentle stream of nitrogen.
10. Derivatize samples with DATAN as described in Subheading 3.2.

3.2 Sample Derivatization

1. Pipette 50 μL of DATAN solution, prepared as described in Subheading 2.4, **step 10**, into each tube to be derivatized, including calibrators, controls, and samples.
2. Cap each tube and heat to 75 °C for 30 min in a heat block to derivatize samples.
3. Cool tubes to room temperature and dry down under a gentle stream of nitrogen.
4. Add 0.5 mL of Optima® LC/MS grade water to each sample residue and vortex to dissolve.
5. Transfer all samples to labeled microfuge tubes and centrifuge in the microfuge for 5 min at 16,100 × *g*.
6. Transfer all samples to labeled autosampler vials and cap (*see* **Note 10**).
7. Transfer vials to the Perkin-Elmer autosampler and analyze via LC-MS/MS.

3.3 LC-MS/MS Analysis

1. Perform liquid chromatography-tandem mass spectrometry analysis using C18 reverse phase separation for the liquid chromatography and multiple reaction monitoring (MRM) in the tandem mass spectrometer at the specified transitions.
2. Prior to analyzing samples, perform the following functions: (a) Turn on the Turbo Ionspray Gas to 7000–7500 mL/min. (b) Equilibrate the column for at least ten column volumes (*see* **Note 11**).
3. The LC-MS/MS method uses the Perkin-Elmer autosampler to inject 20 μL of sample onto the 150 × 3.9 mm (i.d.) C18 column with a 5 μm bead size, at a flow rate of 0.5 mL/min.

The 2HG isomers are separated on the column utilizing a mobile phase gradient that starts at 100% buffer A and drops to 96.5% buffer A and 3.5% buffer B at 3.5 min. This is held for 20 min and then ramps back to 100% buffer A by 23 min, followed by a 7-min re-equilibration at 100% buffer A. This results in a 30-min run time. After passing through the column, half of the column eluent is diverted to waste before the sample is introduced directly into the AB Sciex-3000 tandem MS via an electrospray ionization nebulizer and analyzed in the tandem mass spectrometer.

4. The MS/MS-run parameters for this method are given in Table 1.

5. After the analysis is finished, quantification of the results is performed. Each sample file is examined to ensure that the instrument has properly identified the peaks. L-2HG is always the first peak and D-2HG is the second peak. The quantification transition for both isomers is m/z – 363.2 > m/z – 147.1 and the qualifier transition is m/z – 363.2 > m/z – 129.1. The quantifier transition for the internal standard is m/z – 367.2 > m/z – 151.1 and a qualifier is not used. All three transition peaks must be present in order for the sample to be quantitated. Figure 3 depicts a chromatograph with elevated concentrations of D-2-hydroxyglutaric acid and normal concentrations of L-2-hydroxyglutaric acid.

The concentration calculations are performed as follows: Calibrator concentrations/IS concentrations are graphed on the x-axis.

Table 1
AB Sciex-3000 instrument parameters

Parameter	Setting
Nebulizer gas (NEB)	4
Curtain gas (CUR)	10
Collision gas (CAD)	4
IonSpray voltage (IS)	–4500 V
Temperature (TEM)	500 °C
Declustering potential (DP)	–22
Focusing potential (FP)	–115
Entrance potential (EP)	–11
Collision energy (CE)	–15 (147.1, 151.05); –34 (129.1)
Collision cell exit potential (CXP)	–10

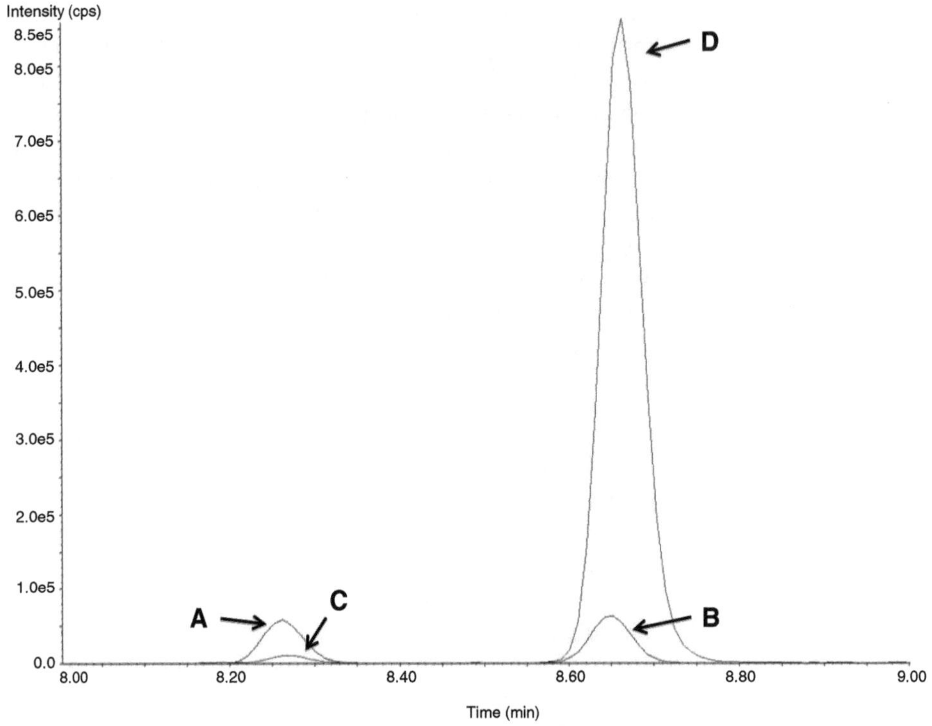

Fig. 3 Representative chromatograph demonstrating elevated D-2-hydroxyglutaric acid. *A* = [D4]-L-2-hydroxyglutaric acid internal standard, *B* = [D4]-D-2-hydroxyglutaric acid internal standard, *C* = L-2-hydroxyglutaric acid, *D* = D-2-hydroxyglutaric acid

Calibrator abundance counts/IS abundance counts are graphed on the *y*-axis; the equation for the resulting line is used by the instrument software to calculate the concentrations of the QCs and samples. The results are divided by the sample volume in mL (0.1) to give 2HG results in ng/mL. Finally, results are reported as numerical data for L-2HG, D-2HG, total 2HG, and the ratio of D,/L-2HG, with the appropriate reference intervals and accompanied by an interpretive comment as shown in Table 2 (*see* **Note 12**).

4 Notes

1. Sonication (VirSonic 50, VirTis Co., Inc., Gardiner, NY) at setting 5 (using a microprobe) for 10–20 s facilitates resuspending the pellet.
2. Discard the acetone washes by evaporating under a hood.
3. All evaporations and dry-down steps must be done under a chemical fume hood.

Table 2
Reference intervals and interpretations for human peripheral blood plasma and bone marrow plasma samples

Reference intervals	
L-2HG	6–147 ng/mL
D-2HG	18–263 ng/mL
Total 2HG	24–410 ng/mL
Ratio D-/L-2HG	0.2–3.8

Result	Interpretation
L-, D-, and total 2HG fall within reference intervals	Normal concentrations of L- and D-2-hydroxyglutarate
L-2HG and total 2HG are elevated; D-2HG is normal. Ratio is low	Markedly increased levels of L-2-hydroxyglutarate suggestive of mutations in L2HGDH (L-2-hydroxyglutarate dehydrogenase)
L-2HG is normal. D-2HG, total 2HG, and ratio are elevated	Markedly increased levels of D-2-hydroxyglutarate suggestive of mutations in IDH1 (isocitrate dehydrogenase 1), IDH2 (isocitrate dehydrogenase 2), or D2HGDH (D-2-hydroxyglutarate dehydrogenase)
Other combinations	Free text interpretation

4. While the contaminating substance will not affect the assay or results, it will cause the weighed concentration of IS to be less than expected when diluted. Additionally, one can compare the abundances of the m/z – 367.2 and m/z – 363.2 base ions and the m/z – 367.2 > m/z – 151.1 and 363.2 > m/z – 147.1 transitions in MRM mode. This will tell you if your DATAN derivatization went to completion. If the reaction is incomplete, more DATAN, higher derivatization temperatures, and/or longer derivatization times may be employed.
5. If using pre-prepared calibrators that have been frozen, bring them to room temperature prior to use.
6. The concentrations are approximate because they are the theoretical concentrations the controls are made to be. Actual measured concentrations are determined by repeated assays.
7. The concentrations for both QCs were chosen because the high values are close to the highest plasma values normally

seen in affected individuals. The low values are both in the normal range.

8. Linearity and lower limit of detection were determined by repeatedly assaying calibration curves using the calibration standards as described above. The ratio of native to isotopic compound abundance was obtained for each calibrator, and the ratios were then plotted against ratio of the known native to the known isotope concentration (ng). It was determined that best linearity was achieved between 1.5 and 15,000 ng/mL, with 1.5 ng/mL being the lowest concentration that could be reliably reproduced.
9. Precisions were determined from repeated analyses at the bottom, middle, and top of the range, and coefficient of variation (CV) was found to range from 0.8 to 31% across the range, with CVs between 0.8 and 1.0% at the high end of the range and CVs of 26–31% at the low end of the concentration range.
10. At this point, the samples are stable for 2 weeks or more if stored in the refrigerator.
11. This equilibration is roughly 70 min which is most easily accomplished by equilibrating for 10 min with buffer A and then running two 30 min water blanks at the start of the run.
12. Total 2HG is calculated by adding L-2HG and D-2HG together. The ratio is calculated by dividing D-2HG results by L-2HG results.

References

1. Struys EA, Verhoeven NM, Jansen EE et al (2006) Metabolism of gamma-hydroxybutyrate to d-2-hydroxyglutarate in mammals: further evidence for d-2-hydroxyglutarate transhydrogenase. Metabolism 55:353–358
2. Struys EA, Verhoeven NM, Ten Brink HJ et al (2005) Kinetic characterization of human hydroxyacid-oxoacid transhydrogenase: relevance to D-2-hydroxyglutaric and gamma-hydroxybutyric acidurias. J Inherit Metab Dis 28:921–930
3. Van Schaftingen E, Rzem R, Veiga-da-Cunha M (2009) L-2-Hydroxyglutaric aciduria, a disorder of metabolite repair. J Inherit Metab Dis 32:135–142
4. Intlekofer AM, Dematteo RG, Venneti S et al (2015) Hypoxia induces production of L-2-Hydroxyglutarate. Cell Metab 22:304–311
5. Oldham WM, Clish CB, Yang Y et al (2015) Hypoxia-mediated increases in L-2-hydroxyglutarate coordinate the metabolic response to reductive stress. Cell Metab 22:291–303
6. Steenweg ME, Jakobs C, Errami A et al (2010) An overview of L-2-hydroxyglutarate dehydrogenase gene (L2HGDH) variants: a genotype-phenotype study. Hum Mutat 31:380–390
7. Topcu M, Jobard F, Halliez S et al (2004) L-2-Hydroxyglutaric aciduria: identification of a mutant gene C14orf160, localized on chromosome 14q22.1. Hum Mol Genet 13:2803–2811
8. Rzem R, Veiga-da-Cunha M, Noel G et al (2004) A gene encoding a putative FAD-dependent L-2-hydroxyglutarate dehydrogenase is mutated in L-2-hydroxyglutaric aciduria. Proc Natl Acad Sci U S A 101:16849–16854
9. Struys EA (2006) D-2-Hydroxyglutaric aciduria: Unravelling the biochemical pathway and the genetic defect. J Inherit Metab Dis 29:21–29
10. Kranendijk M, Struys EA, Gibson KM et al (2009) Evidence for genetic heterogeneity in D-2-hydroxyglutaric aciduria. Hum Mutat 31:279–283

11. Struys EA, Korman SH, Salomons GS et al (2005) Mutations in phenotypically mild D-2-hydroxyglutaric aciduria. Ann Neurol 58:626–630
12. Struys EA, Salomons GS, Achouri Y et al (2005) Mutations in the D-2-hydroxyglutarate dehydrogenase gene cause D-2-hydroxyglutaric aciduria. Am J Hum Genet 76:358–360
13. Nota B, Struys EA, Pop A et al (2013) Deficiency in SLC25A1, encoding the mitochondrial citrate carrier, causes combined D-2- and L-2-hydroxyglutaric aciduria. Am J Hum Genet 92:627–631
14. Kranendijk M, Struys EA, van Schaftingen E et al (2010) IDH2 mutations in patients with D-2-hydroxyglutaric aciduria. Science 330:336
15. Parsons DW, Jones S, Zhang X et al (2008) An integrated genomic analysis of human glioblastoma multiforme. Science 321:1807–1812
16. Yan H, Parsons DW, Jin G et al (2009) IDH1 and IDH2 mutations in gliomas. N Engl J Med 360:765–773
17. Mardis ER, Ding L, Dooling DJ et al (2009) Recurring mutations found by sequencing an acute myeloid leukemia genome. N Engl J Med 361:1058–1066
18. Thol F, Damm F, Wagner K et al (2010) Prognostic impact of IDH2 mutations in cytogenetically normal acute myeloid leukemia. Blood 116:614–616
19. Abbas S, Lugthart S, Kavelaars FG et al (2010) Acquired mutations in the genes encoding IDH1 and IDH2 both are recurrent aberrations in acute myeloid leukemia: prevalence and prognostic value. Blood 116:2122–2126
20. Rakheja D, Konoplev S, Su M et al (2011) High incidence of IDH mutations in acute myeloid leukaemia with cuplike nuclei. Br J Haematol 155:125–128
21. Borger DR, Tanabe KK, Fan KC et al (2012) Frequent mutation of isocitrate dehydrogenase (IDH)1 and IDH2 in cholangiocarcinoma identified through broad-based tumor genotyping. Oncologist 17:72–79
22. Wang P, Dong Q, Zhang C et al (2013) Mutations in isocitrate dehydrogenase 1 and 2 occur frequently in intrahepatic cholangiocarcinomas and share hypermethylation targets with glioblastomas. Oncogene 32:3091–3100
23. Amary MF, Bacsi K, Maggiani F et al (2011) IDH1 and IDH2 mutations are frequent events in central chondrosarcoma and central and periosteal chondromas but not in other mesenchymal tumours. J Pathol 224:334–343
24. Gross S, Cairns RA, Minden MD et al (2010) Cancer-associated metabolite 2-hydroxyglutarate accumulates in acute myelogenous leukemia with isocitrate dehydrogenase 1 and 2 mutations. J Exp Med 207:339–344
25. Dang L, White DW, Gross S et al (2009) Cancer-associated IDH1 mutations produce 2-hydroxyglutarate. Nature 462:739–744
26. Ward PS, Patel J, Wise DR et al (2010) The common feature of leukemia-associated IDH1 and IDH2 mutations is a neomorphic enzyme activity converting alpha-ketoglutarate to 2-hydroxyglutarate. Cancer Cell 17:225–234
27. Choi C, Ganji SK, DeBerardinis RJ et al (2012) 2-hydroxyglutarate detection by magnetic resonance spectroscopy in IDH-mutated patients with gliomas. Nat Med 18:624–629
28. Moroni I, Bugiani M, D'Incerti L et al (2004) L-2-hydroxyglutaric aciduria and brain malignant tumors: a predisposing condition? Neurology 62:1882–1884
29. Ozisik PA, Akalan N, Palaoglu S et al (2002) Medulloblastoma in a child with the metabolic disease L-2-hydroxyglutaric aciduria. Pediatr Neurosurg 37:22–26
30. Haliloglu G, Jobard F, Oguz KK et al (2008) L-2-hydroxyglutaric aciduria and brain tumors in children with mutations in the L2HGDH gene: neuroimaging findings. Neuropediatrics 39:119–122
31. Shim EH, Livi CB, Rakheja D et al (2014) L-2-Hydroxyglutarate: an epigenetic modifier and putative oncometabolite in renal cancer. Cancer Discov 4:1290–1298
32. Flavahan WA, Drier Y, Liau BB et al (2016) Insulator dysfunction and oncogene activation in IDH mutant gliomas. Nature 529:10–114
33. Rakheja D, Medeiros LJ, Bevan S et al (2013) The emerging role of d-2-hydroxyglutarate as an oncometabolite in hematolymphoid and central nervous system neoplasms. Front Oncol 3:169
34. Figueroa ME, Abdel-Wahab O, Lu C et al (2010) Leukemic IDH1 and IDH2 mutations result in a hypermethylation phenotype, disrupt TET2 function, and impair hematopoietic differentiation. Cancer Cell 18:553–567
35. Xu W, Yang H, Liu Y et al (2011) Oncometabolite 2-hydroxyglutarate is a competitive inhibitor of alpha-ketoglutarate-dependent dioxygenases. Cancer Cell 19:17–30
36. Chowdhury R, Yeoh KK, Tian YM et al (2011) The oncometabolite 2-hydroxyglutarate inhibits histone lysine demethylases. EMBO Rep 12:463–469
37. DiNardo CD, Propert KJ, Loren AW et al (2013) Serum 2-hydroxyglutarate levels predict isocitrate dehydrogenase mutations and clinical outcome in acute myeloid leukemia. Blood 121:4917–4924

38. Borger DR, Goyal L, Yau T et al (2014) Circulating oncometabolite 2-hydroxyglutarate is a potential surrogate biomarker in patients with isocitrate dehydrogenase-mutant intrahepatic cholangiocarcinoma. Clin Cancer Res 20:1884–1890
39. Pollyea DA, Kohrt HE, Zhang B et al (2013) 2-Hydroxyglutarate in IDH mutant acute myeloid leukemia: predicting patient responses, minimal residual disease and correlations with methylcytosine and hydroxymethylcytosine levels. Leuk Lymphoma 54:408–410
40. Natsumeda M, Igarashi H, Nomura T et al (2014) Accumulation of 2-hydroxyglutarate in gliomas correlates with survival: a study by 3.0-tesla magnetic resonance spectroscopy. Acta Neuropathol Commun 2(158):2014
41. Andronesi OC, Kim GS, Gerstner E et al (2012) Detection of 2-hydroxyglutarate in IDH-mutated glioma patients by in vivo spectral-editing and 2D correlation magnetic resonance spectroscopy. Sci Transl Med 4:116ra114
42. Janin M, Mylonas E, Saada V et al (2014) Serum 2-hydroxyglutarate production in IDH1- and IDH2-mutated de novo acute myeloid leukemia: a study by the acute leukemia French association group. J Clin Oncol 32:297–305
43. Sellner L, Capper D, Meyer J et al (2010) Increased levels of 2-hydroxyglutarate in AML patients with IDH1-R132H and IDH2-R140Q mutations. Eur J Haematol 85:457–459
44. Kalinina J, Carroll A, Wang L et al (2012) Detection of "oncometabolite" 2-hydroxyglutarate by magnetic resonance analysis as a biomarker of IDH1/2 mutations in glioma. J Mol Med (Berl) 90:1161–1171
45. McGehee E, Rakheja D, Oliver D et al (2016) The importance of plasma D-2HG measurement in screening for IDH mutations in acute myeloid leukaemia. Br J Haematol 173: 323–326
46. Rakheja D, Boriack RL, Mitui M et al (2011) Papillary thyroid carcinoma shows elevated levels of 2-hydroxyglutarate. Tumour Biol 32:325–323
47. Rakheja D, Mitui M, Boriack RL et al (2011) Isocitrate dehydrogenase 1/2 mutational analyses and 2-hydroxyglutarate measurements in Wilms tumors. Pediatr Blood Cancer 56: 379–383
48. Struys EA, Jansen EE, Verhoeven NM et al (2004) Measurement of urinary D- and L-2-hydroxyglutarate enantiomers by stable-isotope-dilution liquid chromatography-tandem mass spectrometry after derivatization with diacetyl-L-tartaric anhydride. Clin Chem 50: 1391–1395
49. Struys EA, Verhoeven NM, Roos B et al (2003) Disease-related metabolites in culture medium of fibroblasts from patients with D-2-hydroxyglutaric aciduria, L-2-hydroxyglutaric aciduria, and combined D/L-2-hydroxyglutaric aciduria. Clin Chem 49:1133–1138
50. Lowry OH, Rosebrough NJ, Farr AL et al (1951) Protein measurement with the Folin phenol reagent. J Biol Chem 193:265–275

Chapter 15

Nanofluidic Allele-Specific Digital PCR Method for Quantifying IDH1 and IDH2 Mutation Burden in Acute Myeloid Leukemia

Daniel H. Wiseman and Tim C.P. Somervaille

Abstract

Precise quantitation of allelic burden for a pathogenic mutation has diverse clinical and research applications but can be difficult to achieve with conventional qPCR-based techniques, especially at lower mutant allele frequencies. Digital PCR overcomes many of the limitations of qPCR and can be highly quantitative even for single-nucleotide variants, with distinct advantages over next-generation sequencing approaches. Here we describe a method combining the principles of TaqMan®-chemistry SNP genotyping with microfluidic digital PCR to generate a highly sensitive, quantitative allele-specific digital PCR assay for the six most common IDH1 and IDH2 mutations encountered in myeloid malignancy. The concept and approach could easily be applied to other suitable SNVs.

Key words Digital PCR, Allelic discrimination, Mutant allele frequency, Acute myeloid leukemia, Isocitrate dehydrogenase

1 Introduction

The metabolic enzymes IDH1 and IDH2 are each mutated in ~10% of patients with acute myeloid leukemia (AML) [1]. Virtually all are single-nucleotide variants (SNVs) involving the arginine hotspots R132 in IDH1 or R140 or R172 in IDH2. Sanger sequencing remains the gold-standard method for detection but is nonquantitative and has limited sensitivity (~10–15%) for the variant allele. The ability to sensitively quantify mutant allele frequency (MAF) in AML can have diverse clinical and research applications. For example, the allelic burden of some mutations may be prognostic [2], and others are validated markers of minimal residual disease (MRD) [3]. Quantitation further enables the researcher to track individual mutations longitudinally and to study the subclonal architecture of malignancy.

Paolo Fortina et al. (eds.), *Acute Myeloid Leukemia: Methods and Protocols*, Methods in Molecular Biology, vol. 1633, DOI 10.1007/978-1-4939-7142-8_15,

Whereas qPCR has high sensitivity for oncogenic fusions and NPM1 (four base pair) insertional mutations [4], designing qPCR assays to quantitate SNVs against a backdrop of wild-type DNA is more challenging. Such assays tend to have lower specificity because, for any mix of wild-type and mutant DNA, the alternate (i.e., majority wild type) sequence will usually also be detected, albeit at much lower (~5%) detection efficiency than for the variant sequence [5]. Various allele-specific qPCR methods for quantifying SNVs have been developed based on the amplification refractory mutation system (ARMS-) or mismatch amplification mutation assay (MAMA-) PCR techniques. Such assays pool distinct primers, specific for each allele, in which the 3′ terminal nucleotide of either forward or reverse primer perfectly matches either the variant or reference base. Typically an additional mismatch is included within 3 bases of the 3′ end to further reduce efficiency for the non-desired allele, and a host of other modifications has been reported to further enhance specificity for the mutant allele by this approach (reviewed in [6]). However, no gold-standard method has emerged, and restrictive design criteria for primer/probe location render some templates unsuitable. Moreover, any conventional qPCR-based approach relies on standard curves for absolute quantitation and is influenced by the exponential amplification kinetics of the PCR. These are potential sources of variability or inaccuracy when quantifying rare targets.

By contrast, digital PCR (dPCR) circumvents several limitations of qPCR and is uniquely suited to quantitation of rare SNVs against a complex DNA background [7]. Conceptually, it relies on the random distribution of DNA molecules in solution. With extensive partitioning and sufficient limiting dilution such that some partitions contain no template, single DNA molecules can be PCR amplified simultaneously in parallel and the products of each individual reaction detected. Enumeration of partitions containing a positive reaction thus provides a binary, absolute, and linear quantitation of target in the whole sample, across a wide dynamic range and without the need for standard curves (Fig. 1) [8]. A Poisson correction compensates for the likelihood that some partitions will contain >1 copy of template [9], extending the dynamic range beyond the total number of partitions [10]. This approach effectively dilutes out background signal and increases the signal-to-noise ratio of low-abundance targets. dPCR thus has the capacity to be precise, reproducible, sensitive for rare variants, and tolerant of inhibitors or suboptimal amplification efficiency [7]. Current dPCR platforms achieve partitioning either by distributing sample into individual chambers of nanofluidic chips or through formation of emulsion droplets containing individual DNA templates. Each platform has advantages and disadvantages: for example, droplet dPCR affords greater partitioning capability, while nanofluidic chips provide consistent sensitivity and capacity to monitor and review real-time amplification data for each individual

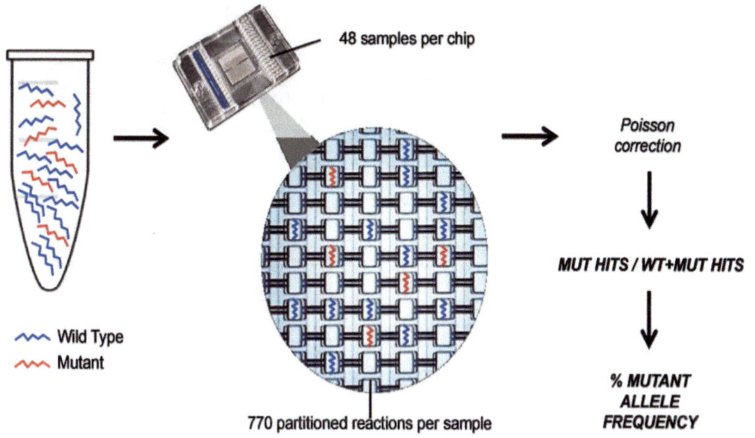

Fig. 1 Nanofluidic digital PCR technique for determining mutant allele frequency using Fluidigm 37K IFC chips

reaction. However, in general there is impressive concordance between the two formats [11].

Here we describe quantitative, allele-specific, nanofluidic dPCR assays for six common IDH1 and IDH2 mutations (IDH1 R132C/R132G/R132H/R132S; IDH2 R140Q; IDH2 R172K) [12]. The method could be easily applied to other SNVs or short indels. Allelic discrimination is achieved within each partition using TaqMan®-based SNP genotyping [13, 14]. Custom-designed assays pool common forward and reverse primers flanking the region containing each SNV, and two minor groove-binding (MGB) probes specific for either wild-type or mutant allele. Probes are 5′-linked to spectrally distinct fluorescent dyes (FAM™ or VIC®) and 3′-linked to a nonfluorescent quencher that suppresses background fluorescence. As polymerase extends along the template strand during each PCR cycle, it cleaves any hybridized probe, separating dye from quencher and emitting fluorescence. The endpoint respective change in fluorescence for each dye indicates the presence of either or both alleles, albeit in a nonquantitative manner (Fig. 2). In the dPCR context, however, the relative proportion of mutant to wild-type DNA can be precisely determined, with high reproducibility and sensitivity to ≤0.1% MAF [12].

2 Materials

2.1 Equipment

1. Fluidigm qdPCR 37K™ integrated fluidic circuit (IFC) chip(s) (Fluidigm). Each chip contains wells for 48 samples each linked by nanofluidic circuitry to 770 separate reaction chambers within which separate real-time PCR amplifications occur. One chip can therefore perform 36,960 separate PCRs (Fig. 3). Store at room temperature.

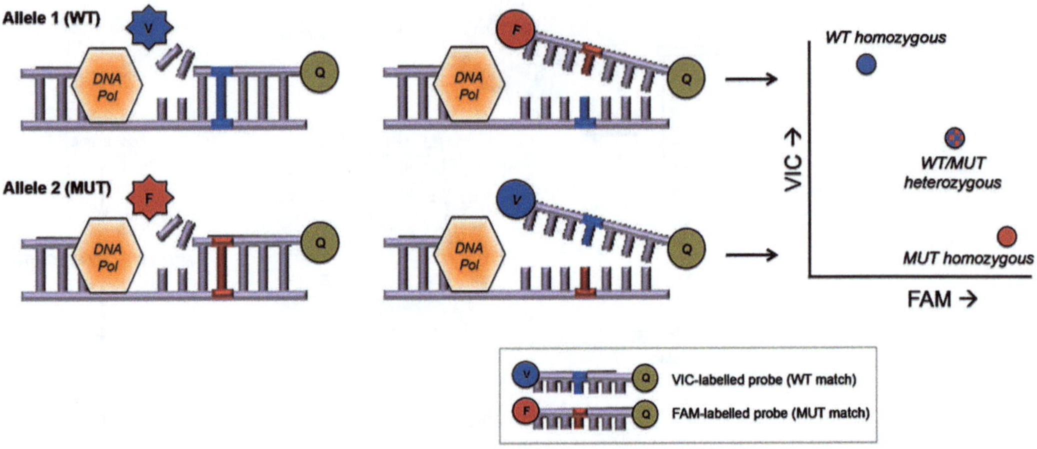

Fig. 2 Allelic discrimination PCR using TaqMan® SNP genotyping assays. *DNA pol* DNA polymerase, *V* VIC® dye, *F* FAM™ dye, *Q* nonfluorescent quencher

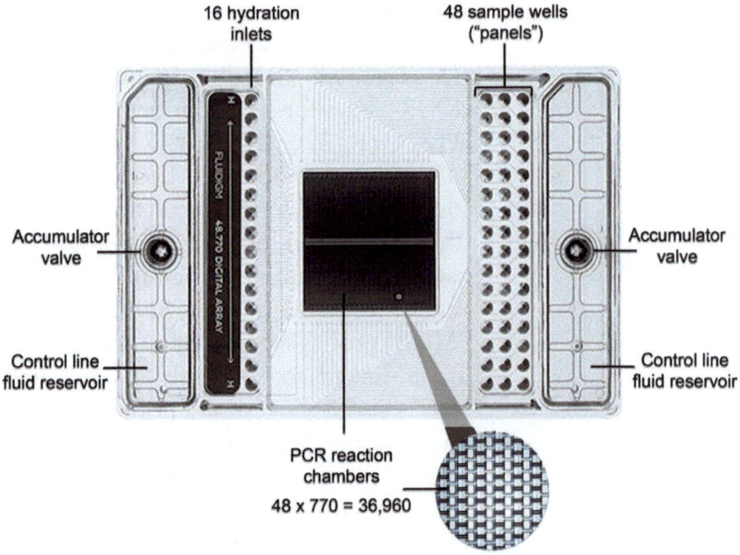

Fig. 3 The Fluidigm 37K™ integrated fluidic circuit chip for digital PCR. The chip consists of 48 panel inlet wells through each of which sample reaction mixes is pressure loaded into 770 chamber partitions

2. IFC Controller Module MX (Fluidigm; *see* **Note 1**). This instrument is required for priming and loading the IFC chip microfluidics. It employs pneumatic pressure to meter samples and reagents and to control valves within the IFC.
3. Biomark™ HD thermal cycler (Fluidigm; *see* **Note 1**).
4. "48.48" prefilled syringes with control line fluid (300 μL) (Fluidigm, Cat #89000020). Store at room temperature.
5. NanoDrop 2000 spectrophotometer.

6. (Optional) Agilent® 2100 Bioanalyzer.
7. Centrifuge suitable for 96-well PCR microplates.
8. Single-channel pipettes (P2; P10; P20; P200).
9. 8-channel pipette (P10).
10. Microcentrifuge tubes (1.5 mL).
11. 25G sterile hypodermic needles.
12. Pressure-sensitive adhesive tape.

2.2 Reagents

1. Genomic DNA. DNA can be extracted with any commercially available kit. We recommend QIAamp® DNA mini (Qiagen). For very low DNA concentrations, a pre-amplification step may be necessary (*see* **Note 2**). Genomic DNA is stored in microcentrifuge tubes or 96-well plates at −20 °C.
2. 20× TaqMan® SNP genotyping assay(s) (Thermo Fisher Scientific; *see* Subheading 3.1). Store aliquots at −20 °C.
3. 20× GE Sample Loading Reagent (Fluidigm, Cat #85000746). Store at −20 °C.
4. 2× TaqMan® Gene Expression Mastermix (Life Technologies, Cat #4369016; *see* **Note 3**). Store at 4 °C.
5. Deionized molecular grade water.

2.3 Software

1. Biomark™ Software Package v4.2.2 (Fluidigm), including:
   - Biomark Data Collection software.
   - Digital PCR Analysis software.
2. Preferred spreadsheet software capable of opening and editing .csv files (e.g., Microsoft Excel (Microsoft))

3 Methods

This method describes dPCR using Fluidigm's suite of nanofluidic chips, modules, and Biomark™ HD thermal cycler. For further method and troubleshooting, consult Digital PCR Analysis User Guide (Fluidigm; PN 68000100; available for download at https://www.fluidigm.com/documents). As with any PCR-based technique, adherence to best practice and avoidance of contamination is critical. Preparation of reaction mixes should be performed in a DNA-free hood in a dedicated PCR pre-amplification area, using a separate sterile tube for each IFC to be loaded. All procedures should be carried out at room temperature unless otherwise stated.

3.1 TaqMan® Assay Purchase, Design, and Validation

Discrimination between wild-type and mutant allele for each individual reaction chamber within the dPCR chip is achieved using allelic discrimination PCR (AD-PCR) with TaqMan® SNP genotyping assays. Large libraries of predesigned, validated assays for recognized SNPs are commercially available from Thermo Fisher Scientific in various formats. Assays comprise pooled:

- Unlabeled forward and reverse PCR primers (900 nM final concentration).
- Single VIC®-MGB-labeled probe detecting the wild-type sequence.
- Single FAM™-MGB-labeled probe detecting the mutant/variant sequence.

Assays are specific for a particular variant, including the respective nucleotide substitution partner. Non-polymorphism variants (not covered by a predesigned SNP assay) will require custom assay design. The example IDH1 and IDH2 assays described in this chapter were designed using the Thermo Fisher Scientific custom design service. Assay IDs and primer/probe sequences are provided in Table 1.

1. TaqMan® Assay Purchase and Design: Go to https://www.thermofisher.com, register, and log in. Search for/navigate to "TaqMan® SNP Genotyping Assays." Use the Assay Search Tool to identify if the variant has a predesigned assay available. If so, proceed to purchase and select the assay size desired (*see* **Note 4**). If no suitable predesigned assay exists, proceed to custom assay design. Choose and submit the DNA sequence for the region of interest containing the SNV, in 5′→3′ orientation (*see* **Note 5**). Indicate the wild-type and variant nucleotides in square brackets separated by a forward stroke, as in the example below (where G is the reference nucleotide, and A is the variant): 5′…GTGAACCAGT[G/A]CCAATATGCC…3′. Proceed to purchase custom assay (as above).
2. TaqMan® SNP genotyping assays are supplied at 40× or 80× concentration (*see* **Note 4**). Upon arrival immediately dilute to 20× concentration with molecular grade ddH_2O and aliquot in 20 μL volumes (each sufficient for a single full IFC chip run). Aliquots should be stored in the dark at −20 °C until use (*see* **Note 6**).
3. (Optional) It is good practice to validate the qualitative performance of new custom assays by AD-PCR to confirm good separation of homozygous wild type from heterozygous mutant (±homozygous mutant) in the relative fluorescence plots (Fig. 4). This can be performed on any standard qPCR thermal cycler. We validated the assays described here on an ABI 7900HT real-time PCR system with SDS software v2.1 (both Applied Biosystems; *see* **Note 7**).

3.2 Preparation of High-Quality Genomic DNA Samples

1. Extract genomic DNA from source cells (e.g., blood or marrow mononuclear cells) using commercial kit and manufacturer's protocol.

Table 1

Primer and probe sequences for the six IDH1 and IDH2 TaqMan® SNP genotyping assays

Mutation	Custom assay ID		Sequence
IDH1 R132C	AHD2BZ0	F primer	5′-CTTGTGAGTGGATGGGTAAAACCTA-3′
		R primer	5′-CACATTATTGCCAACATGACTTACTTGAT-3′
		MUT probe	5′-FAM/AAGCATGACAACCTATG/NFQ-3′
		WT probe	5′-VIC/AAGCATGACGACCTATG/NFQ-3′
IDH1 R132G	AH0JE6I	F primer	5′-CTTGTGAGTGGATGGGTAAAACCTA-3′
		R primer	5′-TGCAAAATCACATTATTGCCAACATG-3′
		MUT probe	5′-FAM/AAGCATGACCACCTATG/NFQ-3′
		WT probe	5′-VIC/AAGCATGACGACCTATG/NFQ-3′
IDH1 R132H	AHCTDTS	F primer	5′-CTTGTGAGTGGATGGGTAAAACCTA-3′
		R primer	5′-CACATTATTGCCAACATGACTTACTTGAT-3′
		MUT probe	5′-FAM/ATCATAGGTCATCATGC/NFQ-3′
		WT probe	5′-VIC/CATCATAGGTCGTCATGC/NFQ-3′
IDH1 R132S	AHFA958	F primer	5′-CTTGTGAGTGGATGGGTAAAACCTA-3′
		R primer	5′-CACATTATTGCCAACATGACTTACTTGAT-3′
		MUT probe	5′-FAM/CCATAAGCATGACTACCTAT/NFQ-3′
		WT probe	5′-VIC/CATAAGCATGACGACCTAT/NFQ-3′
IDH2 R140Q	AHVJL0G	F primer	5′-AAGATGTGGAAAAGTCCCAATGGA-3′
		R primer	5′-TGGGCTCCCGGAAGACA-3′
		MUT probe	5′-FAM/ACTATCCAGAACATCC/NFQ-3′
		WT probe	5′-VIC/CTATCCGGAACATCC/NFQ-3′
IDH2 R172K	AHGJ8CG	F primer	5′-GCTGGACCAAGCCCATCA-3′
		R primer	5′-TCCACCCTGGCCTACCT-3′
		MUT probe	5′-FAM/ATTGGCAAGCACGCC/NFQ-3′
		WT probe	5′-VIC/ATTGGCAGGCACGCC/NFQ-3′

2. Determine the quantity and quality of each genomic DNA sample using an appropriate method (e.g., NanoDrop 2000 spectrophotometer).
3. (Optional) Assess integrity of genomic DNA on an Agilent® 2100 Bioanalyzer, according to the manufacturer's instructions.
4. Dilute DNA to 20 ng/μL with ddH_2O or TE buffer (*see* **Note 8**). Store diluted DNA at −20 °C. Avoid excessive freeze-thaw cycles.

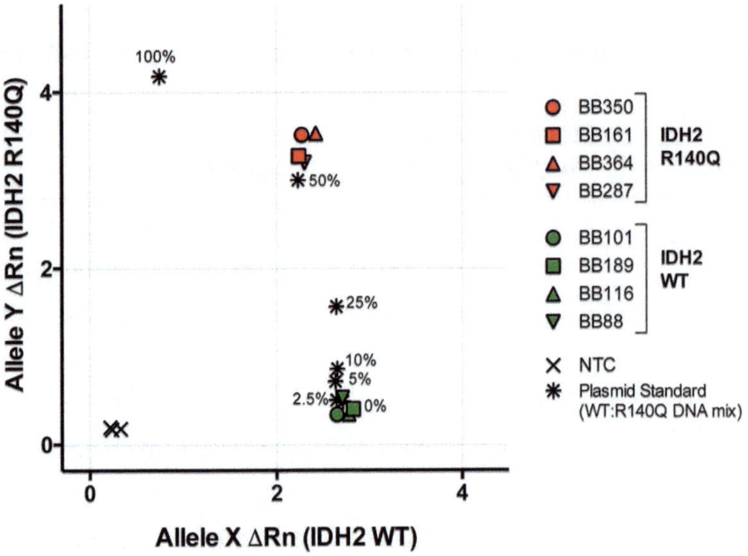

Fig. 4 Example allelic discrimination qPCR cluster plot for TaqMan® SNP genotyping assays. Each pooled assay was validated by endpoint AD-PCR using genomic DNA from ≥3 primary patient samples known to harbor the relevant IDH1 or IDH2 mutation. Representative plots for IDH2 R140Q are shown. Each sample is plotted as the endpoint ratio of corrected fluorescence (ΔRn) for VIC® (wild type; *X*-axis) versus FAM™ (mutant; *Y*-axis) after 40 PCR cycles. Plasmid standards containing the indicated percentage mutant/wild-type DNA mixes are shown. *NTC* no template control

3.3 Planning a 37K™ IFC Chip Run Experiment

1. Select 48 samples for inclusion in each IFC chip to be run. We recommend including each sample in at least duplicate and preferably triplicate wells per IFC chip (*see* **Note 9**).
2. Include appropriate controls, including at least one each of:
   (a) Negative DNA control sample (i.e., a sample confirmed wild type for the mutation of interest).
   (b) No template control (NTC) (i.e., with ddH_2O substituted for DNA template).
3. Design an experiment template, allocating a position for each sample in 96-well plate format. We recommend allocating the 48 wells in the left half of a 96-well plate (i.e., wells A1–H6). This facilitates easy transfer of DNA/reaction mix samples across to the chip using an 8-channel pipette (*see* Subheading 3.6) and automated mapping of sample destination wells using the onboard analysis software (*see* Subheading 3.8).

3.4 Prime a New dPCR 37K™ IFC Chip

1. Carefully remove a new 37K™ IFC chip from its packaging. The chip must be used within 24 h of opening the package.
2. Holding the chip at a ~45° angle with the shorter edge against the work surface, slowly inject control line fluid into each accumulator inlet. Inject a full syringe (300 μL) into each accumulator inlet on the chip (*see* **Note 10**).

3. Remove and discard the blue protective film from underside of the chip.
4. Place the chip into the IFC controller module MX.
5. Follow the on-screen instructions, selecting the "Prime (167×)" script (*see* **Note 11**).

3.5 Prepare 48 Assay Reaction Mixes for DNA Test Samples

1. Table 2 summarizes the relative volumes of each component in the assay reaction mix for each 37K™ IFC chip and sample panel (*see* **Note 12**).
2. In a DNA-free hood, combine the total required volumes of TaqMan® assay, Mastermix, Loading Reagent, and ddH_2O in a 1.5 mL microcentrifuge tube.
3. Pipette 4.2 μL of this reaction mix (i.e., all components excluding DNA) into each of the 48 active wells of a 96-well PCR microplate according to the experiment template designed in Subheading 3.3, **step 3** (i.e., the left half of the plate for a single chip run).
4. Remove the microplate from the DNA-free hood, and add 1.8 μL of DNA (at 20 ng/μL; *see* Subheading 3.2, **step 4**) to the active well corresponding to its location in the experiment template. Each well should now contain 6 μL total volume.
5. Cover microplate with adhesive seal and centrifuge at ≥1000 × *g* for 2 min to collect reaction/DNA mix at the bottom of each well.

Table 2
Reaction mix components and volumes

	Final volume/inlet (μL)	Volume/inlet with overage (μL)	Volume/full IFC chip (μL)
TaqMan® Gene Expression Mastermix (Life Technologies, Cat #4369016)	2.0	3.0	180
20× GE Sample Loading Reagent (Fluidigm, Cat #85000746)	0.4	0.6	36
20× gene-specific TaqMan® assay	0.2	0.3	18
PCR-grade ddH_2O	0.2	0.3	18
DNA	1.2	1.8	n/a
Total	4.0	6.0	252

3.6 Load DNA/Assay Reaction Mixes into 37K™ IFC Chip

1. After "Prime" script has completed, remove the chip from the IFC controller module MX.
2. Prepare 1× GE Sample Loading Reagent from the supplied 20× stock (*see* **Note 13**).
3. Pipette 10 μL of 1× GE Sample Loading Reagent into each of the 16 hydration inlets on the chip. Avoid introducing bubbles into the hydration inlets through careful ± reverse pipetting.
4. Pipette 4 μL of each DNA/assay reaction mix into the 48 sample inlets on the chip, using the pipetting map to guide sample transfer (Fig. 5; *see* **Note 14**).
5. Visualize each sample well to confirm that the reaction mix is covering the inlet channel and is free of bubbles. Small bubbles can be manually cleared using a fresh, sterile 25G hypodermic needle. Take care to avoid cross-contamination of DNA/assay reaction mix between inlet wells.

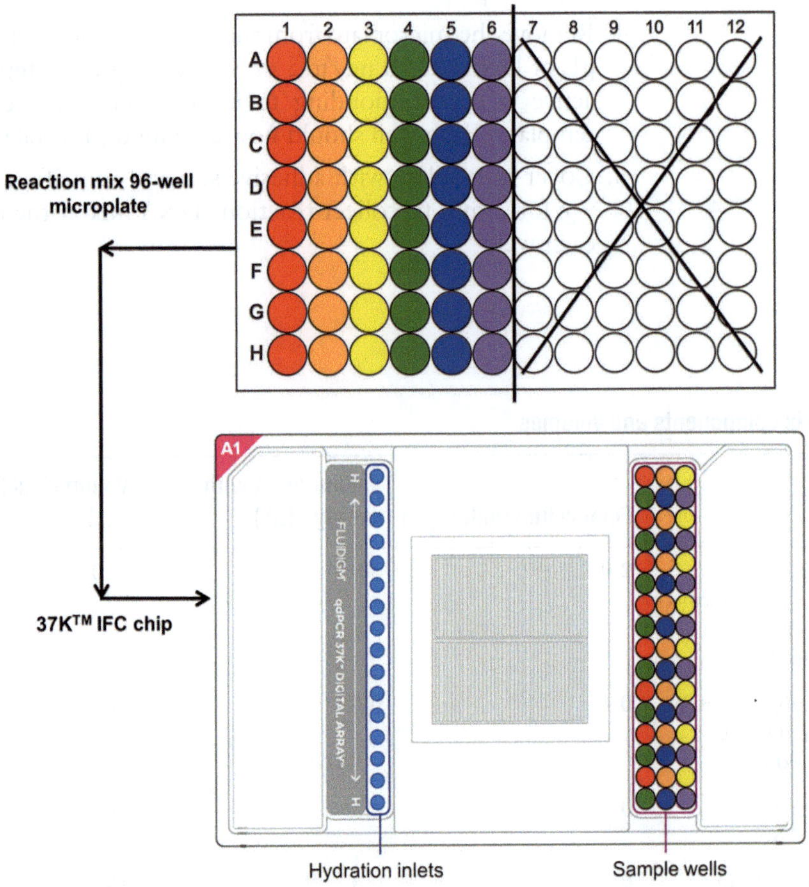

Fig. 5 Pipetting map from the 96-well microplate layout to 37K IFC chip sample panel inlet wells. We recommend transferring samples from the 96-well plate by column, using an 8-channel P10 pipette, to the chip sample wells bearing the matching color

6. Place the IFC chip into MX controller module (or Juno™ system).
7. Follow the on-screen instructions, selecting the "Load (167×)" script (*see* **Note 15**).

3.7 Digital PCR Thermal Cycling

1. After "Load" script has completed, remove the chip from the IFC controller module MX.
2. Remove any dust particles or debris from the IFC surface (*see* **Note 16**).
3. Ensure that the Biomark HD™ and the associated desktop computer terminal are switched on. Launch the **Biomark Data Collection** program on the terminal and select **Start a New Run**. Ensure that the status indicators for the lamp and camera are green.
4. Place the loaded 37K™ IFC chip into the instrument tray. Click **Load**.
5. Verify the IFC chip barcode and that the correct chip type is automatically detected. Click **Next**.
6. Provide a name and select a file storage location for a new IFC chip run. Click **Next**.
7. Choose the application (**Digital PCR**) and passive reference (**ROX**). Check **Select Probes Manually** and choose assay type (**Two Probes**). Select the probe types (**FAM-MGB** and **VIC-MGB**). Click **Next**.
8. Browse for and select the thermal protocol**dPCR Standard v1.pcl** (*see* **Note 17** and Table 3). Confirm **Auto Exposure** is selected. Click **Next**.
9. Verify all selected parameters are correct. Click **Start Run** (*see* **Note 18**).

3.8 Using the Digital PCR Analysis Software

1. Once the thermal cycling run is complete, launch the Digital PCR Analysis software on the Biomark HD™ desktop computer terminal.

Table 3
Real-time PCR thermal cycling conditions for the default protocol "dPCR standard v1.pcl"

Step	Temperature (°C)	Time	Cycles
Initial incubation	50	120 s	1
Initial denaturation	95	10 m	1
Denaturation	95	15 s	40
Annealing/extension	60	60 s	
Hold	4	∞	

2. Click **Open a Chip Run** and locate the saved file containing the run data (file extension .bml). The file opens in the Chip Explorer panel (*see* **Note 19**).
3. Click **Sample and Detector Setup** in the Chip Explorer pane, followed by **New**, to assign the sample identity to each well of the IFC chip used in the test (or **Import**, if recalling a saved layout template). Select Source **96 Wellplate** and Mapping **48.770-SBS94-Left**, to automatically map sample wells from the original reaction mix 96-well microplate to their destination wells in the 37K IFC chip (*see* **Note 20**).
4. Open the sample **Editor** from the taskbar, and label each sample well following the layout of the original reaction mix 96-well microplate template. For each sample specify **Sample Type** ("Unknown" for test samples), the **Sample Name** and specify the identity of the **Detector Name** (e.g., "IDH1 R132H" or "IDH1 wild type"), and **Detector Type** ("Test" for test samples) for the respective probes. There is also an option to specify sample relative concentration to permit onboard analysis of serial tenfold dilutions, if required.
5. Click **Analyze** to initiate sample mapping and to update raw data output. Labeled sample raw data for the full 37K™ IFC chip are now available to view via the Chip Explorer panel (*see* **Note 21**). **Panel Summary** displays output for each of the 48 sample panels on the chip. This can be displayed as a Results Table, containing basic identification and raw data for each sample, or in Heat Map View, which displays each sample/panel as a grid of 770 chambers. Those containing a positive reaction are filled in red (FAM; mutant) or blue (VIC; wild type). It is possible to toggle between heat maps displaying FAM alone, VIC alone, or both together (Fig. 6). Data and amplification curves for each chamber for every panel on the chip can also be viewed individually in the **Panel Details** view.

3.9 Data Analysis and Interpretation

1. **Establish and set optimal analysis settings for the selected assays.** The Digital PCR Analysis software will automatically set default qPCR Analysis Settings, but these may not be optimal for all assays. We recommend determining optimal settings for each custom assay and manually entering these values in the Analysis Settings. Remember to click **Analyze** in the Task panel to apply any changes made and to update results data (*see* **Note 22**).

   Optimization can be determined by detailed inspection of PCR amplification curves for individual sample panels, which display superimposed amplification curves for each individual chamber reaction for either FAM (red) or VIC (blue) or both (Fig. 7). We recommend (a) manual adjustment of baseline correction (if required), (b) adjustment of Ct threshold to eliminate impact of crosstalk between the FAM and VIC filters

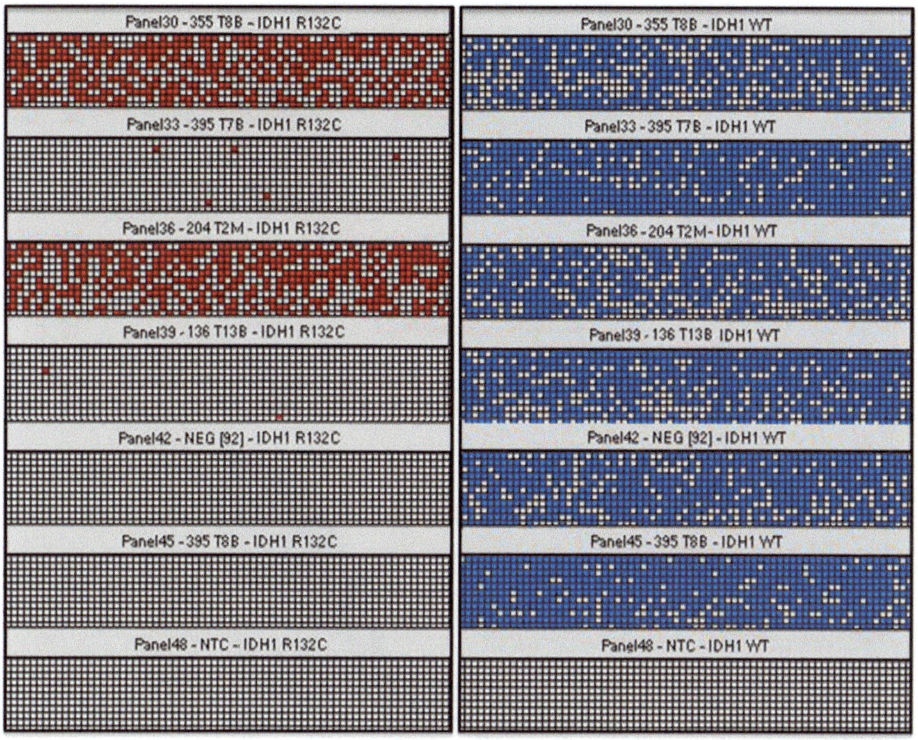

Fig. 6 Example heat map outputs for seven (of 48) representative panels from an IDH1 R132C 37K™ IFC chip digital PCR run. The *left panel* (*red*) indicates the FAM channel (mutant allele), and the *right panel* (*blue*) indicates the VIC channel (wild-type allele). Note the "NEG" (sample known to be wild type; panel 42) and no template (NTC; panel 48) controls

(*see* **Note 23**), and (c) adjustment of Ct threshold and Ct range to establish a suitable threshold to define a "positive" reaction. This should be set at a point that optimally captures every positive (but no negative) reaction amplification curve within the selected Ct range (*see* **Note 24**).

The following **Analysis Settings** are those used within our laboratory and deliver good performance for all of the assays described in this chapter:

Quality threshold:	0.65
Baseline correction:	Linear
Ct threshold method:	User (global) (*see* **Note 25**)
Ct ranges:	15–35
Ct thresholds:	*See* Table 4

2. **Check panel template saturation is within the optimal range for each sample.** The final column in the Panel Summary results table ("All Union") indicates the number of chambers containing a positive reaction for one or both probes (/770) in that panel. For optimal performance of the Poisson correction,

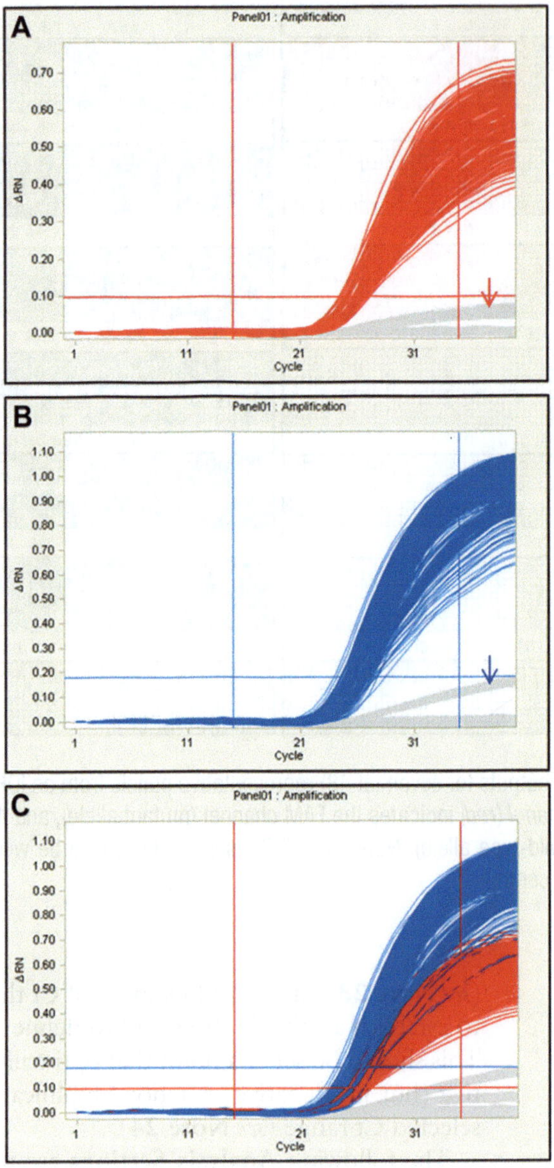

Fig. 7 Example real-time PCR amplification curves for a representative panel from an IDH1 R132C 37K™ IFC chip run. This sample had a calculated mutant allele frequency of 28.6%. Graphs combine the amplification curves from each of 770 individual chamber partition reactions for the FAM (**A**; *red*) and VIC (**B**; *blue*) detector channels. Each curve plotsΔRn (i.e., reporter fluorescence normalized to ROX passive reference signal; *Y*-axis) against PCR cycle number. Crosstalk between the two channels is evident in the *gray traces deviating from baseline* (but these are unequivocally *negative reactions, indicated by arrows*). Ct range and Ct threshold (*vertical and horizontal colored lines*, respectively) were set for each channel to negate the impact of crosstalk while clearly defining all "positive" reactions for each probe. (**C**) Curves for both channels are displayed simultaneously on the same scale. Note that the mutant allele (FAM) assay displays relatively lower amplification efficiency than the wild-type (VIC) assay. Nevertheless, all positive reactions for each probe are clearly captured. This illustrates an important advantage of the binary dPCR output for absolute allele-specific quantitation compared with the "analogue" output of conventional qPCR approaches, in which assay efficiency can directly influence the derived relative quantitation

it is recommended that between 200 and 700 chambers contain a template "hit." With our recommended input DNA concentration of 17–23 ng/µL, this will typically be achieved. However, any samples that appear oversaturated (>700) or too dilute (<200) should be repeated following further dilution or concentration of DNA.

3. **Review IFC chip run controls**. Confirm that the negative/wild-type DNA control samples return zero chambers with FAM (i.e., mutant) targets and that the NTCs return zero chambers with **either** FAM or VIC targets. Otherwise repeat the IFC chip run with fresh reagents as this may indicate DNA contamination that could substantially impact on results.
4. **Inspect raw data**. The Panel Summary results table presents raw data for each sample panel as a separate row in a spreadsheet table. Data for each probe detector are presented in a separate block of columns. Noteworthy data include the actual number of chambers meeting criteria for a positive reaction ("**Count**") for each probe, the Poisson-corrected positive hits (**"Est. Targets")** and the associated 95% confidence interval (lower, "**Est. T-95L**"; upper, "**Est. T-95U**"). The "**Est. Targets**" figure that should be considered the final result for that probe for that assay.
5. **Export raw data**. Raw data for all chambers on the chip ("Detailed") or summaries for each sample panel ("Summary") can be exported as .csv files to a compatible spreadsheet software (e.g., Microsoft Excel) for further analysis. A PDF report can also be exported that includes composite real-time amplification curves for each sample panel.
6. **Calculate mutant allele frequencies (MAFs)**. MAFs are not automatically calculated by the software but are easily derived as the number of estimated targets for mutant (FAM) probe divided by the total number of estimated (FAM + VIC) targets analyzed in any sample panel:

   Mutant allele frequency = Estimated mutant (FAM) targets/ Estimated total (FAM + VIC) targets

   Sensitivity can be extended by including multiple sample replicates in the same chip and manually applying the Poisson correction to the extended and collated dataset for that sample (*see* **Note 26**). Using two panels per sample, these IDH1 and IDH2 assays have been validated as quantitative to ≤0.1% MAF. For any new custom assays, we recommend establishing the lower quantitative limit through testing serial dilutions of known mixes of mutated/wild-type DNA for each SNV of interest (*see* [12]).

Table 4
Recommended Ct thresholds for the six IDH1 and IDH2 dPCR assays

Assay	FAM (mutant) Ct threshold	VIC (wild type) Ct threshold
IDH1 R132C	0.096	0.178
IDH1 R132G	0.05	0.10
IDH1 R132H	0.064	0.10
IDH1 R132S	0.05	0.10
IDH2 R140Q	0.04	0.07
IDH2 R172K	0.056	0.07

4 Notes

1. The Juno™ (Fluidigm) is an alternative system that combines priming, loading, and qPCR in the same instrument. It can therefore replace the IFC Controller Module MX and Biomark™ HD thermal cycling system in this protocol.
2. We recommend diluting genomic DNA to a starting concentration of 17–23 ng/μL but have seen successful panel saturation (i.e., >200 chambers containing template reaction) with DNA concentrations as low as ~5 ng/μL. If sample concentration is below this and further concentration (e.g., by centrifugal evaporation) is not possible, we recommend including a pre-amplification step. We have validated this protocol on DNA samples subjected to multiple whole genome amplification using the REPLI-g mini amplification kit (Qiagen).
3. Other qPCR mastermixes can be substituted but are not supported by Fluidigm. We have also validated 2× TaqMan® Genotyping Mastermix (Life Technologies, Cat #4371355) as an alternative.
4. Thermo Fisher Scientific supplies TaqMan® SNP genotyping assays in three sizes: small (188 μL), medium (625 μL), and large (750 μL). Large assays are manufactured at 80× concentration, and small or medium assays are supplied at 40× concentration. One small assay provides sufficient reagent for ≥20 full IFC chip runs of 48 samples each.
5. It is recommended that submitted template sequences be 300–600 bases in length. Other factors that can influence the assay design success include the presence of polymorphisms close to the region of interest and low complexity or repetitive regions of DNA. In these cases unique primer/probe design may not be possible. We recommend designing assays using FAM™-MGB

and VIC®-MGB probes. Note however that FAM™-TAMRA™ and FAM™-nonfluorescent quenchers are also supported with the Biomark™ HD system. Further, other fluorophores with excitation between 465–505 nm and 510–550 nm and emission between 500–550 nm and 540–600 nm, respectively, should also be compatible. See "Custom TaqMan® Genomic Assays Protocol: Submission Guidelines" (Thermo Fisher Scientific; PN 4367671) for further guidelines and tips on custom assay design. This is available for download at https://tools.thermofisher.com/content/sfs/manuals/cms_042307.pdf.

6. TaqMan® SNP genotyping assays are potentially susceptible to light degradation. Aliquoting and storage in the dark at −20 °C mitigates the need for freeze-thawing and unnecessary light exposure.
7. For more information on the principles of allelic discrimination PCR, a detailed technical method, and a guide to interpreting the results, see "Allelic Discrimination Getting Started Guide" (Applied Biosystems, PN 4364015), available for download at http://www3.appliedbiosystems.com/cms/groups/mcb_support/documents/generaldocuments/cms_042114.pdf.
8. Each sample well inlet on the IFC chip will contain 1.2 μL of DNA sample as part of a combined reaction mix. Poisson distribution estimates of positive targets are accurate and reproducible for between ~230 and 1900 copies per panel ($0.3 < \lambda < 2.5$), which equates to a target range of 200–700 (/770) chambers containing a template reaction [15]. For the assays described in this chapter, we have validated that a starting sample DNA concentration of 17–23 ng/μL will appropriately saturate a sample panel.
9. All wells of a 37K™ IFC chip must be in use before loading and thermal cycling. Batching samples (or increasing number of replicates) will maximize the number of chip wells returning useful data.
10. Ensure that the correct prepackaged control line fluid is used (i.e., "48.48" syringes with 300 μL preloaded fluid). Other kits contain different volumes that will not adequately prime the chip microfluidics. Before loading, use the syringe with shipping cap in place to actuate both accumulator check valves using gentle downward pressure. Only proceed if the poppets depress freely. Before dispensing the control line fluid, visually confirm that the check valve is open. The O-ring seal at the bottom of the valve will be depressed and displaced to the side. Take care to avoid any spillage of control line fluid onto the chip or inlets and to confirm that the O-ring returns to its normal position after removing the syringe tip.

11. The MX "Prime" script runs for approximately 50 min. While the script is running, proceed to prepare the reaction mix (*see* Subheading 3.5). Ensure that the 37K™ IFC chip is loaded (*see* Subheading 3.6) within 60 min of priming.
12. The volumes in Table 2 are calculated for 60 reactions to ensure sufficient overage for accurate pipette transfer from 96-well plate to 37K™ IFC chip. Multiple TaqMan® assays can be used in the same chip (in different sets of wells). Scale down components, maintaining the indicated relative proportions, as appropriate for each assay, or scale up if more than one chip run is planned for the same assay.
13. Diluting 10 μL of the GE Sample Loading Reagent 20× stock with 190 μL PCR-grade ddH_2O will prepare sufficient 1× Loading Reagent for a single full 37K™ IFC chip.
14. Use an 8-channel P10 pipette to transfer DNA/assay reaction mix from each complete column (i.e., rows A–H) of the 96-well microplate into the corresponding inlet wells on the 37K™ IFC chip, according to Fig. 5. Avoid introducing bubbles into the sample inlet wells. This can interfere with sample uptake during pneumatic loading. Reverse pipetting (with slight overage) will avoid bubble contamination and is highly recommended.
15. The "Load" script draws sample through the inlet channels into the microfluidic circuit of the IFC chip and partitions into 770 individual chambers for each sample panel. The script runs for ~40 min. The dPCR thermal cycling run should be commenced within 60 min of chip loading.
16. Gentle application and rapid removal of a pressure sensitive adhesive tape across the IFC chamber surface is a simple and effective method for lifting dust or debris.
17. The dPCR standard thermal cycling protocol in Table 3 provides satisfactory performance for all of the IDH1 and IDH2 assays described in this chapter while permitting simultaneous inclusion of different assays in the same IFC chip run. However, optimal annealing temperature varies from assay to assay and may need optimizing for new custom assays.
18. Thermal cycling for this protocol takes approximately 90 min. FAM™, VIC®, and ROX (passive reference) signals of all chambers for all panels within the IFC chip are automatically detected and recorded at the start of each annealing step and at the end of the program. Real-time PCR data and PCR amplification curves are recorded for each chamber of each sample panel.
19. The first time a chip run .bml file is opened, all data are analyzed, and the chamber-finding algorithm locates the chamber

boundaries of each captured image. It may take several minutes for the .bml file to load. If the algorithm cannot locate the four corner cells of the chip during the first analysis (rare), an error message will appear, prompting the user to manually find them. If this occurs, follow the on-screen instructions (Note: adjusting the contrast slider can aid in visualizing the corner cells).

20. The suggested selections assume that the user has followed the 96-well plate template layout recommended in Subheading 3.3 and the left-to-right pipetting scheme outlined in Subheading 3.6/Fig. 5 when loading the chip with DNA samples.

21. Raw data will initially be presented using the system's default settings, ranges, and thresholds. These may require manually changing (*see* Subheading 3.9). For a detailed software manual, see Fluidigm's Digital PCR Analysis User Guide (PN 68000100; available for download at https://www.fluidigm.com/documents).

22. Once determined the same analysis settings should be employed each time an assay is run. When optimizing parameters for a new assay, we recommend reviewing several chip runs, containing samples with a wide range of MAFs, before confirming settings used to report definitive results.

23. Crosstalk between filters can be observed in the real-time PCR amplification curves for DNA samples containing high allelic burden for one allele as a distinctive and consistent deflection from baseline of a proportional bulk of overtly "negative" chamber amplification curves visible in the opposite probe's detector channel. *See* Fig. 7 for a worked example.

24. Note that since the output for each chamber reaction is a binary readout, the precise positioning of the Ct threshold (in relation to the PCR amplification phases) is less critical than for conventional qPCR. The foremost consideration is establishing a Ct threshold and range that will reliably and reproducibly distinguish positive from negative reaction chambers. Hence this approach is more permissive to (modest) deviations from optimal in assay amplification efficiency and annealing temperature compared with conventional qPCR.

25. The "User" (versus "Auto") settings allow thresholds for each probe type to be set manually. We have observed improved performance of the assays with manually determined Ct thresholds, based on the individual amplification kinetics and efficiency curve morphologies for each probe/assay. "Global" applies the specified Ct threshold to all sample panels on the chip simultaneously. The option exists to manually adjust the threshold for each probe in each panel individually ("User [Detectors]" setting). However, even when including several

assays with different optimal settings within the same chip, we find that setting a "Global" threshold for each assay's settings separately, and saving and exporting the data for the entire chip, before repeating with each other assay's settings, is faster and more efficient.

26. The sensitivity of dPCR is highly dependent on the total number of sample partitions. Whereas droplet dPCR can generate many thousands of individual droplet partitions, nanofluidic platforms are inherently limited by the number of chambers for each sample panel in the chip (i.e., 770 for the 37K™ IFC chips). This is counterbalanced by several advantages of the Fluidigm system, including consistent and reproducible run sensitivity, and access to real-time PCR data for each individual reaction. This offers greater control over defining thresholds for a positive reaction and monitoring and optimizing assay performance. Moreover, the sensitivity of nanofluidic dPCR can be improved by increasing the number of panels allocated to a particular sample on the same chip, thus expanding the number of chamber partitions by 770 for each additional panel allocated. To deepen sensitivity (rather than simply provide technical replicates), the Poisson correction must be applied manually on the expanded dataset, using the following calculation:

    Estimated targets in panel = $\mathrm{LN}((y - x)/y) \times (-y)$,

    where x = count of positive targets and y = total number of chambers across which the sample is partitioned (i.e., 770 × number of panels allocated to that sample). Since each chamber on a chip contains a fixed volume (0.75 nL for the 37K™ IFC chip), this effectively becomes equivalent to distributing a larger starting sample across a greater number of partitions, deepening sensitivity accordingly. This affords a degree of control over balancing sensitivity requirements against throughput and overall cost, as demanded by different circumstances.

    For further explanation as to the derivation of this calculation, see Fluidigm's technical note "Calculating Copy Number Using a 12.765 Digital ArrayTM IFC" (PN 68000119). For a detailed explanation of Poisson distribution mathematics as applied to dPCR (beyond the scope of this article), *see* [9].

References

1. Losman JA, Kaelin WG (2013) What a difference a hydroxyl makes: mutant IDH, (R)-2-hydroxyglutarate, and cancer. Genes Dev 27:836–852
2. Thiede C, Steudel C, Mohr B et al (2002) Analysis of FLT3-activating mutations in 979 patients with acute myelogenous leukemia: association with FAB subtypes and identification of subgroups with poor prognosis. Blood 99:4326–4335
3. Grimwade D, Freeman SD (2014) Defining minimal residual disease in acute myeloid leukemia: which platforms are ready for "prime time"? Blood 124:3345–3355
4. Schnittger S, Kern W, Tschulik C et al (2009) Minimal residual disease levels assessed by

NPM1 mutation-specific RQ-PCR provide important prognostic information in AML. Blood 114:2220–2231

5. Roma C, Esposito C, Rachiglio AM et al (2013) Detection of EGFR mutations by TaqMan mutation detection assays powered by competitive allele-specific TaqMan PCR technology. Biomed Res Int 2013:385087
6. Matsuda K, Sugano M, Honda T (2012) PCR for monitoring of minimal residual disease in hematologic malignancy. Clin Chim Acta 413:74–80
7. Huggett JF, Foy CA, Benes V et al (2013) The digital MIQE guidelines: minimum information for publication of quantitative digital PCR experiments. Clin Chem 59:892–902
8. Vogelstein B, Kinzler KW (1999) Digital PCR. Proc Natl Acad Sci U S A 96:9236–9241
9. Dube S, Qin J, Ramakrishnan R (2008) Mathematical analysis of copy number variation in a DNA sample using digital PCR on a nanofluidic device. PLoS One 3:e2876
10. Bhat S, Herrmann J, Armishaw P et al (2009) Single molecule detection in nanofluidic digital array enables accurate measurement of DNA copy number. Anal Bioanal Chem 394:457–467
11. Huggett JF, Cowen S, Foy CA (2015) Considerations for digital PCR as an accurate molecular diagnostic tool. Clin Chem 61:79–88
12. Wiseman DH, Struys EA, Wilks DP et al (2015) Direct comparison of quantitative digital PCR and 2-hydroxyglutarate enantiomeric ratio for IDH mutant allele frequency assessment in myeloid malignancy. Leukemia 29:2421–2423
13. Shen GQ, Abdullah KG, Wang QK (2009) The TaqMan method for SNP genotyping. Methods Mol Biol 578:293–306
14. Schleinitz D, Distefano JK, Kovacs P (2011) Targeted SNP genotyping using the TaqMan® assay. Methods Mol Biol 700:77–87
15. Whale AS, Cowen S, Foy CA et al (2013) Methods for applying accurate digital PCR analysis on low copy DNA samples. PLoS One 8:e58177

Chapter 16

Isolation of Biologically Active Exosomes from Plasma of Patients with Cancer

Chang-Sook Hong, Sonja Funk, and Theresa L. Whiteside

Abstract

A method for exosome isolation from human plasma was developed for rapid, high-throughput processing of plasma specimens obtained from patients with cancer. This method removes the bulk of plasma proteins associated with exosomes and can be used for comparative examinations of exosomes and their content in serial specimens of patients' plasma, allowing for monitoring changes in exosome numbers, profiles, and functions in the course of cancer progression or during therapy. The plasma-derived exosomes can be recovered in quantities sufficient for the characterization of their morphology by transmission electron microscopy (TEM), size and concentration by qNano, protein/lipid ratios, nucleic acid extraction, molecular profiling by Western blots or immune arrays, and functional assays.

Key words Plasma exosomes, Isolation, Cancer, Size exclusion chromatography, Exosome functions, Exosome cargo

1 Introduction

Exosomes have been traditionally isolated by a series of differential centrifugations aimed at removing first the cell debris and then larger **EVs** followed by ultracentrifugation of smaller exosomes at 100,000 × *g* for 2–3 h and by flotation on a sucrose density gradient to obtain purified exosomes [1]. More recently, this time-consuming ultracentrifugation has been replaced by a variety of other methods, which aim at a more rapid high-throughput isolation of purified exosomes with a defined size and molecular content from body fluids [2]. We have modified a previously described size exclusion chromatography (SEC) approach [3] to be able to reliably and readily recover morphologically intact functionally competent exosomes from small volumes (1 mL) of plasma by "mini-SEC" in patients with cancer [2]. The methodology of exosome isolation from plasma by mini-SEC is described below.

Paolo Fortina et al. (eds.), *Acute Myeloid Leukemia: Methods and Protocols*, Methods in Molecular Biology, vol. 1633, DOI 10.1007/978-1-4939-7142-8_16, © Springer Science+Business Media LLC 2017

2 Materials

2.1 Plasma of Cancer Patients or Healthy Donors

1. Plasma is obtained from venous blood samples by centrifugation at 1000 × *g* for 10 min. Collect clear plasma and aliquot into 2 mL cryovials. Store specimens frozen at −80 °C until exosome isolation.

3 Methods

Prepare all solutions at room temperature before experiments unless specified. Perform all steps in a laminar flow hood. Columns for exosome isolation are set up on clean benches. All solutions are sterile and no sodium azide is added. Dispose of waste materials following the institutional guidelines. Details are as follows:

3.1 Exosome Isolation from Plasma (Fig. 1)

1. Thaw frozen plasma and centrifuge at 2000 × *g* for 10 min and transfer clear plasma into new tubes. Recentrifuge at 10,000 × *g* for 30 min and save clarified plasma. Filter the plasma with a 0.22 μm-pore Millipore filter (*see* **Note 1**).
2. Wash Sepharose 2B solution (**Sigma-Aldrich**, 60–200 μm bead diameter) with 1× PBS three times before preparing SEC columns.
3. Set up a disposable 1.5 cm × 12 cm mini-column (Bio-Rad, Hercules, CA, USA, Econo-Pac columns) on the ring stand and mark at the 10 mL line, which will be the column bed volume. Place a 50 mL Falcon tube for waste collection at the bottom of the stand.

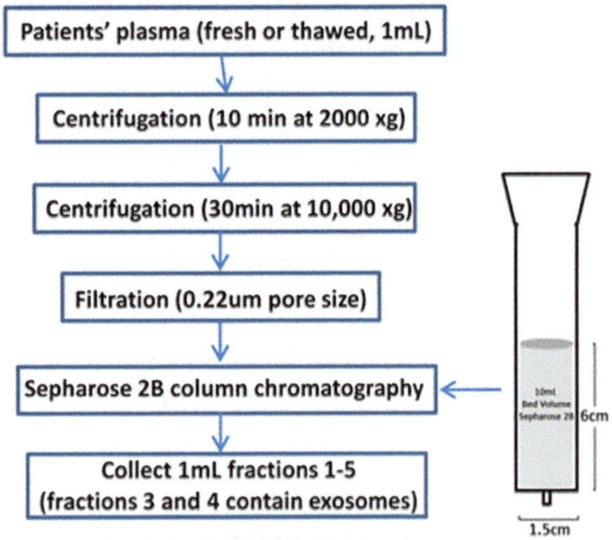

Fig. 1 Schema of the exosome isolation procedure from plasma

4. Load prewashed Sepharose 2B slurry into the column and allow PBS to flow through the column by gravity to a waste tube. Let the gel settle up to the 10 mL line. After dripping stops, close the outlet with a yellow cap and insert a porous frit, which are both provided along with the Econo-Pac columns, on the top of the gel (*see* **Note 2**) and then wash the column with 20 mL of 1× PBS. Now the column is ready to be used for exosome processing.
5. Load 1 mL of the ultrafiltrated plasma from **step 1** of Subheading 3.1 on top of the column and let it flow through the column.
6. After dripping stops, add 1 mL of 1× PBS to the column and let it flow through the column to the waste tube. This is fraction #1.
7. Repeat **step 6** of Subheading 3.1 for fraction #2. Then replace the waste tube with a clean 15 mL Falcon tube for collecting exosome fractions.
8. Add 1 mL of 1× PBS and collect fraction #3. Then replace the fraction #3 tube with a new 15 mL falcon tube and add 1 mL PBS to the column and collect fraction #4.
9. Repeat **step 8** of Subheading 3.1 to collect fraction #5 (*see* **Note 3**). After fraction #5, stop collecting fractions and discard the column.

3.2 Exosome Concentration

Concentrate fractions #3 or #4 using 100K Amicon Ultra 0.5 mL centrifugal filter (EMD Millipore, Billerica, MA, USA) by centrifugation at 5000 × *g* for 1–10 min, depending on the final concentration for downstream analysis (*see* **Note 4**).

3.3 Protein Measurements

Measure protein concentration in fractions #3 and #4 using a BCA protein assay kit (Pierce Biotechnology, Rockford, IL, USA) according to the manufacturer's instructions.

3.4 Particle Size and Concentration Measurements

Tunable Resistive Pulse Sensing (TRPS) by qNano (Izon, Cambridge, MA, USA) is used to measure the size distribution and concentration of particles in fractions #3 and #4. The procedures are performed according to the manufacturer's instructions (*see* **Note 5**).

3.5 Transmission Electron Microscopy

TEM procedures and imaging of exosomes usually are performed in imaging facilities and details have been published elsewhere. Briefly:

1. Put 2 μL of fractions #3 or #4 on a copper grid coated with 0.125% Formvar in chloroform.
2. Stain the grids with 1% (v/v) uranyl acetate in ddH_2O.
3. Image exosomes immediately with a JEM 1011 transmission electron microscope.

3.6 Western Blot of Exosomes

Approximately 10 μg of exosome proteins, either from fraction #4 or after concentration from Subheading 3.2, can be separated on SDS-PAGE gels and transferred into an Immobilon membrane. Then it can be analyzed by Western blots with antibodies of exosomal markers, CD9, CD63, or TSG101, and other cancer markers (Fig. 2).

3.7 Functional Studies

Exosomes isolated by SEC are biologically active and relatively free of plasma components and thus optimal for studies of their effect on immune cells. In Fig. 3, the effects of exosomes isolated from plasma of a normal donor (ND) or from plasma of head and neck cancer patients on primary $CD4^{+}$ T cells or $CD8^{+}$ Jurkat cells are shown (*see* **Note 6**).

3.8 Peripheral Blood Mononuclear Cell (PBMC) Isolation and Culture

Primary $CD4^{+}$ and $CD8^{+}$ T cells can be isolated from whole blood of NDs as follows:

1. Centrifuge venous blood samples at 1000 × *g* for 10 min to separate plasma (upper level) from other blood components (lower level).
2. Take off and save plasma for exosome isolation.
3. Dilute the pellet in PBS and load the solution on a Ficoll-Hypaque gradient.
4. Centrifuge at 900 × *g* for 30 min.
5. Collect the PBMC layer located at the PBS/plasma interface.
6. Wash PBMC in PBS at 1000 × *g* for 10 min.
7. Resuspend PBMC at 2–3 × 10^6 PBMC/mL in RPMI MV- (Lonza RPMI 1640, 10% (v/v) FBS that is exosome-depleted (**Gibco**), 100 IU/mL penicillin, 100 μg/mL streptomycin, and 2 mM/L L-glutamine) and plate for 2–3 h to remove plastic-adherent monocytes.

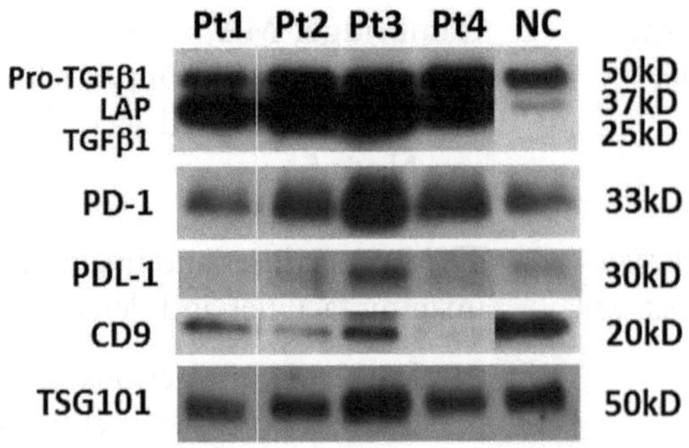

Fig. 2 Western blot analysis of exosomes isolated from plasma of AML patients and a normal donor. Each lane was loaded with 10 μg exosomal protein

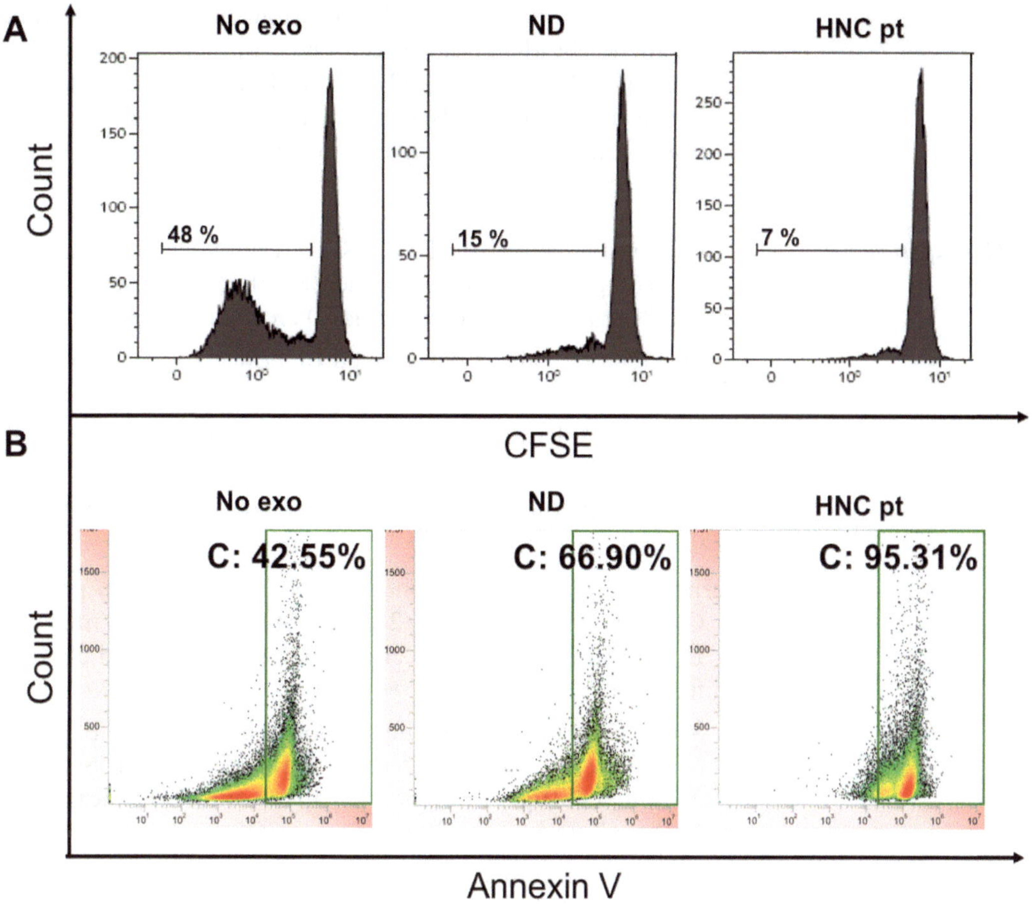

Fig. 3 Functional assays. (**a**) Proliferating CFSE+ CD4+ T cells are inhibited by exosomes isolated from plasma of NDs and HNC patients. (**b**) Apoptosis in CD8+ Jurkat cells is induced by exosomes of NDs and HNC patients

3.9 Primary CD4+ and CD8+ T Cell Isolation

1. Centrifuge PBMC at 500 × *g* for 10 min.
2. Cell separation can be performed using negative or positive isolation kits for CD4+ and CD8+ T cells on an autoMACS cell separator (Miltenyi Biotec, San Diego, CA, USA) following the manufacturer's instructions. We prefer negative isolations because the cell purity is higher.

3.10 CFSE-Based Proliferation Assay with CD4+ T Cells (Fig. 3a)

1. Label primary CD4+ T cells of healthy volunteers with 1.5 μM CFSE (i.e., CellTrace Proliferation Kit, **Thermo Scientific**) in 0.1% BSA in PBS for 10 min at 37 °C [5].
2. Quench staining with an equal volume of exosome-depleted FBS and wash two times in RPMI MV-.
3. Activate CFSE-labeled CD4+ T cells at a ratio of 10^5 cells/100 μL in a 96-well plate with CD3/28 (i.e., plate-bound CD3 and CD28 in solution, 2 μg/mL) and IL-2 (i.e., 150 IU/mL, **PeproTech**) for 24 h. Also, plate resting CFSE+ T cells at the same concentration as controls.

Alternatives for T cell activation are CD3/28-coated magnetic beads (bead-to-cell-ratio of 1:2, Miltenyi) or Immunocult Human CD3/28T cell activator (25 μL/mL, **Stemcell)**. In our hands, the human T cell activator (Stemcell) was the most reliable, simplest, and cleanest (no beads) way of T cell activation.

3.11 Experimental Setup

1. On day 1, co-incubate 10^5 CFSE$^+$ T cells with exosomes (2–3 μg in 50 μL PBS) or no exosomes (50 μL PBS). Resting CFSE$^+$ T cells that were cultured on day 0 are another control.
2. Proliferation can be determined by flow cytometry on day 4 or 5.
3. Annexin V-based apoptosis assay with CD8$^+$ Jurkat cells (Fig. 3b).
4. Plate CD8$^+$ Jurkat cells (10^5 cells in 100 μL RPMI MV- per 96-well for 24 h).

Alternatively, isolate (*see* Subheading 3.7) and activate primary CD8$^+$ T cells with CD3/28 (i.e., Stemcell 25 μL/mL) and IL-2 (150 IU/mL) in a cell incubator at 37 °C and 5% CO_2 for 48 h.

5. Set up experiment by adding exosomal fraction #4 (i.e., 50 μL of 2–3 μg) to your CD8$^+$ cells. Appropriate controls are no exosomes (50 μL PBS) as a negative control and heat-killed CD8$^+$ cells (56 °C for 30 min) as a positive control.
6. Incubate for 24 h at 37 °C and 5% CO_2.
7. Apoptosis can be detected using an Annexin V apoptosis detection kit (Beckman Coulter) by flow cytometry.

4 Notes

1. Frozen vs. fresh plasma: We compared exosome isolation from frozen/thawed plasma to fresh plasma [4]. We observed that frozen/thawed plasma decreased the yield of exosomes compared to fresh samples, but biological activity of exosomes was not affected.
2. Inserting the frit on top of Sepharose 2B gel: Porous frits are included in the preparation of SEC columns. After Sepharose 2B gel is settled up to the 10 mL bed volume, using a tweezer slowly push the frit into the column. It is important to level the frit on the top of the gel. This step may affect exosome fractionation.
3. Fractions 3, 4, and 5: Since the procedure is based on size exclusion chromatography, the earlier fractions contain larger molecules than the later fractions. Fraction #3 contains a very

low protein concentration (often below detection level of BCA assay). Nevertheless, TEM and particle analysis by qNano show exosome presence in fraction #3. Fraction #5 has a high protein concentration but contains aggregates of serum proteins and exosomes, as seen by TEM. Fraction #4 is the major fraction containing unclustered morphologically intact exosomes as seen shown by TEM at the highest concentrations by qNano analyses (Figs. 4, 5, and 6).

4. Exosome concentration: Protein concentrations in fractions #3 and #4 vary widely among different plasma samples and cancer types. Therefore, depending on the analyses, the recovered

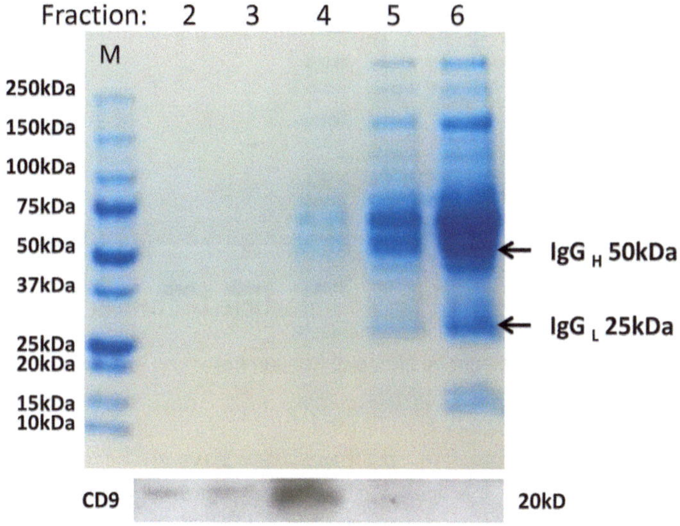

Fig. 4 Protein contents in the fractions recovered after SEC. An aliquot (50 μL) of each fraction was separated by SDS-PAGE gels and stained with Coomassie blue and analyzed by Western blotting. CD9 is used as an exosomal marker

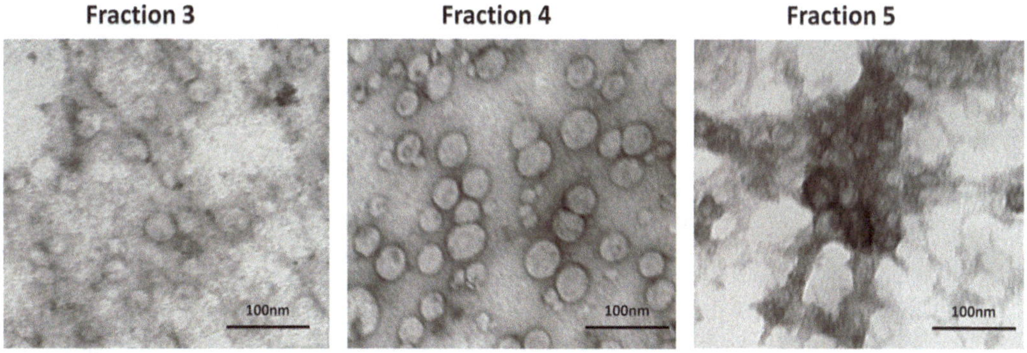

Fig. 5 Transmission electron microscopy (TEM) of fractions #3, #4, and #5 recovered after SEC of plasma obtained from a patient with AML

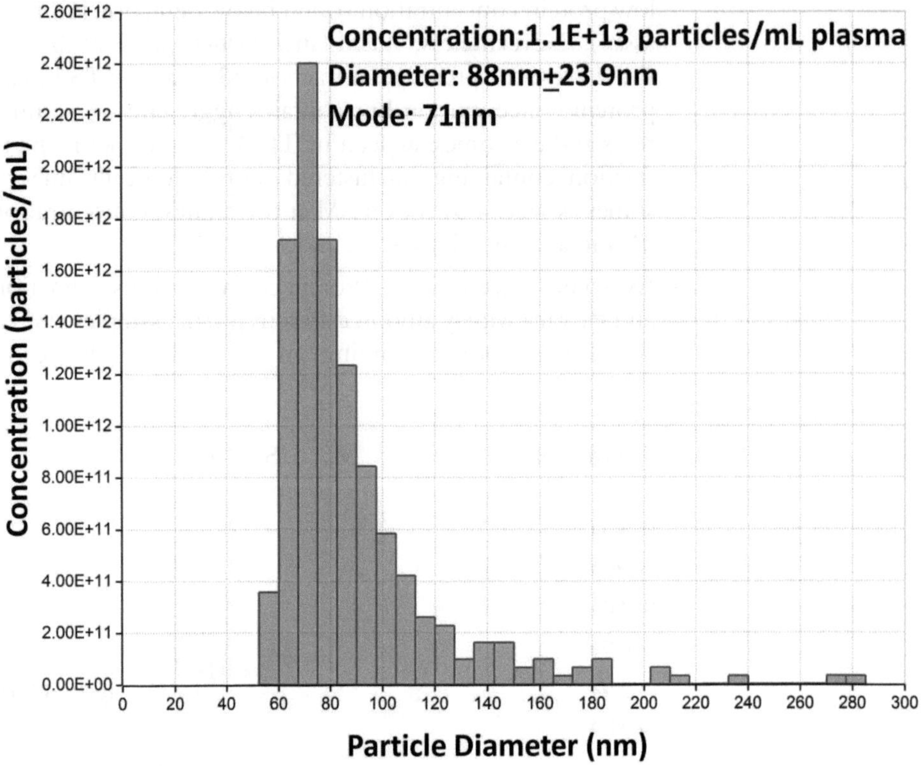

Fig. 6 Particle measurement by qNano of fraction #4

fractions may have to be concentrated. Protein spin-column concentrators, such as 300K MWCO Vivaspin 500 (Sartorius Corp, New York, NY, USA) or 100K MWCO Amicon Ultra 0.5 mL centrifugal filter (EMD Millipore, Billerica, MA, USA), work fine for concentrating exosomes. The concentrating procedure further removes contaminating serum proteins. However, while 300K MWCO removes more contaminants, it may also lead to a loss of smaller exosomes.

5. Particle quantification by qNano: Measuring the size distribution and concentration of exosomes, especially plasma-derived exosomes which are opsonized with immunoglobulins, is often difficult. These exosomes have a tendency to form aggregates of varying sizes. Thus, we routinely add 0.03% Tween 20 to the collected fractions in order to prevent/dissolve the aggregates before placing exosomes in the nanopore (NP150), which is used to measure exosomes. We have used a smaller nanopore (NP100), but it tended to clog, creating problems. Also, we use the reagent kit provided by Izon to coat the nanopore and prevent protein binding to the pore. The calibration particles, which are included in the Izon kit, are measured directly before and after experimental samples under identical

conditions, and the size and concentration of the particles are determined using the Izon software (version 3.2).

6. For all functional assays, the amount of exosomes added should be titrated. However, in our hands about 2–3 μg exosomal protein from SEC fraction #4 (ca. 50 μL) showed reproducible and significant in vitro immune reactivity.

Acknowledgments

The development of the method was in part supported by NIH grants RO-1CA168628 and R21-CA205644 to TLW.

References

1. Thery C, Amigorena S, Raposo G, Clayton A (2006) Unit 3.22 Isolation and characterization of exosomes from cell culture supernatants and biological fluids. Curr Protoc Cell Biol. doi:10.1002/0471143030.cb0322s30
2. Hong CS, Funk S, Muller L, Boyiadzis M, Whiteside TL (2016) Isolation of biologically active and morphologically intact exosomes from plasma of patients with cancer. J Extracell Vesicles 5:29289
3. Taylor DD, Chou IN, Black PH (1983) Isolation of plasma membrane fragments from cultured murine melanoma cells. Biochem Biophys Res Commun 113(2):470–476
4. Muller L, Hong CS, Stolz DB, Watkins SC, Whiteside TL (2014) Isolation of biologically-active exosomes from human plasma. J Immunol Methods 411:55–65
5. Saze Z, Schuler PJ, Hong CS, Cheng D, Jackson EK, Whiteside TL (2013) Adenosine production by human B cells and B cell-mediated suppression of activated T cells. Blood 122:9–18

Chapter 17

Generating and Expanding Autologous Chimeric Antigen Receptor T Cells from Patients with Acute Myeloid Leukemia

Saad S. Kenderian, Carl H. June, and Saar Gill

Abstract

Adoptive transfer of genetically engineered T cells can lead to profound and durable responses in patients with hematologic malignancies, generating enormous enthusiasm among scientists, clinicians, patients, and biotechnology companies. The success of adoptive cellular immunotherapy depends upon the ability to manufacture good quality T cells. We discuss here the methodologies and reagents that are used to generate T cells for the preclinical study of chimeric antigen receptor T cell therapy for acute myeloid leukemia (AML).

Key words Chimeric antigen receptor, Acute myeloid leukemia, T cell expansion, CAR T cells, Adoptive T cell therapy, Synthetic biology

1 Introduction

Genetic material encoding a chimeric antigen receptor (CAR) or transgenic T cell receptor (TCR) can be easily transferred into primary human T cells ex vivo using viral or nonviral approaches, and the T cells can then be further propagated in order to generate large numbers of tumor antigen-recognizing effector and memory cells [1]. The treatment of B-cell malignancies using this approach is particularly advanced. Here, autologous or allogeneic peripheral blood mononuclear cells are removed by leukapheresis and can be further enriched by elutriation or by positive selection using magnetic beads. The resultant product is initially composed of a mixture of lymphocytes, but a pure CD3+ T cell product composed of both CD4 and CD8 cells is usually generated within 7–9 days (occasionally longer) by exposing the lymphocytes to stimulatory anti-CD3/CD28 beads, agonistic anti-CD3 antibodies, interleukin-2, interleukin-7, interleukin-15, artificial antigen presenting cells, or a combination of these. Notably, the transduction of an anti-CD19 CAR into the T cells effectively leads to an ex vivo

Paolo Fortina et al. (eds.), *Acute Myeloid Leukemia: Methods and Protocols*, Methods in Molecular Biology, vol. 1633,
DOI 10.1007/978-1-4939-7142-8_17,

selection procedure, as the T cells are immediately functional once the CAR is expressed. Hence, an ex vivo "purge" occurs when anti-CD19 CAR T cells are exposed to CD19-bearing cells in the product [1–8]. Notably, T cell expansion and gene transfer methodology vary significantly between institutions and indeed may need to be adapted for different disease states [4–6, 9].

The successful application of CART cell therapy in acute myeloid leukemia (AML) would represent a significant advance in the field. Treatment of AML has minimally changed over the last few decades and prognosis remains very poor [10]. Since virtually all antigens expressed by AML blasts are also present on normal myeloid progenitors and since the functional avidity of CAR T cells appears to be stronger than that of the soluble antibodies on which they are based, we expect that treatment with CAR T cells will result in significant marrow toxicity regardless of prior clinical experience with antibodies. Several groups have developed CAR T cells directed against AML antigens, such as CD123 [11, 12], CD33 [13, 14], Le-Y [15], CD44v6 [16], and NKG2D [17]. These CAR T cells resulted in potent anti-leukemic activity and disease eradication in preclinical models at the cost of permanent myeloablation in humanized xenografts in some models [11, 13]. Several methods are being employed to avoid this permanent unwanted toxicity and to increase the therapeutic index of CART cell therapy. Examples of such approaches include RNA modification [13] that results in transient expression of CARTs and the use of suicide genes. Notably, in the case of mRNA electroporation into expanded T cells, gene transfer does not occur until the end of the manufacturing period and therefore there is no ex vivo purge [18].

In this chapter, we share our observations and protocols for optimizing T cell expansion and generation of CAR T cells in patients with AML for preclinical experiments. We outline our methods and protocols of T cell expansion, T cell enrichment, generation of permanently modified lentivirally (LV) transduced-CART and transiently modified RNA-electroporated CAR T cells from AML patients.

2 Materials

2.1 Primary AML Samples

1. De-identified viably cryopreserved primary human AML specimens are obtained from institutional repositories under IRB-approved protocols.
2. Normal donor peripheral blood mononuclear cells (PBMCs) are obtained from institutional repositories under IRB-approved protocols, or collected fresh. PBMCs are isolated from peripheral blood by Ficoll density gradient (Thermo Fischer Scientific, Waltham, MA, USA).

2.2 T Cell Expansion

1. T cell Media (TCM): X-vivo 15 media (Fisher Scientific), human serum 5% (Gemini Bio-product, Inc., West Sacramento, CA, USA), penicillin, streptomycin (10,000 U/mL, Thermo Fisher Scientific), and glutaMAX (100×, Thermo Fisher Scientific).
2. Anti-human antibodies are purchased from Biolegend (San Diego, CA, USA), eBioscience (San Diego, CA, USA), or BD Biosciences (San Jose, CA, USA). Live Dead fixable aqua detection reagent is from Life Technologies (Frederick, MD, USA).
3. Anti-CD3/CD28 Dynabeads (Life Technologies).
4. Surface expression of CAR is detected by staining with an Alexa Fluor 647-conjugated goat anti-mouse F(ab')2 antibody from Jackson Immunoresearch (West Grove, PA, USA) if the CAR is based on a murine single chain variable fragment. If the CAR is based on a human or humanized single chain variable fragment, an anti-human IgG(H + L) antibody (Jackson Immunoresearch) may be used instead.
5. Anti-PE, or anti-CD4 and anti-CD8 microbeads (Miltenyi, San Diego, CA, USA).
6. Fetal bovine serum (90%) with 10% DMSO.
7. Flow buffer is PBS, 2% FBS, 0.02%NaN_3. PBS (Invitrogen), FBS (Gemini), and sodium azide (Ricca Chemical Company).

2.3 RNA-Modified CART Cell Production

1. mMESSAGE mMachineT7 ULTRA Transcription Kit (Life Technologies).
2. RNeasy plus mini kit (Qiagen, Inc., Hilden, Germany).
3. OptiMEM (Life Technologies).
4. ECM830 Electro Square Wave Porator (Harvard Apparatus BTX, Holliston, MA, USA).
5. Gene pulser/Micropulser Cuvettes, 0.2 cm gap sterile electroporation cuvette (Bio-Rad Laboratories, Hercules, CA, USA).

3 Methods

3.1 Expanding T Cells from AML Patients

1. Thaw frozen PBMCs from AML patients using warm TCM, spin at 500 g for 7 min to remove DMSO, and resuspend in TCM. Plate at a concentration of 1×10^6 cells/mL and rest overnight in incubator at 37 °C, 5% CO_2 (*see* **Note 1**).
2. Take an aliquot for flow cytometry, stain with CD45, CD3, and live/dead staining. Acquire using a cytometer to determine the percentage and total number of T cells.
3. Prepare CD3/CD28 Dynabeads: Calculate the number of beads needed to reach a 3:1 ratio of beads to total PBMCs.

Resuspend beads well by gently pipetting up and down for a minute. Do not vortex. Add the required volume of beads to a total of 1 mL TCM in a 1.5 mL tube and gently resuspend to wash. Place the tube in magnet (e.g., DynaMag-2, Thermo Fisher Scientific) and wait for 1 min. Remove media without disturbing the beads. Repeat the washing steps three times. After washings, resuspend beads in 500–1000 μL of TCM.

4. Add beads to cells already plated at 1 × 10^6 cells/mL if using a flask. If planning to use multiple individual wells of a plate, add the beads to the cells in a conical tube, then distribute 1 mL aliquots of the cell/bead mixture. Keep in incubator at 37 °C, 5% CO_2. The day of stimulation (adding beads to cells) represents day 0.
5. Beginning on day 3, count cells using Coulter multi-sizer every other day. Feed cells with TCM to bring the final concentration to 1 × 10^6 cells/mL (*see* **Notes 2** and **3**).
6. Remove beads on day 6 as follows: gently resuspend cells by pipetting up and down several times, collect the cells, and place in a 15 mL or 50 mL conical tube. Put the tube in a magnet (e.g., DynaMag-15, Thermo Fisher Scientific), and wait for 2 min to allow the beads to migrate to the side. Remove cell suspension from the middle of the tube by aspirating with a pipette. Count using Coulter multi-sizer and plate in new flasks at 1 × 10^6 cells/mL in warm TCM.
7. Record counts and mean cell volume (MCV) and graph to generate expansion curves (Fig. 1). MCV increases as T cells become

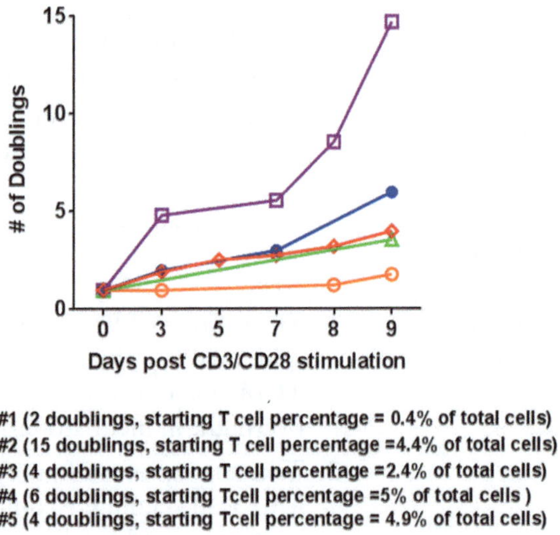

Fig. 1 Expansion curves and number of doublings after expansion of 5 primary AML samples. AML samples were expanded as outlined in Subheading 3.1 of this chapter

activated, then reaches its maximum between day 5 and 7 post-activation, and then declines as T cells start resting down.

8. When MCV reaches 300 fL, cells are adequately rested (typically within 9–14 days) and can be used or frozen for future experiments. Freeze cells at up to 10 × 10^6/mL in 90% fetal bovine serum with 10% DMSO in rate-controlled manner. Recovery upon subsequent thawing should be higher than 75%.
9. Figure 1 represents T cell expansion kinetics from 5 AML patients (*see* **Notes 4** and **5**).

3.2 Enrichment of T Cells Prior to T Cell Expansion in AML Patients

1. We have found that the presence of residual AML blasts impairs T cell expansion. T cells were separated from AML by flow cytometric sorting to a purity of 100%. Then T cells were mixed with AML cells at different ratios (Fig. 2a), stimulated and expanded (as described in Subheading 3.1). There was a significant improvement in T cell expansion when AML cells were depleted.
2. To enrich for T cells in primary AML samples, CD3/CD28 Dynabeads or CD4/CD8 positive selection can be performed.

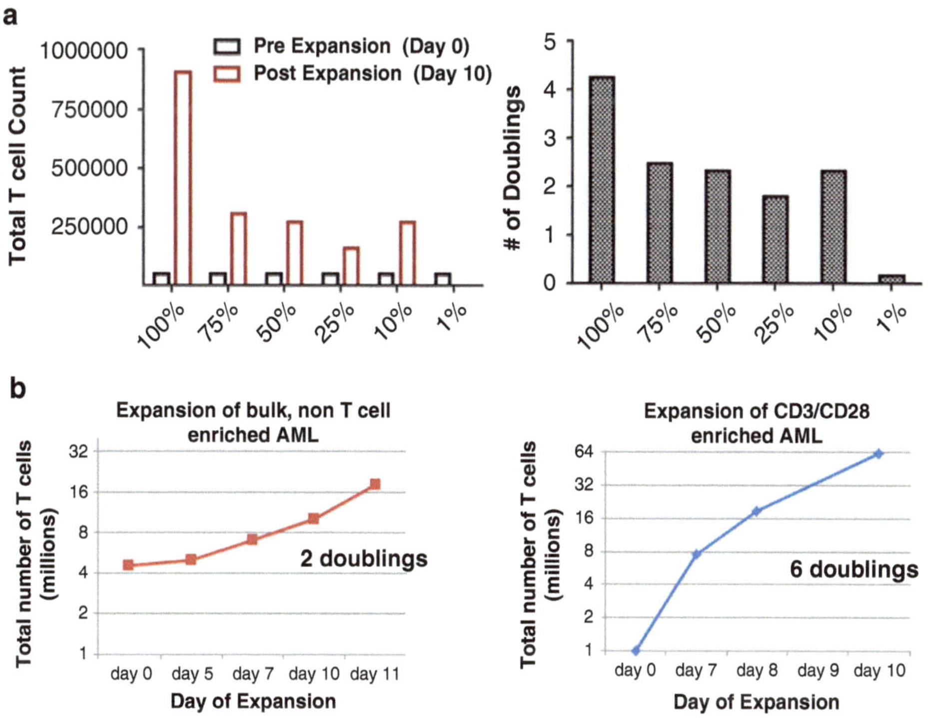

Fig. 2 (**a**) T cells were separated by flow cytometry sorting to >99% purity. T cells were then mixed with AML blasts at the indicated percentages on *x*-axes and expanded in culture as outlined in Subheading 3.1. (**a** *1*) Shows the total number of T cells pre (*black*) and post (*red*) expansion. (**a** *2*) Shows the number of doublings plotted against the percentage of T cells in culture. (**b**) T cell expansion curves of bulk unselected AML (*left*) or CD3/CD28 enriched AML growth before (**a**) and after (**b**) CD3/CD28 selection (purity 90%)

3. Enrichment of T cells using CD3/CD28 beads: Thaw, plate AML samples at 1 × 10^6 cells/mL, and rest overnight (as described in Subheading 3.1). Count, prepare, and wash beads (as described in Subheading 3.1). Add beads to cells, place cells in a 15 mL or 50 mL conical tube, and incubate while rotating for 45 min at room temperature. T cells will be tightly bound to beads during this time. Place tube in a magnet and wait for 1 min. Beads (and T cells that are attached to them) will migrate to the side. Gently aspirate media from the center of the tube (this media contains mostly AML cells at this time, rather than T cells that will be bound to CD3/CD28 Dynabeads). Resuspend beads (and attached T cells) in TCM, count with Coulter multi-sizer, and plate at 1 × 10^6 cells/mL. Take an aliquot for flow cytometry (as described in Subheading 3.1). Continue T cell expansion as described in Subheading 3.1. Figure 2b represents an example of T cell expansion curve after CD3/CD28 enrichment.
4. Enrichment of T cells using CD4/CD8 positive selection: thaw, plate AML samples at 1 × 10^6 cells/mL, and rest overnight at 37 °C in an incubator (as described in Subheading 3.1). Stain with CD4 and CD8 antibodies conjugated to PE and then use MACS enrichment with anti-PE microbeads according to the manufacturer's instructions. Following T cell selection, stimulate and expand T cells as discussed in Subheading 3.1.

3.3 Generating Lentiviral-CART from AML Patients

1. The CAR lentivirus plasmid is generated as previously described [19].
2. The CAR lentivirus is generated by transfection of 293 T cells with the specific plasmid and the supernatant is frozen at −80 °C as previously described [19].
3. Start T cell expansion as described in Subheadings 3.1 and 3.2.
4. On day 1, transduce T cells with lentivirus. Thaw frozen lentiviral supernatant gradually at room temperature for 20–30 min. Add previously titrated lentiviral supernatant to T cells dropwise at a multiplicity of infection (MOI) of 3.0. Resuspend by gently swirling the plate.
5. On day 6, check CAR expression by flow cytometry. Take an aliquot of T cells, wash once with flow buffer, stain with anti-CAR antibody and live/dead staining, wash twice, then stain with mouse anti-human CD45, and CD3. Acquire on a cytometer to determine the transduction efficiency. We typically obtain a transduction efficiency of 50–75% (*see* **Note 6**).
6. Continue the rest of expansion as outlined in Subheading 3.1.
7. Figure 3 represents an example of CD123 directed CAR T cells generated from an AML patient. Introducing the CAR transgene provides an expansion advantage to the T cells (Fig. 3a) (*see* **Note 7**).

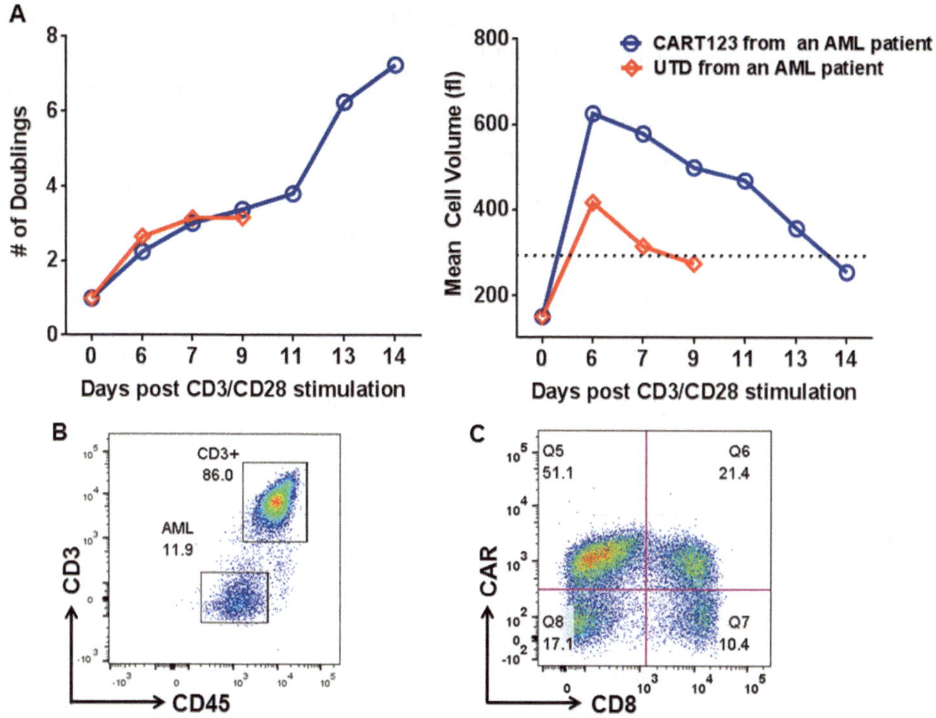

Fig. 3 (**A**) Expansion and cell volume curves of T cells from AML samples after transduction with CD123-chimeric antigen receptor. Transduction with CD123-CAR and generation of CART123 result in eradication of residual AML and increase proliferation of T cells. (**B**) Flow plot of a final T cell expansion product of an AML patient (untransduced T cells). Note that there are residual leukemic cells. (**C**) Flow plot of a final T cell expansion product of an AML patient (CD123 directed CARTs). Note the transduction efficiency is 72.5%

3.4 Generating RNA-Modified CAR T Cells from AML Patients

1. Plate AML samples and start T cell expansion as described in Subheading 3.1.
2. The CAR lentivirus construct is subcloned into the pDA vector as previously described [18].
3. RNA is generated by in vitro transcription using mMESSAGE mMachineT7 ULTRA Transcription Kit. RNA is purified using the RNeasy Mini Kit as previously described.
4. When the MCV falls under 300 fL, T cells can be electroporated with RNA or frozen in fetal calf serum with 10% DMSO for future use.
5. Electroporation of T cells: if using frozen expanded T cells, thaw in warm TCM, spin at 500 g for 7 min to remove DMSO, and rest overnight in incubator at 37 °C, 5% CO_2. From now on, carry out all procedures on ice.
6. Transfer cells to a conical 50 mL tube and wash with cold OptiMEM three times. Spin at 500 g for 7 min between washes. After the third wash, aspirate the supernatant completely, and

resuspend in cold OptiMEM up to 300 × 10^6 cells/mL. Transfer T cells to bullet tubes (100 μL) (30 × 10^6 T cells) to each bullet tube. Add RNA (1 μg for each 1 × 10^6 T cells) and resuspend gently by pipetting up and down several times. Transfer cells plus RNA from each bullet tube to a cuvette and keep on ice.

7. Turn on the ECM830 Electro Square Wave Porator, set the machine to 500 V and 700 μs (*see* **Note 8**). Place the cuvette in the machine, tighten firmly in place and pulse. Wash cuvette three times with 1 mL of warm TCM and transfer cells to a six-well plate. Feed with TCM to bring the concentration to 2 × 10^6 cells/mL. Rest in incubator at 37 °C, 5% CO_2.
8. Rest cells for 2–4 h post electroporation. Then cells can be used or frozen for future experiments (*see* **Note 9**).

4 Notes

1. For small-scale expansions we prefer to rest PBMC or T cells at 1 mL in individual wells of a 24 well tissue culture plate. Larger volume work is typically carried out in T25–T150 flasks (Corning).
2. Expect a drop-off in live cell number if counting before day 3.
3. The media will start to change color, representing metabolic activity of the T cells, around day 3 (Fig. 4).
4. Expansion kinetics are variable between patients and the average number of doublings after T cell expansion from AML patients is 4.
5. When T cells are stimulated and expanded from AML patients, the final product may contain residual leukemia cells (Fig. 3b).
6. Staining for CAR needs to be performed first if the CAR is based on an anti-mouse scFv. Sample needs to be washed twice before surface staining is performed.
7. Transducing with myeloid directed CAR construct (such as CART123 or CART33) at the beginning of culture results in

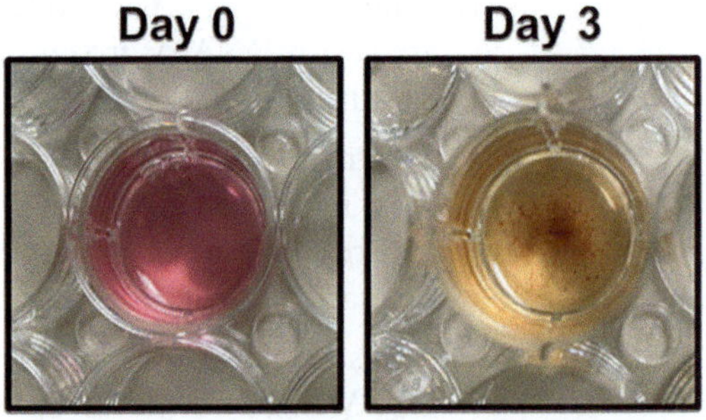

Fig. 4 An example of changes in T cell expansion media between day 0 and 3 of expansion

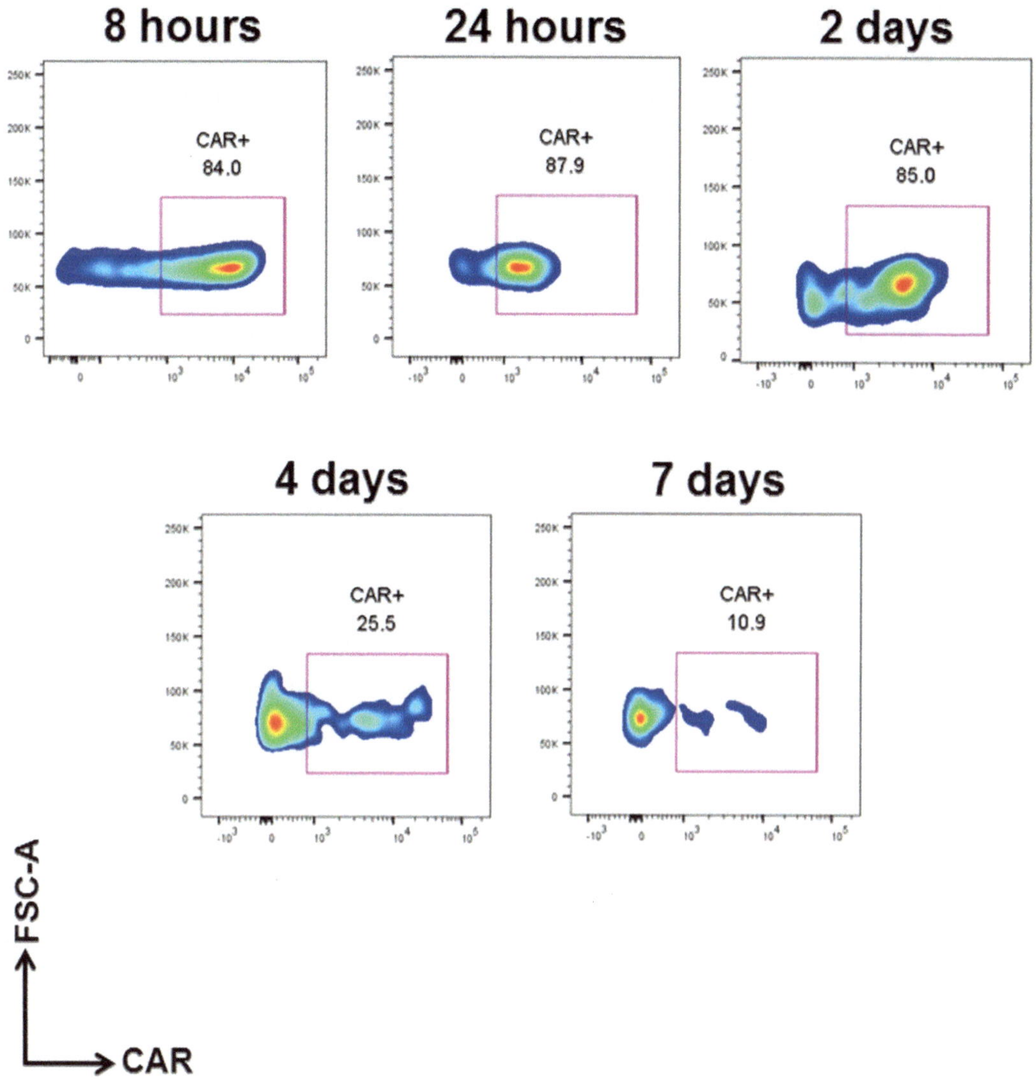

Fig. 5 Expression of CD33 directed chimeric antigen receptor at different time points (as indicated) after RNA electroporation of T cells. Maximum expression of CAR is 24 h after electroporation and declines over a period of 5–7 days

eradiation of the residual leukemia in culture, whereas with a strategy that incorporates gene transfer at the end of culture there may be residual leukemia cells at the end of culture (Fig. 3b).

8. Users are advised to titrate machine settings.
9. CAR can be detected on the surface of the electroporated T cells within an hour, and typically achieves maximal median fluorescence intensity (MFI) within 24–48 h. If the T cells are not exposed to antigen, the CAR MFI will diminish gradually over approximately 5–7 days (Fig. 5) [18].

Acknowledgments

This work was partly supported by grants from the University of Pennsylvania-Novartis Alliance (Carl June/Saar Gill), Leukemia Lymphoma Society (Carl June/Saar Gill), and the Predolin foundation (Saad Kenderian).

References

1. Maus MV, Grupp SA, Porter DL, June CH (2014) Antibody-modified T cells: CARs take the front seat for hematologic malignancies. Blood 123(17):2625–2635
2. Sadelain M, Brentjens R, Riviere I (2013) The basic principles of chimeric antigen receptor design. Cancer Discov 3(4):388–398
3. Kalos M, June CH (2013) Adoptive T cell transfer for cancer immunotherapy in the era of synthetic biology. Immunity 39(1):49–60
4. Maude SL, Frey N, Shaw PA, Aplenc R, Barrett DM, Bunin NJ et al (2014) Chimeric antigen receptor T cells for sustained remissions in leukemia. N Engl J Med 371(16):1507–1517
5. Davila ML, Riviere I, Wang X, Bartido S, Park J, Curran K et al (2014) Efficacy and toxicity management of 19-28z CAR T cell therapy in B cell acute lymphoblastic leukemia. Sci Transl Med 6(224):224ra225
6. Lee DW, Kochenderfer JN, Stetler-Stevenson M, Cui YK, Delbrook C, Feldman SA et al (2015) T cells expressing CD19 chimeric antigen receptors for acute lymphoblastic leukaemia in children and young adults: a phase 1 dose-escalation trial. Lancet 385(9967): 517–528
7. Kenderian SS, Ruella M, Gill S, Kalos M (2014) Chimeric antigen receptor T-cell therapy to target hematologic malignancies. Cancer Res 74(22):6383–6389
8. Gill S, Maus MV, Porter DL (2016) Chimeric antigen receptor T cell therapy: 25 years in the making. Blood Rev 30(3):157–167
9. Porter DL, Hwang WT, Frey NV, Lacey SF, Shaw PA, Loren AW et al (2015) Chimeric antigen receptor T cells persist and induce sustained remissions in relapsed refractory chronic lymphocytic leukemia. Sci Transl Med 7(303): 303ra139
10. Thein MS, Ershler WB, Jemal A, Yates JW, Baer MR (2013) Outcome of older patients with acute myeloid leukemia: an analysis of SEER data over 3 decades. Cancer 119(15): 2720–2727
11. Gill S, Tasian SK, Ruella M, Shestova O, Li Y, Porter DL et al (2014) Preclinical targeting of human acute myeloid leukemia and myeloablation using chimeric antigen receptor-modified T cells. Blood 123(15):2343–2354
12. Mardiros A, Dos Santos C, McDonald T, Brown CE, Wang X, Budde LE et al (2013) T cells expressing CD123-specific chimeric antigen receptors exhibit specific cytolytic effector functions and antitumor effects against human acute myeloid leukemia. Blood 122(18):3138–3148
13. Kenderian SS, Ruella M, Shestova O, Klichinsky M, Aikawa V, Morrissette JJ et al (2015) CD33 specific chimeric antigen receptor T cells exhibit potent preclinical activity against human acute myeloid leukemia. Leukemia 29(8):1637–1647
14. Pizzitola I, Anjos-Afonso F, Rouault-Pierre K, Lassailly F, Tettamanti S, Spinelli O et al (2014) Chimeric antigen receptors against CD33/CD123 antigens efficiently target primary acute myeloid leukemia cells in vivo. Leukemia 28(8):1596–1605
15. Ritchie DS, Neeson PJ, Khot A, Peinert S, Tai T, Tainton K et al (2013) Persistence and efficacy of second generation CAR-T cell against the LeY antigen in acute myeloid leukemia. Mol Ther 21(11):2122–2129
16. Casucci M, Nicolis di Robilant B, Falcone L, Camisa B, Norelli M, Genovese P et al (2013) CD44v6-targeted T cells mediate potent antitumor effects against acute myeloid leukemia and multiple myeloma. Blood 122(20):3461–3472
17. Spear P, Barber A, Rynda-Apple A, Sentman CL (2013) NKG2D CAR T-cell therapy inhibits the growth of NKG2D ligand heterogeneous tumors. Immunol Cell Biol 91(6): 435–440
18. Zhao Y, Moon E, Carpenito C, Paulos CM, Liu X, Brennan AL et al (2010) Multiple injections of electroporated autologous T cells expressing a chimeric antigen receptor mediate regression of human disseminated tumor. Cancer Res 70(22):9053–9061
19. Milone MC, Fish JD, Carpenito C, Carroll RG, Binder GK, Teachey D et al (2009) Chimeric receptors containing CD137 signal transduction domains mediate enhanced survival of T cells and increased antileukemic efficacy in vivo. Mol Ther 17(8):1453–1464

Index

Paolo Fortina et al. (eds.), *Acute Myeloid Leukemia: Methods and Protocols*, Methods in Molecular Biology, vol. 1633, DOI 10.1007/978-1-4939-7142-8, © Springer Science+Business Media LLC 2017

MIX
Papier aus verantwortungsvollen Quellen
Paper from responsible sources
FSC® C105338

If you have any concerns about our products,
you can contact us on
ProductSafety@springernature.com

In case Publisher is established outside the EU,
the EU authorized representative is:
Springer Nature Customer Service Center GmbH
Europaplatz 3, 69115 Heidelberg, Germany

Printed by Libri Plureos GmbH
in Hamburg, Germany